# ELECTROPHYSIOLOGY – FROM PLANTS TO HEART

Edited by **Saeed Oraii**

**Electrophysiology – From Plants to Heart**
Edited by Saeed Oraii

**Published by InTech**
Janeza Trdine 9, 51000 Rijeka, Croatia



**Publishing Process Manager** Dejan Grgur

**Technical Editor** Teodora Smiljanic

**Cover Designer** InTech Design Team

Additional hard copies can be obtained from orders@intechopen.com

Electrophysiology – From Plants to Heart, Edited by Saeed Oraii
p. cm.
ISBN 978-953-51-0006-5

For EU product safety concerns:
IN TECH d.o.o., Prolaz Marije Krucifikse Kozulić 3, 51000 Rijeka, Croatia,
info@intechopen.com or visit our website at intechopen.com.

# Meet the editor

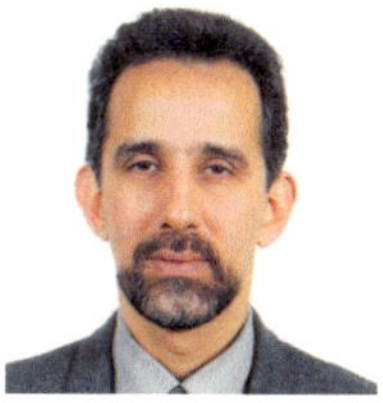

Dr Saeed Oraii received his MD from the Teheran University of Medical Sciences in 1987. He also received a board certification in Cardiology from the Iran University of Medical Sciences in 1995, and in Electrophysiology from the Pacemaker and Electrophysiology Board, Iranian Heart Association in 2001. He is a member of the Iranian Heart Association, Iranian Atherosclerosis Society, and the Heart Rhythm Society. Dr Oraii currently works at the Tehran Arrhythmia Center.

# Contents

# Preface

Enormous progress has been made in the science of Electrophysiology over the last two centuries or more. William Gilbert, the physician of Queen Elizabeth I, first introduced the term "electrica" in the year 1600, for objects that hold static electricity. He derived it from the Greek word for amber (electra). The introduction of "bioelectricity" however, dates back to the works of Luigi Galvani in 1787, and his observations that a frog nerve-muscle preparation could be contracted by delivering electrical impulses.

From 1825, the development of sensitive galvanometers by Leopoldo Nobili made it possible to record charges and currents within the animal cells. Further investigations into the nature of "animal electricity" led to the demonstration of the resting heart muscle electrical currents by Carlo Matteucci in 1838, and this can truly be considered as the birth of cardiac electrophysiology.

In 1877, Augustus Desiree Waller was the first to record electric potentials associated with the beating heart from the body surface: the first human electrocardiogram. This was made possible by the invention of a capillary electrometer by Thomas Goswell, a technician in his laboratory.

During subsequent years, the outstanding evolution of recording techniques paved the way for better understanding of electrophysiological phenomena within the human organs, including the cardiovascular, ophthalmologic and neural systems. In the field of cardiac electrophysiology, the development of more and more sophisticated recording and mapping techniques made it possible to elucidate the mechanism of various cardiac arrhythmias. This has even led to the evolution of techniques to ablate and cure most complex cardiac arrhythmias. Nevertheless, there is still a long way ahead and this book can be considered a valuable addition to the current knowledge in subjects related to bioelectricity from plants to the human heart.

**Saeed Oraii**
Cardiologist, Interventional Electrophysiologist, Cardiology Department - Shahid Rajaii Heart Hospital, Iran University of Medical Sciences, Tehran, Iran

1

# Electrophysiology of Woody Plants

Luis A. Gurovich
*Universidad Católica de Chile*
*Chile*

## 1. Introduction

A fundamental property of all living organisms is related to the continuous gathering of environmental information and the expression of physiological responses aimed to optimize its performance under new environmental conditions. In order to keep homeostasis, plants need to continuously gather information about its environment and to react physiologically, in order to synchronize its normal biological functions. Plant cells become bio - electrochemically excited under the influence of environmental changes and the conduction of these electric potential modifications to distant plant organs have been widely reported. Electrochemical phenomena in plants have attracted researchers since the eighteenth century (Bertholon, 1783; Burdon-Sanderson, 1873; Darwin, 1875; Lemström, 1904; Bose, 1926); however, only in the last decade numerous papers related to plant electrophysiology have been published (for a comprehensive review on the subject see Volkov´s book *"Plant Electrophysiology, Theory and Methods"*, 2006). Detection of electrical potentials in plants indicates that electrical signaling is a major system to transmit information over long distances throughout its organs. The reason why plants have developed pathways for electrical signal transmission is probably related to its need to respond rapidly to environmental stress factors (Fromm & Lautner, 2007). Electrophysiological studies of long-distance signals in plants and animals contribute to our knowledge of the living world by revealing important similarities and crucial differences between plants and animals, in an area that might be directly related to their different capacities to respond to environmental change.

The existence of electrophysiological mechanisms for information perception, transmission and processing between different plant organs and tissues, allowing the expression of fast and accurate physiological reactions to specific biotic or abiotic stimuli, is expressed by means of real-time detectable *action* (APs) and *variation* (VPs) potentials (Datta & Palit, 2004; Gil et al., 2008; Lautner et al., 2005; Oyarce & Gurovich, 2010; Volkov et al., 2009; Wang et al., 2009). An additional type of electric potential in plants has been proposed by Zimmermann et al. (2009), to be called *system* potential. In addition to APs that occur also in animals and lower plants (Trebacz et al., 2005) higher plants feature an additional, unique, hydraulically propagated type of electric signals VPs, called also *slow wave potentials* (Stahlberg et al., 2005).

Several models have been proposed to explain the onset of plant cell electric excitation, resulting from external stimuli (Wayne, 1993; Fromm & Lautner, 2007). All plant cells are surrounded by a plasma membrane (Murphy et al., 2010), composed of a lipid bilayer, with a variety of molecular structures embedded in it, known generically as *ion channels* and *electrogenic pumps* (Hedrich & Schroeder, 1989). Electrochemical excitation is caused by ionic fluxes through the cell plasma membrane (Knudsen, 2002; Blatt, 2008), creating an electric charge modification in the membrane itself, as well as a differential charge on either side. This trans - membrane potential is the difference in voltage (or electrical potential difference) between the interior and exterior of a cell ($V_{interior} - V_{exterior}$). Plant plasma membranes always maintain a potential, the cell interior being more negative than the exterior, arising mainly from the activity of electrogenic pumps. As an example, $H^+$-transporting ATPases (Sze et al., 1999) pump protons out of the cell, thus maintaining a pH gradient across the plasma membrane. This process is involved in the simultaneous symport of carbohydrates and amino acids into the cell, which are produced at different plant tissues as photosynthetic derivatives. Other electrogenic ion pumps described for plant cell plasma membranes are related to ion and solute fluxes, underpinning inorganic mineral nutrient uptake; they trigger rapid changes in secondary messengers such as cytosolic-free $Ca^{+2}$ concentrations, and also power the osmotic gradients that drive cell expansion (Schroeder & Thuleau 1991; Gelli & Blumwald, 1997; Zimmermann et al., 1997; Bonza et al., 2001; Sanders, 2002; Blatt, 2008; Lautner & Fromm, 2010). The $K^{+1}$-transporting ATPase, also embedded in the cell plasma membrane, enables the onset of different ion concentrations (and therefore electrical charge) on the intracellular and extracellular sides of the membrane (Maathuis & Sanders, 1997).

Ion channels, when active, partially discharge the plasma membrane potential, while the electrogenic pumps restore and maintain it (Fromm & Spanswick, 1993; Neuhaus & Wagner, 2000). The plasma membrane potential has two basic functions. First, it allows a cell to function as a *battery*, providing power to operate the variety of electrogenic pumps embedded in its lipid bilayer. Second, in electrically excitable cells, it is used for transmitting signals between different parts of a cell or to other plant cells, tissues or organs. Opening or closing of ion channels at one point in the membrane produces a local and transient change in the membrane potential, which causes an electric current to flow rapidly to other points in the membrane and eventually, to the plasma membrane of surrounding cells. In non-excitable cells, and in excitable cells in their baseline state, the membrane potential is held at a relatively stable value, called the *resting potential*, characterized by its absence of fluctuations; the resting potential varies from −20 mV to −200 mV according to cell type. Opening and closing of ion channels can induce a departure from the resting potential, called a *depolarization* if the interior voltage rises, or a *hyperpolarization* if the interior voltage becomes more negative. In excitable cells, a sufficiently large depolarization can evoke an action potential (AP), in which the membrane potential very rapidly undergoes a significant, measurable change, often briefly reversing its sign; AP are short-lasting, all-or-nothing events.

Change in trans - plasma membrane potential creates a *wave of depolarization*, which affects the adjoining resting plasma membranes, thus generating an *impulse*. Once initiated, these impulses can propagate to adjacent excitable cells. Electrical signals can propagate along the plasma membrane (Van Bel & Ehlers, 2005; Volkov et al., 2011) on short distances through plasmodesmata and on long distances in plant phloematic tissue (Ksenzhek & Volkov, 1998; Volkov, 2000; Volkov, 2006; Volkov et al., 2011).

Research on the subject of electrochemical phenomena in plants is generically known as *plant electrophysiology* (Volkov, 2006); this knowledge is the basis of a newly developed discipline in the field of plant physiology: *plant neurobiology* (Brenner et al, 2006; Stahlberg, 2006; Baluška & Mancuso, 2008; Barlow, 2008). Plant neurobiology is aimed at establishing the structure of information networks that exist within the plant, which is expressed as responses to environmental stimuli by means of electrochemical signals (Baluška et al., 2004; Trewavas, 2005). These signals seem to complement other plant signals: hydraulic, mechanical, volatile and hormonal, already well documented in plant science (Fromm & Lautner, 2007; Gil et al., 2009; Dziubinska et al., 2003).

Research on plant electrophysiology specifically focused on woody plants like poplar and willow trees, have been seldom reported (Fromm & Spanswick, 1993; Lautner et al, 2005; Gibert et al., 2006). In fruit bearing deciduous and perennial plant species, electrophysiology studies are very limited as well, although it is in such plants that the need for rapid and efficient signals other than chemical and hydraulic signaling becomes more obvious (Gil et al., 2008; Nadler et al. 2008; Gurovich & Hermosilla, 2009; Oyarce & Gurovich, 2011). These studies have associated the effect of water stress, deficit irrigation, light cycles and mechanical or heat injury with electrical signaling in several fruit bearing tree species. Electrical signaling has been also associated to conditions of differential soil water availability; the use of real-time information on tree electrochemical behavior, as early indicator of biotic or abiotic induced water stress conditions, can provide a strategy to quantitatively relate plant physiological reactions to environmental changes and eventually, for the auto-programmed operation of pressurized irrigation systems, aimed to prevent water stress conditions in irrigated trees (Oyarce and Gurovich, 2010).

Additional applications of electrical signals in plants have been postulated, including its eventual use as environmental biosensors (Davies, 2004; Volkov & Brown, 2006) as well as to correlate sap flow based ET measurements with plant electrical behavior has been proposed (Gibert et al., 2006). Artificially applied electric potential differentials between plant organs under field conditions may enhance water use efficiency in woody plants, through its controlled influence on stomata conductance and plant internal water flux (Gil et al., 2008; Jia & Zhang, 2008; Gil et al., 2009; Gurovich, 2009).

## 2. History of plant electrophysiology

For a long time, plants were thought to be living organisms whose limited ability to move and respond was related to its relative limited abilities of sensing (Trewawas, 2003), with the exception only for plants with rapid and/or purposeful movements such as *Mimosa pudica* (also called *the* sensitive plant), *Drosera* (sundews), *Dionea muscipula* (flytraps) and tendrils of climbing plants. These sensitive plants attracted the attention of outstanding pioneer researchers such as Burdon-Sanderson (1873, 1899), Pfeffer (1873), Haberlandt (1914), Darwin (1896) and Bose (1926). They found plants not only to be equipped with various mechano-receptors that exceeded the sensitivity of a human finger, but also its ability to trigger action potentials (APs) that implemented these movements.

The discovery that common plants had propagating APs just as the "sensitive" plants (Gunar & Sinykhin 1962, 1963; Karmanov et al., 1972) was a scientific breakthrough with important consequences, correcting the long-held belief that normal plants are less sensitive and responsive as compared to the so-called "sensitive plants." Also, it led to studies aimed to understand the meaning of the widely distributed electrical signals in different plant tissues (Pickard, 1973), which carry important messages with a broader relevance than the established induction of organ movements in "sensitive plants".

The first known recording of a plant AP was done on leaves of the Venus flytrap (*Dionea muscipula* Ellis) in 1873 by Burdon-Sanderson, measuring the voltage difference between adaxial and abaxial surfaces of a *Dionea* leaf half, while stimulating the other half mechanically by touching the hairs (Burdon-Sanderson 1873, 1899). The trap closure in *Dionea* has been considered as a model case, showing comparable roles of APs in plants and nerve–muscle preparations of animals (Simons, 1992). Bose (1926) proposed that vascular bundles act analogous to nerves, by enabling the propagation of an excitation that moved from cell to cell. A comprehensive review of the early development of plant electrophysiology is provided by Stahlberg (2006).

For many years, the application of external electrodes to the surface of plant and animal organs was the only available technique for measuring potentials. The introduction of microelectrodes, like KCl-filled glass micropipettes with a tip diameter small enough to be inserted into living cells (Montenegro et al., 1991), enabled to record intracellular, *i.e.* real, membrane potentials (Vm). This technique was first adopted for giant cells from charophytic algae such as *Chara* and *Nitella*. Later on, it was complemented with precise electronic amplifiers and voltage clamp circuits, monitoring the activity of ion channels by direct measurement of ion currents instead of voltages. Parallel voltage (V) and current (I) measurements allowed I-V-curves, used to differentiate between the action of an ion channel (ohmic or parallel changes in I and V) or ion pump (non-ohmic relation between V and I changes) (Higinbotham, 1973).

As a next step to improve recording possibilities, the *patch clamp* technique was developed; by going from single cells to isolated membrane patches, one can record the current of as small a unit as a single ionic channel. Initially developed for animal cells, this technique was rapidly adopted for plant cell studies (Hedrich & Schroeder 1989). Voltage clamp techniques were introduced to demonstrate the contribution of various ion currents involved in the AP in *Chara* cells (Lunevsky et al. 1983; Wayne 1994). To this day, charophytic algae have served as important research models for higher plant cells electric behavior studies.

Additional studies made considerable progress in linking electrical signals with respiration and photosynthesis (Lautner et al, 2005; Koziolek et al. 2003), phloem transport (Fromm & Eschrich, 1988; Fromm & Bauer, 1994) and the rapid, plant-wide deployment of plant defenses (Wildon et al. 1992; Malone et al. 1994; Herde et al. 1995, 1996; Volkov & Haak 1995; Stankovic & Davies, 1996, 1998; Volkov, 2000). The significant development of plant neurobiology in the last decade is mostly related to electrophysiology based research, as an integrated view of plant signaling and behavior (Brenner et al., 2006; Baluška & Mancuso 2008; Barlow, 2008).

## 3. Hormonal and hydraulic physiological signals in woody plants

Hydraulic and hormonal signals in woody plants complement signaling electrophysiology in plants, playing a significant role in the dynamics of information processes integrating the plant responses to the environment.

Hydraulic pressure signals are propagating changes in water pressure inside plant tissues (Malone, 1996); plant tissues have plenty of hydraulic connections (mainly xylematic vessels) which provide a pathway for long-distance transmission of hydraulic signals. Pressure waves can be relatively quick and fast, as they can diffuse through the plant at the speed of sound (~1500 m $s^{-1}$ in water), but, to be physiologically important, a hydraulic signal must cause a significant change in turgor pressure inside a cell. As plant cells can be elastic, their turgor will change only when a significant influx (or efflux) of water occurs: the needed flux is strictly linked with the hydraulic capacitance of the cell, a widely variable property related to plant water potential and plant cell wall elasticity. Thus, hydraulic signals must involve massive water mass flow; for example, to increase the turgor pressure in leaf cells by 1 bar, a net water influx equivalent to 1–5% of the total volume of a leaf must occur (Malone 1996). For a detailed review on plant hydraulic signaling, see Mancuso & Mugnai (2006).

Many chemicals are critical for plant growth and development and play an important role in integrating various stress signals and controlling downstream stress responses, by modulating gene expression machinery and regulating various transporters/pumps and biochemical reactions. These chemicals include calcium ($Ca^{+2}$), cyclic nucleotides, polyphosphoinositides, nitric oxide (NO), sugars, abscisic acid (ABA), jasmonates (JA), salicylic acid (SA) and polyamines. Significant research in chemical signaling in plants has been aimed to understand the ability of plants respond to abscisic acid (ABA), often called the *stress hormone*. This hormone controls many of the adaptive responses that plants have evolved to conserve water when they perceive a reduced supply of this commodity. Stomata closure, reduced canopy area, and increased root biomass are three of the major adaptive processes regulated by ABA that can potentially be manipulated to improve crop water use efficiency (Wilkinson & Hartung, 2009; Jiang & Hartung, 2008). A comprehensive review on chemical signaling under abiotic stress environment in plants has been recently published by Tuteja & Sopory (2008).

## 4. Facts and hypothesis about electrical signals in woody plants

Rapid plant and animal responses to environmental changes are associated to electrical excitability and signaling, using the same electrochemical pathways to drive physiological responses, characterized in animals by movement (physical displacement) and in plants by continuous growth. In plants and animals, signal transmission can occur over long and short distances and correspond to intra and intercellular communication mechanisms, which determine the physiological behavior of the organism. Electrical pulses can be monitored in plants as *signals*, which are transmitted through excitable phloematic cell membranes, enabling the propagation of electrical pulses in the form of a depolarization wave or "action potential" AP. (Dziubinska et al., 2001; Fromm & Spanswick, 2007). At the onset of a change in the environmental conditions, plants respond to these stimuli at the site of occurrence and bioelectrical pulses are distributed throughout the entire plant, from roots to shoots and vice versa. A working model (Figure 1) to define plant behavior has been adapted from work published by Volkov & Ranatunga, 2006 and Gibert et al., 2006.

Two different types of electrical signals have been reported in plants: AP (Fromm, 2006), which is a rapid propagating electrical pulse, travelling at a constant velocity and maintaining a constant amplitude, and VP (slow wave or "variation potential"), corresponding to a long range of a variation pulse (Stahlberg et al., 2006), which varies with the intensity of the stimulus, and its amplitude and speed decrease with increasing distance from its generation site (Davies, 2004, 2006). AP is an all-or-none depolarization that spreads passively from the excited cellular membrane region to the neighboring non-excited region. Excitation in plant cells depends on $Ca^{+2}$ depolarization and Cl- and K+ repolarization, that spreads passively from the excited cellular membrane region to the neighboring non-excited region (Brenner et al., 2006). A similitude on electrical signal transmission between animal and plant organs has been postulated by Volkov & Ranatunga (2006), using the model presented in Figure 2.

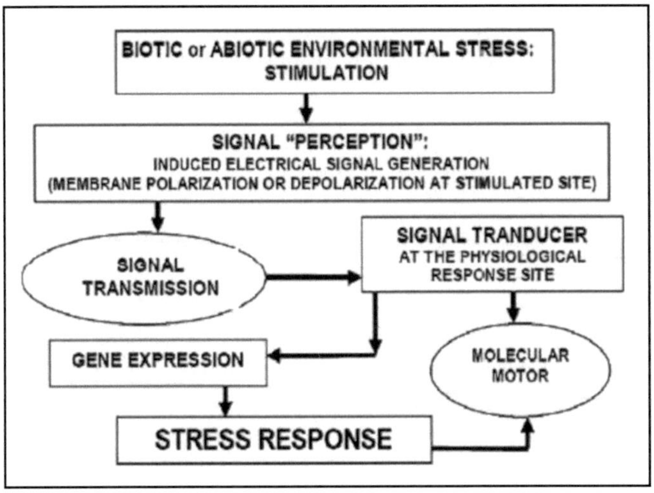


Fig. 1. Proposed mechanism of electric potential signals in plants *(Adapted from Volkov & Ranatunga, 2006 and Gibert et al., 2006).*

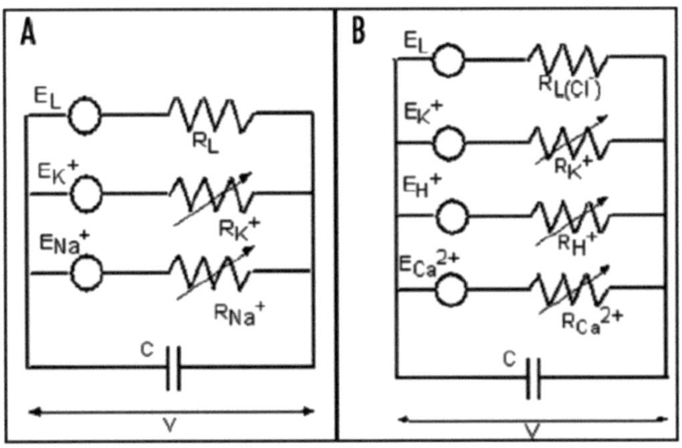


Fig. 2. The Hodgkin-Huxley (HH, 1952) equivalent circuit for an axon (A) and the modified HH circuit for sieve tubes in phloem (B) (*Volkov & Ranatunga, 2006*).

Electrical conduction rate of most of the plant action potentials studied so far is in the range of 0.01-0.2 m $s^{-1}$, i.e. much slower than the conduction velocity of action potentials in animal nerves, which is between 0.4 and 42 m $s^{-1}$ (van Bel & Ehlers 2005). Usually, the receptor potential lasts as long as the stimulus is present, being an electrical replica of the initial stimulus. If the stimulus is sufficiently large to cause the membrane potential to depolarize below a certain threshold, this will cause an action potential to be generated. It shows a large transient depolarization which is self perpetuating and therefore allows the rapid transmission of information over long distances.

Action potentials can propagate over short distances through plasmodesmata, and after it has reached the sieve element/companion cell (SE/CC) complex (Figure 3), it can travel over long distances along the SE plasma membrane in both directions.

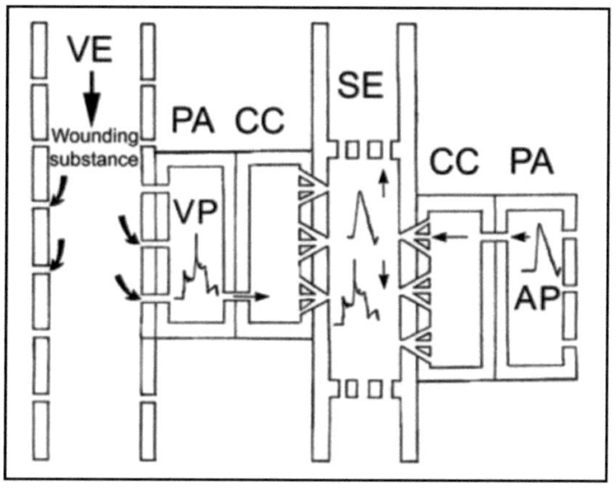


Fig. 3. Action and variation potentials in plants. (*After Lautner et al. 2005; Fromm & Lautner, 2007*).

In contrast, a VP is generated at the plasma membrane of parenchyma cells (PAs) adjacent to xylem vessels (VEs) (Figure 3) by a hydraulic wave or a wounding substance. Because VPs were measured in SEs, it is suggested that they also can pass through the plasmodesmal network and can reach the phloem pathway. However, in contrast to APs, their amplitude will be reduced with increasing distance from the site of generation.

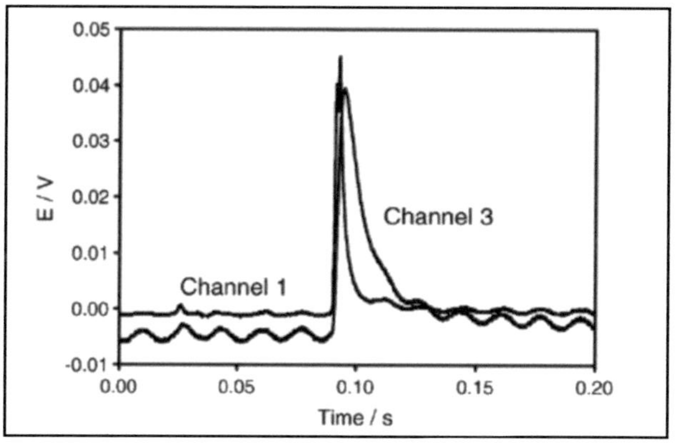


Fig. 4. An action potential recorded in Aloe vera spp. (*After Volkov et al., 2007*).

Action potentials (AP) induced in leaves of an Aloe vera spp. plant by thermal shock (flame) are described by Volkov et al., 2007 (Figure 4). Measurements were recorded at 500,000 scans/second and 2,000,000 scans/sample. Channel 1 is located on the leaf treated by thermal shock and channel 2 is located on a different leaf of the same plant. Distance between Ag/AgCl electrodes for each channel was 1 cm.

Stankovic et al. (1998) provide data on APs and VPs measured in *Helianthus annuus* stems by extracellular electrodes (Figure 5). The AP was elicited by electrical stimulation (±), and the VP by wounding (*W*).

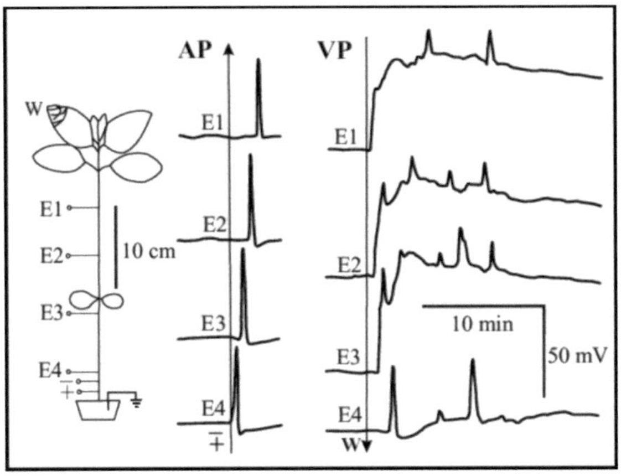


Fig. 5. Action potentials (*APs*) and variation potentials (*VPs*) recorded in the stem of *Helianthus annuus* by extracellular electrodes, *E1–E4*. *Vertical arrows* indicate the moment of stimulation. *Arrowheads* point to the direction of propagation. (*After Stankovic et al., 1998*).

After a transient change in the membrane potential of plant cells (depolarization and subsequent repolarization), VPs and APs make use of the vascular bundles to achieve a potentially systemic spread through the entire plant. The principal difference used to differentiate VPs from APs is that VPs show longer, delayed repolarizations, as shown in Figure 6.

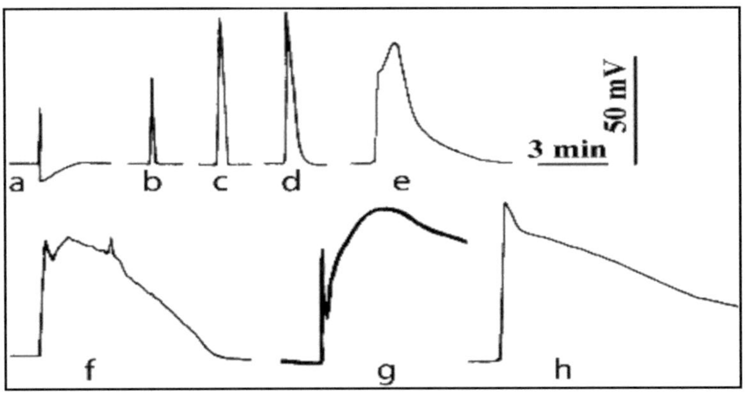


Fig. 6. APs (a to e) and VP (f to h) in plants (*After Stahlberg et al., 2006*).

VPs repolarizations show a large range of variation that makes a clear distinction to APs difficult; however, VPs and APs do differ more clearly in two aspects: a. the causal factors stimulating their appearance - the ionic mechanisms of their depolarization and repolarization phases - and b. the mechanisms and pathways of signal propagation. The generation of APs occurs under different environmental and internal influences, like touch, light changes, cold treatment or cell expansion that trigger a voltage-dependent depolarization spike in an all-or-nothing manner. The depolarizations of a VP arise with an increase in turgor pressure cells experience as a result of a hydraulic pressure wave, that spreads through the xylem conduits after rain, embolism, bending, local wounds, organ excision or local burning. While APs and VPs can be triggered in excised organs, VPs depend on the pressure difference between the atmosphere and an intact plant interior. High humidity and prolonged darkness will also suppress VP signaling.

The ionic mechanism of the VP is thought to involve a transient shutdown of a P-type $H^+$-ATPase in the plasma membrane and differs from the mechanism underlying APs. Another defining characteristic of VPs is the hydraulic mode of propagation, that enables them — but not APs — to pass through killed or poisoned areas. Unlike APs they can easily communicate between leaf and stem. VPs can move in both directions of the plant axis, while their amplitudes show a decrement of about 2.5% $cm^{-1}$ and move with speeds that can be slower than APs in darkness and faster in bright light. The VPs move with a rapid pressure increase, establishing an axial pressure gradient in the xylem. This gradient translates distance (perhaps via changing kinetics in the rise of turgor pressure) into increasing lag phases for the pressure-induced depolarizations in the epidermis cells. VPs are not only ubiquitous among higher plants but represent a unique, defining characteristic without parallels in lower plants or animals (Stahlberg et al., 2005; Baluska, 2010).

Electric signals in different fruit bearing trees and other plants species are evaluated at the present, and the effects of different environmental stimuli on its magnitudes and interpretation is a major subject of research. Also, the large number of experiences, yet to be published and now on the peer review referral process in several scientific journals is indicative of a major breakthrough in our knowledge of plant electrical physiology. As an example, data on the effects of tipping and shoot removal in apple trees (Gurovich, Rivera & García, 2011, Figure 7), and dark - light cycles in olive trees (Gurovich and Cano, 2011, Figure 8) are presented below.

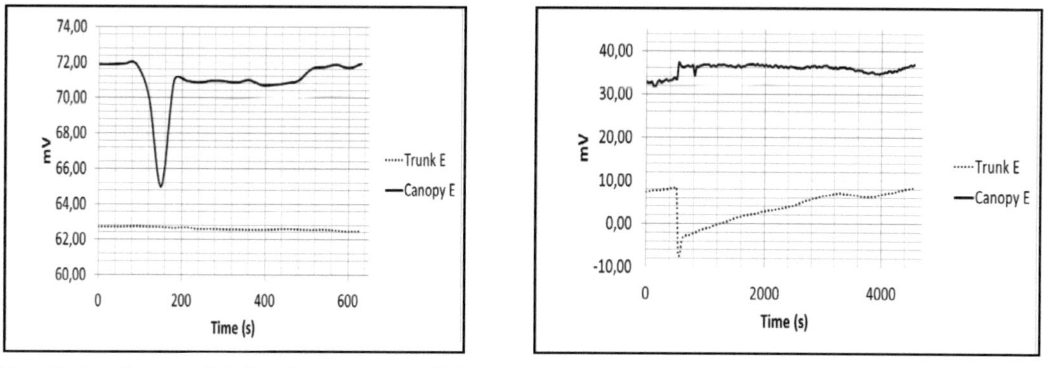


Fig. 7. Apple tree (*Malus domestica* Borkh), cv. Granny Schmidt electric behavior after tipping (A) and basal shoot removal (B). Electrodes are separated by 35 cm. (*After Gurovich, Rivera & García, 2011, unpublished data*).

In Figure 7A an electrical pulse is transmitted from the tree distal upper tipped point down to the microelectrode located 50 cm in the trunk, within the canopy, with a 3 s delay, and led to a maximal EP reduction of 6.93 ± 1.2 mV in 15 s, with an almost complete EP recovery in 90 s; however, no changes in the EP were measured at the base of the trunk. Elimination of a basal shoot from the rootstock (Figure 7 B) resulted in a EP 15.76 mV reduction, measured with a microelectrode located 5 cm above the rootstock - tree grafting area and a slight increase of 3.88 mV measured at the canopy.

Olive plants kept for 48 hr in total darkness were cyclically illuminated every 5 min for 1000 s periods and EP was measured at the root, rootstock, grafted tree and 2 shoots (Figure 8). A sharp reduction in EP values (on average 50 mV, with a polarity change) take place 3 to 5 s after each illumination cycle, with a slow EP recovery when dark conditions are restored. This behavior is much intense in shoots than in roots, grafted tree and rootstock, and each electric impulse travels throughout the whole plant with similar patterns and velocities.

## 5. Plant electrophysiology research technology and applications

Two techniques for the measurement of electrical currents in plant studies have been developed: a. non invasive surface recording and b. measurements using inserted thin metal electrodes (Fromm & Lautner, 2007). At different positions of the plant, from roots to fruits, electrodes are connected by insulated cables to a high - input impedance multichannel electrometer and a reference electrode is inserted in the soil. When all channels are stabilized electrically, the effect of many treatments on plant electric behavior can be evaluated, such as electrical stimulation at different organs in the symplastic continuum, to study its transmission dynamics within the plant, resulting from environmental stimuli like light - darkness sequences, drought - irrigation cycles, heat pulses at a specific leaf, localized chemical product applications, variable wind speed and air relative humidity conditions, or plant organ mechanical wounding, like trunk girdling, pruning, leaf and fruit thinning or root excision by underground tillage.

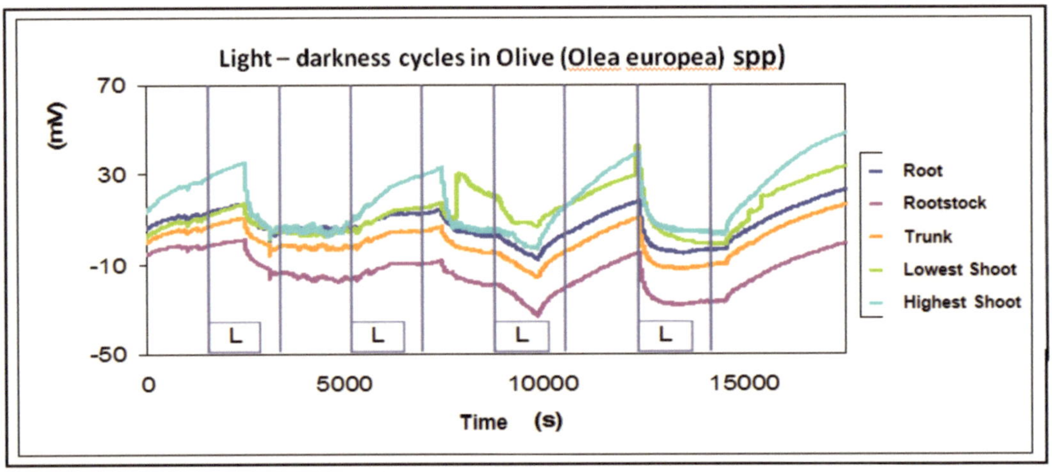


Fig. 8. Electrical behavior of Olive (*Olea europea*) trees) in alternate dark - light cycles (average values from 10 plants) (*After Gurovich & Cano, 2011, unpublished data*). L = light period at constant 45 watt $m^{-2}$, at the canopy top).

Several micro-electrodes have been used for electrophysiological studies in plants. In most of our publications, electrical potentials are monitored continuously using own designed nonpolarizable Ag/AgCl microelectrodes inserted into different positions along the trunk; microelectrode characteristics have been reported by Gurovich & Hermosilla (2009), Gil et al. (2009), Oyarce & Gurovich (2011), and consist on a 0.35 mm-diameter silver wire (99.99% Ag), chlorated in a solution of HCl 0.1N for 30 s using a differential voltage of 2.5 V, to obtain an Ag/AgCl coating, which is inserted in a stainless steel hypodermic needle, 0.5 mm in diameter, filled with a KCl 3M solution; both needle ends are heat-sealed with polyethylene. Electrodes were inserted into the trunk using a low velocity electric microdriller, with a barbed microreel, penetrating the phloematic and cambium tissue; needle tip was further inserted into the xylematic tissue, 0.5-0.75 cm, by mechanical pressure. Each Ag/AgCl microelectrode was referenced to an identical microelectrode installed in the sand media, within the root system (Figure 9).

In our work on electrophysiology, EP real time measurements are implemented using a multi channel voltmeter (Model 2701, Keithley Instruments, including a 20 channel switch module Keithley, model 7700), measuring DC and AC voltage in the range from 100 mV to 1000 V, in testing intervals from 1 to 100 ms. Signals obtained are analyzed with the software ExceLINX-1, an utility provided by Microsoftc Excel. All EP measurements are made by keeping the trees within a Faraday-type electromagnetic insulation cage, installed in the laboratory to control constant light and temperature conditions (Figure 10).

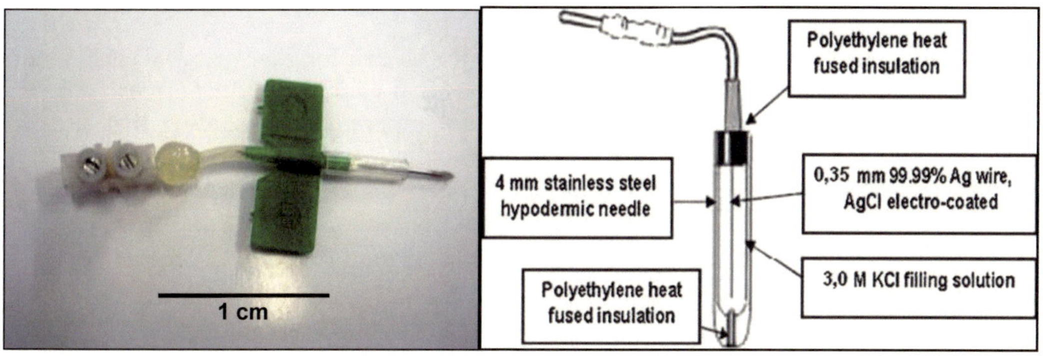


Fig. 9. The Ag/AgCl microelectrode construction.

## 6. Research on plant electrophysiology of woody plants

Trees live in a continuously changing environment and although not all parts of the tree are exposed to the same stimuli at the same time, tree organs respond in a coordinated fashion, for example, by fast stomata closing under even mild water stress buildup, demonstrating the existence of communication between various regions of the tree. For years, researchers have concentrated their efforts on the study of chemical (hormonal) signals in trees, and very seldom considering that plants simultaneously show distinct electrical and hydraulic signals, which correlate to water stress conditions and other physiological stimuli as well. Considering the large leaf area of a tree, very large amounts of chemicals would need to be synthesized, transported and be perceived at the canopy, in order to respond to a signal coming from the roots.

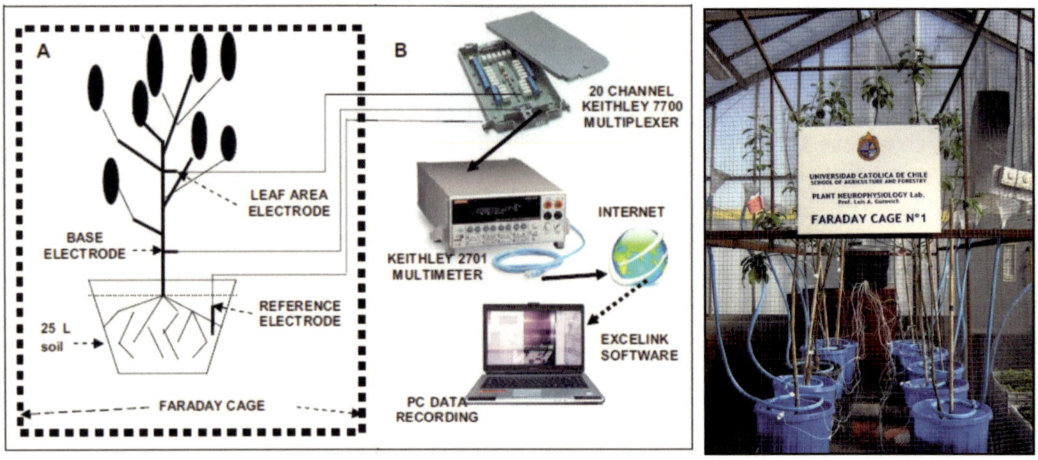


Fig. 10. Schematic diagram of the digital acquisition system for recording voltage differences between the base of the trunk and the canopy. (*After Gurovich and Hermosilla, 2009*).

Limited reaearch has been reported on signaling in woody trees (*Tilia* and *Prunus*, Boari & Malone 1993; *Salix*, Fromm & Spanswick 1993; Grindl et al., 1999; Oak, Morat et al., 1994; Koppan et al., 2000, 2002; *Vitis*, Mancuso,1999; *Poplar*, Gibert et al., 2006) although it is in such plants that the need for rapid and efficient signals other than chemicals becomes more obvious.

Gibert et al., 2006 present relevant information on the electric long term (2 year) behavior of a single poplar tree, focused on the spatial and temporal variations of the electric potential distribution (Figure 11), with its correlation to air temperature, concluding that seasonal fluctuations of EP trends may be correlated to sap flow patterns, largely influenced by seasonal sap constituents and concentrations.

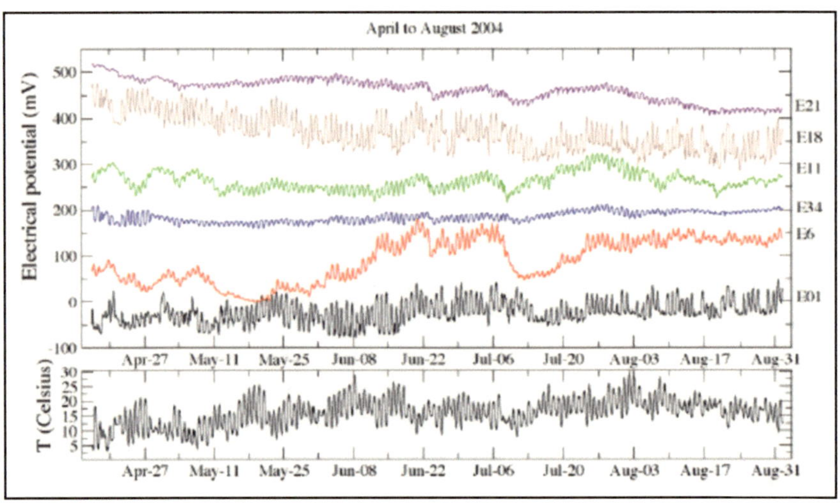


Fig. 11. Top: potential signals for the December 2003–April 2004 period, expressed as relative potential values *(see Gibert et al., 2006, Fig. 1 for electrode location)*. Bottom: outdoor temperature measured near the tree. Tick marks fall at midday.

Recent studies have associated the effect of water stress build-up, irrigation and light with electrical signaling in fruit bearing tree species including avocado (*Persea americana* Mill.), blueberry (*Vaccinium spp.*), lemon (*Citrus limon* (L.) Buró) and olive (*Olea europaea* L.) (Gil et al., 2008; Gurovich & Hermosilla, 2009; Oyarce & Gurovich, 2010, 2011). Some results are included below as examples on this research line, aimed to develop new real - time plant stress sensors based on tree electric behavior, for the automation of irrigation systems operation, optimizing water and energy efficiency in fruit production.

Electric potential (EP) differences have been detected between the base of the stem and leaf petiole and between the base of the stem and the leaf area, located in the upper half of the tree canopy, in response to drought, irrigation and diurnal light and dark cycles (Figure 12). Orders of magnitude of the observed EP variation in those studies were similar to values observed by other authors (Fromm, 2006; Davies, 2006). Electric potential variations observed in avocado trees in response to decreased soil water content have been associated with a decrease in stomata conductance (gs) (Gil et al., 2009), indicating that stomata closure might be induced or at least associated with an electrical signal that travels through the phloem at a speed of 2.4 cm min$^{-1}$. Larger changes in electric potential behavior have been detected in response to drought compared to watering. Thus, an extra-cellular electrical signal appears to be involved in root to leaf communication, initiating stomata closure at a very early stage of drought stress. These drought-induced electrical signals were also related to changes in gs, in concordance to other studies published by Fromm & Fei (1998).

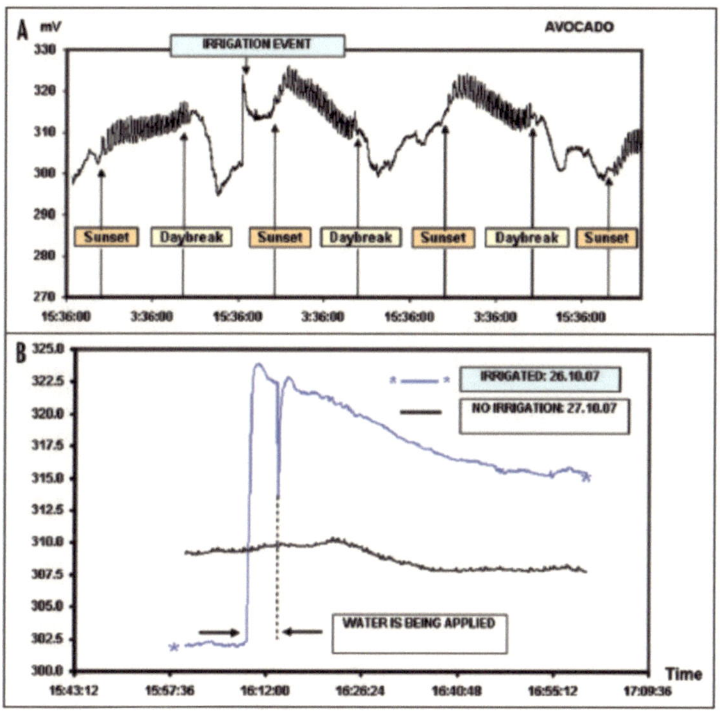


Fig. 12. Electrical potential responses of avocado plants to light and dark and irrigation. (A) EP responses according to the day time. (B) Effect of irrigation on EP behavior *(Adapted from Gurovich & Hermosilla 2009).*

According to Gurovich & Hermosilla (2009) effects of sunset, daybreak and water application are clearly reflected as fast changes in the EP between the base and leaf area electrode locations on the trunk or stem (Figure 12). Electrical potential fluctuations during light and dark periods may be due to differential sap flow velocity at different times of the day as a result of stomata closure during the night. Electrical potential values were reduced during the initial hours after daybreak, and started to increase after midday, as a result of transient water stress conditions; the first dark hours after sunset resulted in rapid increases of voltages and after midnight these increases tended to slow down. Also, a small but consistent increase in voltage was detected about 1-2 hours before daybreak. Explanations for this behavior may also be related to circadian rhythms detected in plants, but need further study to be fully understood (Dodd et al, 2005: Horta et al., 2007).

The effects of irrigation and day – night cycles on the electric behavior of avocado trees has been reported also by Oyarce & Gurovich (2010) under controlled conditions (Figure 13) EP vary in daily cycles throughout the measurement period: during the morning (2:00 to 7:59 AM), the mean 4-day EP average is in the range -89.991 ± 0, 46 mV at 25 cm and -121.53± 0.5 mV at 85 cm above the ground, respectively. During the afternoon (14:00 at 19:59 PM), EP values rise, reaching mean values of -79.71 ± 2.16 mV at 25 cm and -104.05 ± 1.21 mV at 85 cm above the ground, respectively, and maximum values of -76.16 ± 20 mV at 17:10 PM (25 cm) and -101.35 ± 5.05 mV at 18:30 PM (85 cm). These values indicate the existence of significant differences in EP between the periods compared (see Oyarce & Gurovich, 2010, Table 2). The effect of irrigation applied every day at 11:00 AM is clearly expressed by a significant decrease in EP, of the order of 7.10 ± 1.56 mV and 7.53 ± 1.39 mV, for micro electrodes inserted in the tree trunk at 25 and 85 cm above the soil surface respectively, representing specific characteristics of an action potential (AP). The recovery of EP values measured before irrigation requires an average period of 16 minutes. On the fourth day, irrigation applied at 15:35 PM did not induce changes in the electrical potential probably due to a low atmospheric demand at that time.

Oyarce & Gurovich (2011) examined the nature and specific characteristics of the electrical response to wounding in the woody plant Persea americana (avocado) cv. Hass. Under field conditions, wounds can be the result of insect activity, strong winds or handling injury during fruit harvest. Evidence for extracellular EP signaling in avocado trees after mechanical injury is expressed in the form of variation potentials. For tipping and pruning, signal velocities of 8.7 and 20.9 cm/$s^{-1}$, respectively, are calculated, based on data measured with Ag/AgCl microelectrodes inserted at different positions of the trunk (Figure 14 *a* to *d*). EP signal intensity decreased with increasing distance between the tipping and pruning point and the electrode. Recovery time to pre-tipping or pre-pruning EP values was also affected by the distance and signal intensity from the tipping or pruning point to the specific electrode position.

A significant EP signal, corresponding to a variation potential, is generated as a response of tipping or pruning avocado plants (Figure 14 a to d); the signal was transmitted along the tree trunk at a specific velocity, which is dependent on the distance to the mechanical injury. Mancuso (1999) reported a propagation velocity of the front of the main negative-going signal(VP) of 2.7 mm $s^{-1}$, while an AP propagated along the shoot with a velocity of about 100 mm $s^{-1}$. The EP signal intensity also decreases with distance between the mechanical injury sites to the electrode position in the trunk. Several physiological explanations for this

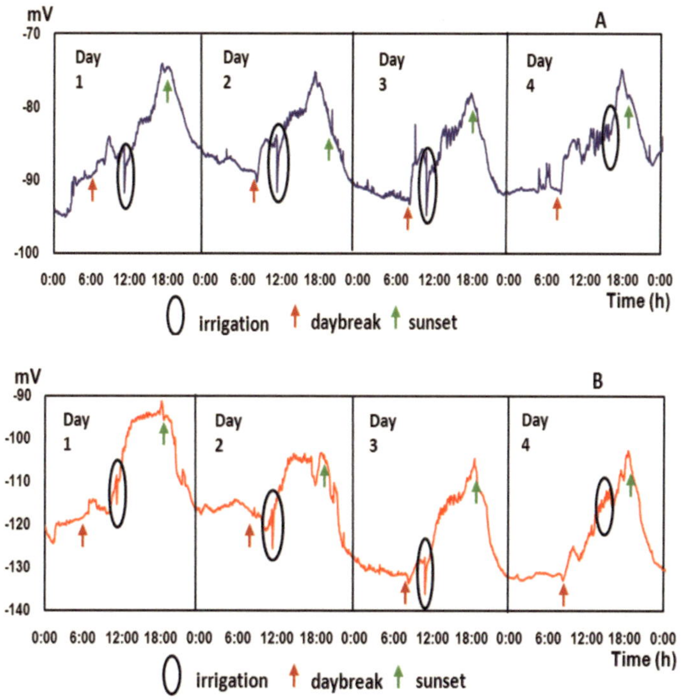


Fig. 13. Electric potentials (EP) in avocado trees during 4 irrigated days. (Average values for 7 trees). Micro electrodes inserted at 25 (A) and 85 (B) cm above the soil surface. (*Adapted from Oyarce & Gurovich, 2010*).

behavior have been proposed by Trewavas & Malho (1997), Zimmermann et al. (1997), Stankovic et al. (1998), Volkov & Brown (2006), Volkov et al. (2008), Baluska et al. (2004); Brenner et al. (2006). All these authors agree with the idea that a certain stimuli receptor must be present at the cell membrane, and that a transient polarization, induced by specific ion fluxes through this membrane, is the ultimate agent of the EP signal generation.

Results presented in these papers indicate a clear and rapid mechanism of electrical signal generation and transmission in woody plants, positively correlated to the intensity and duration of stimuli, such as light intensity, water availability and mechanical injury. The electrical signal is generated in a specific organ or tissue and is transmitted rapidly in the form of AP or VP to other tissues or organs of the plant. The measurement of electrical potentials can be used as a tool for real-time measurement of plant physiological responses, opening the possibility of using this technology as a tool for early detection of stress and for the operation of automatic high frequency irrigation systems.

## 7. Electrophysiology of some plant tropisms

Sedimenting amyloplasts act as statoliths in root and shoot cells specialized for gravisensing; also different auxins are involved in the gravi - stimulated differential growth known a *gravitropism*. However, no comprehensive explanation is available related to gravity signal perception and its transduction pathways in plants from the sedimenting statoliths to the motoric response of organ bending (Baluska et al., 2006).

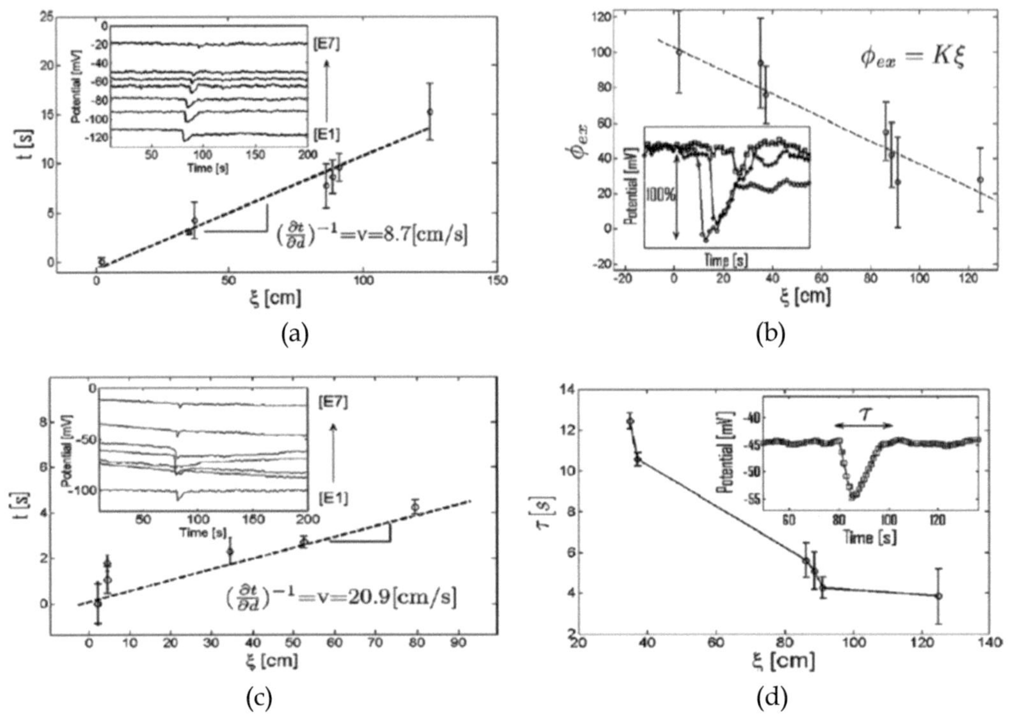


Fig. 14. *a*) Average EP speed of transmission along the trunk, as a result of tipping (n = 5 plants), t (s) = time at which the electrode detected the electric signal, ξ (cm) = distance of electrodes from the tipping point. Error bars represents ±1 std. dev. *b*) Relative intensity of EP as a result of tipping (n = 5 plants). ϕ ex = relative intensity of the signal (%), ξ (cm) = distance from the electrode to the tipping point. Error bars represents ±1 std. dev.
*c*) Average EP speed of transmission along the trunk after pruning, measured above and below the pruned branch (n = 5 plants), t (s) = time at which the electrode detected the electric signal, ξ (cm) = distance of electrodes from the pruning point. Error bars represents +1 std. dev. *d*) Recovery time of the pre-tipping EP potential (n = 5 plants), τ = recovery time signal, ξ (cm) = distance from the electrode to the tipping point. Error bars represents ±1 std. dev (*after Oyarce & Gurovich, 2011*).

Bioelectrochemical signaling in green plants induced by photosensory systems have been reported by Volkov et al., (2004). The generation of electrophysiological responses induced by blue and red photosensory systems was observed in soybean plants. A phototropic response is a sequence of the following four processes: reception of a directional light signal, signal transduction, transformation of the signal into a physiological response, and the production of a directional growth response. It was found that the irradiation of soybean plants at 450±50, 670, and 730 nm induces APs with duration times and amplitudes of approximately 0.3 ms and 60 mV. Plants respond to light ranging from ultraviolet to far-red using specific photoreceptors and natural radiation simultaneously activates more than one photoreceptor in higher plants; these receptors initiate distinct signaling pathways leading to wavelength-specific light responses. Three types of plant photoreceptors that have been identified at the molecular level are phototropins, cryptochromes, and phytochromes respectively.

## 8. Plant electrophysiology modulated by neurotransmitters, neuroregulators and neurotoxins

Plants produce a wide range of phytochemicals that mediate cell functions and translate environmental cues for survival; many of these molecules are also found as neuro - regulatory molecules in animals, including humans. For example, the human neurotransmitter melatonin (N-acetyl-5-methoxytryptamine) is a common molecule associated with timing of circadian rhythms in many organisms, including higher plants. Its major concentrations are located within the phloem conducting vessels and it has been suggested that its action is centered in the electrochemical processes involved in plasmodesmata synaptic - like contacts. Plant synapse has been proposed, since actin cytoskeleton-based adhesive contacts between plant cells resemble the neuronal and immune synapses found in animals (Baluska et al., 2005). A comprehensive review of neurotransmitters in plants is provided by V. V. Roschina in the book *"Neurotransmitters in plant life"* (2001).

Whereas glutamate and glycine were shown to gate $Ca^{+2}$-permeable channels in plants, glutamate was reported to rapidly depolarize the plant cell plasma membrane in a process mediated by glutamate receptors (Baluška, 2010; Felle & Zimmermann, 2007); plant glutamate receptors have all the features of animal neuronal glutamate receptors, inducing plant APs (Stolarz et al., 2010) . These publications strongly suggest that glutamate serves as a neurotransmitter-like in cell-to-cell communication in plants too. Whereas glutamate might represent a plant excitatory transmitter, gamma-aminobutyric acid (GABA) seems to act as an inhibitory transmitter in plants, as it does similarly in animal neurons. For instance, it is well documented that GABA is rapidly produced under diverse stress situations and also that GABA can be transported from cell-to-cell across plant tissues (Bouche et al., 2003).

Many fascinating questions in future research will define the role of neurotransmitters, neuroregulators and neurotoxins in the growth and development of plants. As newer technologies emerge, it will become possible to understand more about the role of neurological compounds in the inner workings of plant metabolism, plant environment interactions and plant electrophysiology. However, signaling molecules, by their nature, are short lived, unstable, difficult to detect and quantify, because they are highly reactive, and present in small concentrations within plant tissues.

## 9. Electrophysiological control of cyclical oscillations in plants.

Sanchez et al. (2011) reviewed the interaction between the circadian clock of higher plants to that of metabolic and physiological processes that coordinate growth and performance under a predictable, albeit changing environment. The circadian clock of plants and abiotic-stress tolerance appear to be firmly interconnected processes, by means of electrophysiological signaling (Volkov et al., 2011). Time oscillations (circadian clocks) in plant membrane transport, including model predictions, experimental validation, and physiological implications has been reported by Mancuso & Shabala (2006) and Shabala et al., (2008).

## 10. Conclusions

Plants have evolved sophisticated systems to sense environmental abiotic and biotic stimuli for adaptation and to produce signals to other cells for coordinated actions, synchronizing their normal biological functions and their responses to the environment. The synchronization of internal functions based on external events is linked with the phenomenon of excitability in plant cells. The generation of electric gradients is a fundamental aspect of long-distance signal transduction, which is a major process to account for tree physiology. Outstanding similarities exist between AP in plants and animals and the knowledge about AP and VP/SWP mechanisms in plants, its physiological consequences and its technological applications is accumulating, but there is still a broad margin for questions and speculations to further elucidate the concepts described in this review; thus, an interesting challenge to understand the complex regulatory network of electric signaling and responses is still an open question. Future improvements in research methods and instruments will reveal more aspects of the signal complexity, and its physiological responses in plants.

Our future knowledge on the subject will help us considering electrical signals in plants as normal phenomena, to be used as a real - time communication mechanism between the plant physiologist and the plant, for example, for the early detection of plant stress, to enable proper and automatic modulation of the tree microenvironment, in order to optimize the agronomic performance of fruit bearing or wood producing trees. Also, highly modulated external electric impulses, to be applied on trees at specific intensities, durations and phenology timings, to modify water use efficiency or photosynthetic efficiency, could be developed from this knowledge.

## 11. References


Baluška, F. (2010). Recent surprising similarities between plant cells and neurons. Plant Signaling and Behavior 5: 87–89.

Baluška, F.; Mancuso, S.; Volkmann, D. & Barlow, P. (2004). Root apices as plant command centers: the unique 'brain-like' status of the root apex transition zone. Biologia Bratislava, 59: 7-19.

Baluška, F.; Volkmann, D. & Menzel, D. (2005). Plant synapses: actin-based domains for cell-to-cell communication. Trends Plant Science 10:106–111.

Baluška, F. & Mancuso, S. (2008). Plant neurobiology: from sensory biology, via plant communication, to social plant behavior. In: "Neuroscience today: neuronal functional diversity and collective behaviors". Guest editors: F. Tito Arecchi, Riccardo Meucci, Walter Sannita, Alessandro Farini. Cognitive Processing 12: 3 - 7.

Baluška, F.; Barlow, P.; Volkmann, D, & Mancuso, S. (2006). Gravity related paradoxes in plants: can plant neurobiology provide the clue? In: Biosemiotics in Transdisciplinary Context. Witzany G (ed), Umweb, Helsinki

Barlow, P. W. (2008). Reflections on plant neurobiology. Biological Systems 92: 132-147

Bertholon, M. L. (1783). De l'Electricite des Vegetaux: Ouvrage dans lequel on traite de l'electricite de l'atmosphere sur les plantes, de ses effets sur l'economie des vegetaux, de leurs vertus medicaux. P.F. Didotjeune, Paris

Blatt, M. R. (2008). Ion Transport at the Plant Plasma Membrane. In: eLS. John Wiley & Sons Ltd, Chichester.

Boari, F. & Malone, M. (1993). Wound-induced hydraulic signals: Survey of occurrence in a range of species. J Experimental Botany 44: 741-746.

Bonza, M. C.; Luoni, L. & De Michelis, M. I. (2001). Stimulation of plant plasma membrane $Ca^{2+}$-ATPase activity by acidic phospholipids. Physiologia Plantarum 112: 315–320.

Bose, J. C. (1926). The Nervous Mechanism of Plants, pp. 123–134. Longmans, Green & Co., London, UK.

Bouche, N.; Lacombe, B. & Fromm, H. (2003). GABA signaling: a conserved and ubiquitous mechanism. Trends Cell Biology 13: 607–610

Brenner, E. D.; Stahlberg, R.; Mancuso, S.; Vivanco, J.; Baluska, F. & Volkenburgh, E. V. (2006). Plant neurobiology: an integrated view of plant signaling. Trends Plant Science 11: 413-419.

Burdon-Sanderson, J. (1873). Note on the electrical phenomena which accompany irritation of the leaf of *Dionaea muscipula*. Proceedings of the Royal Society of London 21: 495–496.

Darwin, C. (1875). Insectivorous Plants. J. Murray, London

Darwin, C. (1896). The power of movements in plants. Appleton, New York

Davies, E. (2004). New functions for electrical signals in plants. New Phytologist 161: 607–610.

Davies, E. (2006). Electrical signals in plants: Facts and hypothesis. In: A. Volkov (Ed.), Plant Electrophysiology: Theory and Methods. Springer-Verlag, Heideberg, Germany ISBN: 3-540-32717-7

Datta, P. & Palit, P. (2004). Relationship between environmental factors and diurnal variation of bioelectric potentials of an intact jute plant. Current Science 87: 680–3.

Dodd, A. N.; Salathia, N.; Hall, A.; Kévei, E.; Tóth, R.; Nagy, F.; Hibberd, J. M.; Millar, A. J. Webb, A. A. (2005). Plant circadian clocks increase photosynthesis, growth, survival, and competitive advantage. *Science* 309: 630-633.

Dziubinska, H.; Trebacz, K. & Zawadski, T. (2001). Transmission route for action potentials and variation potentials in Helianthus annuus L. J Plant Physiology 158: 1167–1172.

Dziubinska, H.; Filek, M.; Koscielniak, J. & Trebacz, K. (2003). Variation and action potentials evoked by thermal stimuli accompany enhancement of ethylene emission in distant non-stimulated leaves of Vicia faba minor seedlings. J Plant Physiology 160: 1203-1210.

Felle, H. H. & Zimmermann, M. R. (2007). Systemic signaling in barley through action potentials. Planta 226: 203–214.

Fromm, J. (2006). Long-Distance electrical signaling and physiological functions in higher plants. In: A. Volkov. (Ed.), Plant Electrophysiology: Theory and Methods. Springer-Verlag, Heidelberg, Germany. ISBN: 3-540-32717-7

Fromm, J. & Eschrich, W. (1988). Transport processes in stimulated and non-stimulated leaves of *Mimosa pudica*. I. The movement of 14C-labelled photoassimilates. Trees 2: 7–17.

Fromm, J. & Spanswick, R. (1993). Characteristics of action potentials in willow (Salix viminalis L.) J Experimental Botany 44: 1119-1125.

Fromm, J. & Bauer, T. (1994). Action potentials in maize sieve tubes change phloem translocation. J Experimental Botany 45: 463–469.

Fromm, J. & Fei, H. (1998). Electrical signaling and gas exchange in maize plants of drying soil. Plant Science 132: 203–13.

Fromm, J. & Lautner, S. (2007). Electrical signals and their physiological significance in plants. Plant, Cell and Environment 30: 249–257.

Fromm, J. & Spanswick, R. (2007). Characteristics of action potentials in willow(Salix viminalis L.). J Experimental Botany 44: 1119–1125.

Gelli, A. & Blumwald, E. (1997). Hyperpolarization-activated $Ca^{2+}$- permeable channels in the plasma membrane of tomato cells. J Membrane Biology 155: 35-45.

Gil, P. M.; Gurovich, L. & Schaffer, B. (2008). The electrical response of fruit trees to soil water availability and diurnal light-dark cycles. Plant Signaling and Behavior 3: 1026–1029.

Gil, P. M.; Gurovich, L.; Schaffer, B.; Alcayaga, J.; Rey, S. & Iturriaga, R. (2008). Root to leaf electrical signaling in avocado in response to light and soil water content. J Plant Physiology 165: 1070-1078.

Gil, P. M.; Gurovich, L.; Schaffer, B.; García, N. & Iturriaga, R. (2009). Electrical signaling, stomatal conductance, ABA and Ethylene content in avocado trees in response to root hypoxia. Plant Signaling and Behavior 4: 100-108.

Gibert, D.; Le Mouel, J. L.; Lambs, L.; Nicollin, F. & Perrier, F. (2006). Sap flow and daily electric potential variations in a tree trunk. Plant Science 171: 572–584

Gindl, W.; Loppert, H. G, & Wimmer, R. (1999). Relationship between streaming potential and sap velocity in Salix Alba L, Phyton 39: 217–224.

Gunar, I. & Sinykhin, A. M. (1962). A spreading wave of excitation in higher plants. Proc. Academy Science USSR (Botany) 142: 214–215.

Gurovich, L. (2009). Real-Time Plant Water Potential Assessment Based on Electrical Signaling In Higher Plants Joint International Meeting. VII. International World Computers in Agriculture and American Society of Agricultural and Biological Engineers Annual Meeting Proc., paper N° 095875.

Gurovich, L. & Hermosilla, P. (2009). Electric signaling in fruit trees in response to water applications and light-darkness conditions. J Plant Physiology 166:290–300.

Haberlandt, G. (1914). Physiological plant anatomy. Macmillan, London

Hedrich, R. & Schroeder, J. I. (1989). The Physiology of Ion Channels and Electrogenic Pumps in Higher Plants. Annual Review of Plant Physiology and Plant Molecular Biology 40: 539-569

Herde, O.; Atzorn, R.; Fisahn, J.; Wasternack, C.; Willmitzer, L. & Peña-Cortés, H. (1996). Localized wounding by heat initiates the accumulation of proteinase inhibitor II in abscisic acid-deficient plants by triggering jasmonic acid biosynthesis. Plant Physiology 112: 853-860.

Herde, O.; Fuss, H.; Peña-Cortés, H.; & Fisahn, J. (1995). Proteinase inhibitor II gene expression induced by electrical stimulation and control of photosynthetic activity in tomato plants. Plant Cell Physiology 36: 737-742.

Higinbotham, N. (1973). Electropotentials of plant cells. Annual Review of Plant Physiology 24: 25–46.

Hodgkin, A. & Huxley, A. F. (1952). A quantitative description of membrane current and its application to conduction and excitation in nerve. J Physiology (London) 117: 500-544.

Jia, W. & Zhang, J. (2008). Stomatal movements and long-distance signaling in plants. Plant Signaling and Behavior 3: 772-777.

Jiang, F. & Hartung, W. (2008). Long-distance signalling of abscisic acid (ABA): the factors regulating the intensity of the ABA signal. J Experimental Botany 59: 37–43.

Karmanov, V. G.; Lyalin, O. O. & Mamulashvili, G. G. (1972). The form of action potentials and cooperativeness of the excited elements in stems of winter squash. Soviet Plant Physiology 19: 354–420.

Knudsen, O. S. (2002). Biological Membranes: Theory of Transport, Potentials and Electric Impulses. Cambridge University Press. ISBN: 0521810183

Koppan, A.; Szarka, L. & Wesztergom, W. (2000). Annual fluctuation in amplitudes of daily variations of electrical signals measured in the trunk of a standing tree, C.R. Academie Science. Paris 323: 559–563.

Koppan, A.; Fenyvesi, L.; Szarka, L. & Wesztergom, W. (2002). Measurement of electric potential difference on trees. Acta Biologica Szegediens 46: 37–38.

Koziolek, C.; Grams, T. E. E.; Schreiber, U.; Matyssek, R. & Fromm, J. (2003). Transient knockout of photosynthesis mediated by electrical signals. New Phytologist 161: 715–722.

Ksenzhek, O. S. & Volkov, A. G. (1998). Plant Energetics. Academic Press, San Diego, USA. ISBN: 97-807794

Lautner, S.; Grams, T. E.; Matyssek, R. & Fromm, J. (2005). Characteristics of electrical signals in poplar and responses in photosynthesis. Plant Physiology 138: 2200-2209.

Lautner, S. & Fromm, J. (2010). Calcium-dependent physiological processes in trees. Plant Biology 12: 268–274.

Lemström, K. (1904). Electricity in Agriculture and Horticulture, Electrician Publications, London.

Lunevsky, V. Z.; Zherelova, O. M.; Vostrikov, I. Y. & Berestovsky, G. N. (1983). Excitation of Characeae cell membranes as a result of activation of calcium and chloride channels. J Membrane Biology 72: 43–58.

Maathuis, F. J. M. & Sanders, D. (1997). Regulation of $K^+$ absorption in plant root cells by external $K^+$: Interplay of different plasma membrane $K^+$ transporters. J Experimental Botany 48: 451-458.

Malone, M. (1996). Rapid, long-distance signal transmission in higher plants. Advances Botanical Research 22: 163–228.

Malone, M.; Alarcon, J. J. & Palumbo, L. (1994). An hydraulic interpretation of rapid, long-distance wound signaling in tomato. Planta 193: 181–185.

Mancuso, S. & Mugnai, S. (2006). Long distance transmission in Trees. In: Communications in Plants: Neuronal aspects of plant life. F. Baluska, S. Mancuso and D. Volkmann Eds. Springer. ISBN: 10 3-540-28475-3

Mancuso, S. & Shabala, S. (2006). Rhythms in Plants. Springer Verlag. ISBN: 978-3-642-08774-5

McClung, C. R. (2001). Circadian rythms in plants. Annual Review of Plant Physiology and Plant Molecular Biology 52: 139-162.

Montenegro, M. I.; Queiros, M. A, & Daschbach, J. L. (1991). Microelectrodes: theory and applications. Kluwer Academic, Dordrecht. ISBN: 0-7923-1229-5

Morat, P.; Le Mouel, J. L. & Granier, A. (1994). Electrical potential on a tree. A measurement of the sap flow? C.R. Academie Science Paris 317: 98–101.

Murphy, A. S.; Peer, W. & Burkhard, S. (2010). The plant plasma membrane. Springer ISBN: 9783642134302

Nadler, A.; Raveh, E.; Yermiyahu, U.; Lado, M.; Nasser, A.; Barak, M. & Green, S. Detecting water stress in trees using stem electrical conductivity measurements. (2008). J Soil Science Society America 72: 1014–1024.

Neuhaus, H. K. & Wagner, R. (2000). Solute pores, ion channels, and metabolite transporters in the outer and inner envelope membranes of higher plant plastids Biochimica et Biophysica Acta 1465: 307 - 323.

Oyarce, P. & Gurovich, L. (2010). Electrical signals in avocado trees. Responses to light and water availability conditions. Plant Signaling and Behavior 5: 34-41.

Oyarce, P. & Gurovich, L. (2011). Evidence for the transmission of information through electric potentials in injured avocado trees. J Plant Physiology 168: 103-108.

Pfeffer, W. (1921). Osmotische Untersuchungen; Studien zur Zellmechanik. Engelmann, Leipzig

Pickard, B. (1973). Action potentials in higher plants. Botanical Review 39: 172–201.

Roschina, V. V. (2001). Neurotransmitters in plant life. Enfield: Science Publishers, Inc. ISBN 1-57808-142-4

Sanchez, A.; Shin, J. & Davis, S, J. (2011). Abiotic stress and the plant circadian clock. Plant Signaling and Behavior 6: 223–231.

Sanders, D.; Pelloux, J.; Brownlee, C. & Harper, J. F. (2002). Calcium at the Crossroads of Signaling. Plant Cell 14: 401-417.

Shabala, S.; Shabala, L.; Gradmann, D.: Chen, Z.; Newman, I. & Mancuso, S. (2006). Oscillations in plant membrane-transport activity: model predictions, experimental validation, and physiological implications. J Experimental Botany 57: 171–184.

Simons, P. (1992). The action plant. Movement and nervous behavior in plants. Blackwell, Oxford. ISBN: 978-0631138990

Schroeder, J. & Thuleau, P. (1991). Ca2+ Channels in Higher Plant Cells. The Plant Cell 3: 555-559.

Stahlberg, R. (2006). Historical overview on plant neurobiology. Plant Signaling and Behavior 1: 6-8.

Stahlberg, R.; Cleland, R. E. & Van Volkenburgh, E. (2005). Slow wave potentials - a propagating electrical signal unique to higher plants. In: Baluska, F.; Mancuso, S. Volkmann, D. eds. Communications in Plants. Neuronal Aspects of Plant Life. Berlin: Springer. ISBN: 978-3-540-28475-8

Stankovic, B.; Witters, D. L.; Zawadzki, T. & Davies, E. (1998). Action potentials and variation potentials in sunflower: An analysis of their relationship and distinguishing characteristics. Physiologia Plantarum 103: 51–58,

Stankovic, B. & Davies, E. (1996). Both action potentials and variation potentials induce proteinase inhibitor gene expression in tomato. Federation of European Biochemical Societies Letters 390: 275-279.

Stankovic, B. & Davies, E. (1998). The wound response in tomato involves rapid growth and electrical responses, systemically up-regulated transcription of proteinase inhibitor and calmodulin and down-regulated translation. Plant and Cell Physiology 39: 268-274.

Stolarz, M.; Król, E.; Dziubinska, H. & Kurenda, A. (2010). Glutamate induces series of action potentials and a decrease in circumnutation rate in Helianthus annuus. Physiologia Plantarum 138: 329–338.

Sze, H.; Xuhang, Li. & Palmgren, M. G. (1999). Energization of Plant Cell Membranes by H+ Pumping ATPases: Regulation and Biosynthesis. The Plant Cell 11: 677–689.

Trebacz, K.; Dziubinska, H. & Krol, E. (2005). Electrical signals in long-distance communication in plants. In: Baluska, F.; Mancuso, S. & Volkmann, D. eds. Communications in Plants. Neuronal Aspects of Plant Life. Berlin: Springer. ISBN: 978-3-540-28475-8

Trewavas, A. J. (2003). Aspects of plant intelligence. Annals of Botany 92: 1–20.

Trewavas, A. J. (2005). Green plants as intelligent organisms. Trends in Plant Science 10: 413-419.

Trewavas, A. J. & Malho, R. (1997). Signal perception and transduction: the origin of the phenotype. Plant Cell 9: 1181-1195.

Tuteja, N.; Sudhir, K. & Sopory, S. K. (2008). Chemical signaling under abiotic stress environment in plants. Plant Signaling and Behavior 3: 525-536.

Van Bel, A. J. & Ehlers, K. (2005). Electrical signalling via plasmodesmata. In: Plasmodesmata, (K.J. Oparka, ed.) Blackwell Publishing, Oxford. ISBN: 9781405125543

Volkov, A. G. (2000). Green plants: Electrochemical interfaces. J Electroanalitical Chemistry. 483: 150-156.

Volkov, A. G. (2006). Plant electrophysiology: theory and methods Volkov, A.G. Springer Distribution Center GmbH ISBN: 9783540327172

Volkov, A. G.; Dunkley, T. C.; Morgan, S. A.; Ruff, D.; Boyce, Y. L. & Labady, A. J. (2004). Bioelectrochemical signaling in green plants induced by photosensory systems. Bioelectrochemistry 63: 91-94.

Volkov, A. G. & Haack, R. A. (1995). Insect induces bioelectrochemical signals in potato plants. Bioelectrochemical Bioenergy 35: 55–60.

Volkov, A. G. & Ranatunga, R. D. (2006). Plants as Environmental Biosensors. Plant Signaling and Behavior 1: 105 - 115.

Volkov, A. G. & Brown, C. L. (2006). Electrochemistry of plant life. In: Plant Electrophysiology: Theory and Methods. A. G. Volkov Ed. ISBN: 978-3-540-32717-2

Volkov, A. G.; Lang, R. D. & Volkova-Gugeshashvili, M. I. (2007). Electrical signaling in Aloe vera induced by localized thermal stress- Bioelectrochemistry 71: 192–197.

Volkov, A. G.; Adesina, T.; Markin, V. & Jovanov, E. (2008). Kinetics and mechanism of Dionaea muscipula trap closing. Plant Physiology 146: 694–702.

Volkov, A. G.; Carrell, H, & Markin, V. S. (2009). Biologically closed electrical circuits in Venus Flytrap. Plant Physiology 149: 1661–1667.

Volkov, A. G.; Baker, K.; Foster, J. C.; Clemmons, J.; Jovanov, E, & Markin, V. S. (2011). Circadian variations in biologically closed electrochemical circuits in Aloe vera and Mimosa pudica. Bioelectrochemistry 81: 39-45.

Volkov, A. G.; Wooten, J. D.; Waite, A. J.; Brown, C. R. & Markin, V. S. (2011). Circadian rhythms in electrical circuits of *Clivia miniata.* J Plant Physiology. In press. doi:10.1016/j.jplph.2011.03.012

Wang, P.; Dong-Mei, Z.; Lian-Zhen, Li. & Dan-Dan, Li. (2009). What role does cell membrane surface potential play in ion-plant interactions. Plant Signaling and Behavior. 4: 42–43.

Wayne, R. (1993). Excitability in plant cells. American Scientist 81:140-151.

Wayne, R. (1994). The excitability of plant cells: with a special emphasis on Characea internode cells. Botanical Review 60: 265-367.

Wildon, D. C.; Thain, J, F.; Minchin, P. E.; Gubb, I. R.; Reilly, A. J.; Skipper, Y. D.; Doherty, H. M.; O'Donnell, J. P. & Bowles, D. J. (1992). Electrical signalling and systemic proteinase inhibitor induction in the wounded plant. Nature 360: 62–65.

Wilkinson, S. & Hartung, W. (2009). Food production: reducing water consumption by manipulating long-distance chemical signaling in plants. J Experimental Botany 60: 1885–1891.

Zimmermann, S.; Nürnberger, T.; Frachisse, J. M.; Wirtz, W.; Guern, J.; Hedrich, R. & Scheel, D. (1997). Receptor-mediated activation of a plant $Ca^{+2}$-permeable ion channel involved in pathogen defense. Proc. National Academy Science USA 94: 2751–2755.

Zimmermann, M. R.; Maischak, H.; Mithofer, A.; Boland, W. & Felle, H. (2009). System potentials, a novel electrical long-distance apoplastic signal in plants, induced by wounding. Plant Physiology 149: 1593–1600.

2

# Pacemaker Currents in Dopaminergic Neurones of the Mice Olfactory Bulb

Angela Pignatelli, Cristina Gambardella,
Mirta Borin, Alex Fogli Iseppe and Ottorino Belluzzi
*Università di Ferrara, Dip. Biologia ed Evoluzione,*
*Sezione di Fisiologia & Biofisica – Centro di Neuroscienze,*
*Ferrara*
*Italy*

## 1. Introduction

In the olfactory bulb (OB) dopaminergic (DA) neurones constitute a fraction of the cells occupying the most external (glomerular) layer (Halász et al.1977). In this region, populated by three types of interneurons, periglomerular (PG) cells, short-axon cells and external tufted (ET) cells (Halász1990) - often collectively referred to as juxtaglomerular cells - an estimated 10% of the neurones in adulthood are positive for tyrosine hydroxylase (TH) (McLean and Shipley1988; Kratskin and Belluzzi2003), the rate limiting enzyme for dopamine synthesis. Dopaminergic neurones in the glomerular layer include PG cells (Gall et al.1987; Kosaka et al.1985) and a fraction of ET cells (Halász1990). Several studies have focused on the role of dopamine in the olfactory bulb, using immunohistochemical (Baker et al.1983; Guthrie et al.1991), behavioral (Doty and Risser1989), and electrophysiological techniques (Nowycky et al.1983; Ennis et al.2001; Davila et al.2003). The more complete description of the functional properties of DA neurons in the OB is probably the paper of Pignatelli (Pignatelli et al.2005), but it was incomplete, as it did not consider the contribution of the inward rectifier currents, a lacuna which is filled in the present work.

A property shared by many DA neurons in the CNS is their capacity to generate rhythmic action potentials even in the absence of synaptic inputs (Grace and Onn1989; Hainsworth et al.1991; Yung et al.1991; Feigenspan et al.1998; Neuhoff et al.2002). In this paper we show for the first time that DA cells in the glomerular layer of the olfactory bulb possess a pacemaker activity, and we provide an explanation for the ionic basis of rhythm generation in these cells.

There is an additional reason to study the functional properties of DA neurones in the OB other than their role in olfaction. The olfactory bulb is one of the rare regions of the mammalian CNS in which new cells, derived from stem cells in the anterior subventricular zone, are also added in adulthood (Gross2000). In the OB, these cells differentiate in interneurones in the granular and glomerular layers. Among these cells there are DA neurones (Betarbet et al.1996; Baker et al.2001), and this has raised a remarkable interest because, for their accessibility, they could provide a convenient source of autologous DA neurons for transplant therapies in neurodegenerative diseases, like Parkinson's disease.

## 2. Results

### 2.1 Localisation and general properties of TH-GFP cells

Generation of transgenic mice (TH-GFP/21-31) was described in previous papers (Sawamoto et al.2001; Matsushita et al.2002). The transgene construct contained the 9.0-kb 5'-flanking region of the rat tyrosine hydroxylase (TH) gene, the second intron of the rabbit β-globin gene, cDNA encoding green fluorescent protein (GFP), and polyadenylation signals of the rabbit β-globin and simian virus 40 early genes.

Cells expressing the GFP transgene under the TH promoter (TH-GFP) occurred primarily in the glomerular layer of the main olfactory bulb (Fig. 1A,B). The intraglomerular processes of these cells displayed high levels of TH-GFP expression, and their intertwine delimitates the glomeruli, with the soma of GFP+ cells laying around them.

Recordings with the patch-clamp technique in the whole-cell configuration were obtained from 368 DA cells in the glomerular layer following the procedures described in Pignatelli et al., 2005.

Cell dimensions were rather variable, as shown in Fig. 1C. Previous studies have suggested that there are two populations of DA neurones in the adult OB, based on size or location (Halász1990; Baker et al.1983). In fact, the distribution of the mean cell diameter of GFP+ cells could be best fitted with two Gaussian curves, identifying two subpopulations with average sizes of 5.67 ± 0.96 µm and 9.48 ± 2.39 µm ($R^2$ = 0.991); the same result could be obtained from the analysis of the membrane capacitances, whose frequency distribution could be best fitted by two Gaussians (5.41 ± 1.5 pF and 10.63 ± 3.45 pF, $R^2$ = 0.975, not shown). However, we found no significant differences in the properties of the two populations.

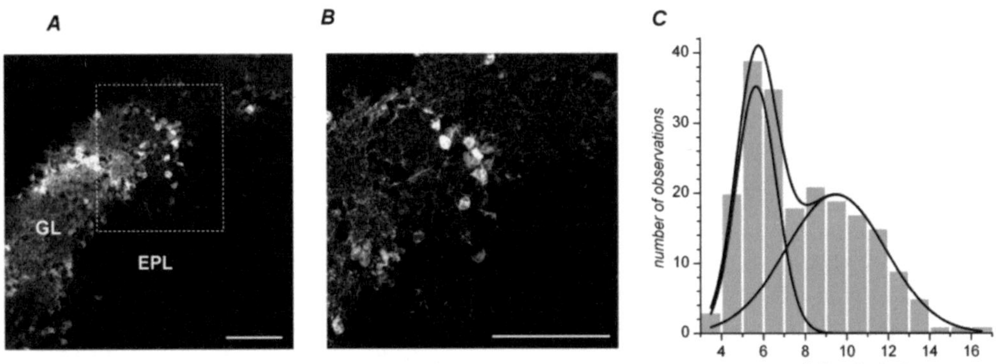


Fig. 1. Morphological properties of TH-GFP cells. A, B - Expression pattern of the TH-GFP transgene in the glomerular layer of the main olfactory bulb in a coronal section. Scale bar 50 µm. C - Frequency distribution of the soma diameter of the cells used in this study. The distribution could be best fitted by two Gaussian curves, identifying two distinct subpopulations of cells.

About 80% of DA neurones were spontaneously active. In the cell-attached configuration, action currents were recorded across the patch, usually structured in a regular, rhythmic pattern (Fig. 2A) with an average frequency of 7.30 ± 1.35 Hz (n = 31).

After disruption, about 60% of the cells continued to fire spontaneous action potentials under current-clamp condition (Fig. 2B) without any significant alteration of the firing frequency (7.84 $\pm$ 2.44 Hz, n = 14). Interspike intervals were rather constant in most of the cells (Fig. 2C), and irregular in others for the presence of sporadic misses. Occasionally, especially in isolated cells (see below), the firing was structured in bursts. We found no correlation of the firing frequency with cell size.

This spontaneous activity was completely blocked by TTX (0.3 μM) or by $Cd^+$ (100 μM), but persisted after block of glutamatergic and GABAergic synaptic transmission with kynurenate 1 mM and bicuculline (10 μM), suggesting that it was due to intrinsic properties of the cell membrane and was not driven by external synaptic inputs, as it resulted even more obviously by the observation that spontaneous activity was maintained also in dissociated cells (Fig. 2D).

Occasionally we did observe spontaneous synaptic currents, which were completely blocked by a mixture of 1 mM kynurenate and 10 μM bicuculline (not shown), and which were not further investigated for the purpose of this study.

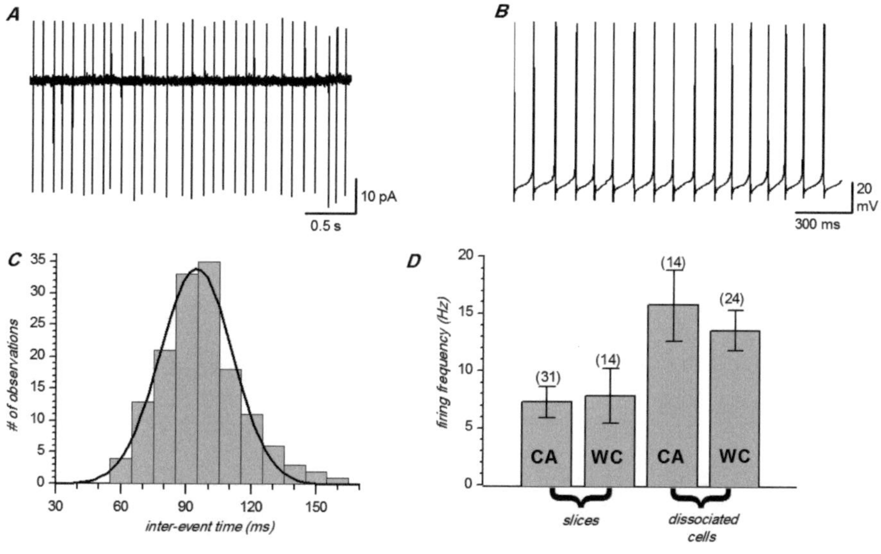


Fig. 2. Spontaneous activity in DA neurones in thin slices. A - Action currents in cell-attached mode B - Action potentials in whole-cell mode C - Frequency distribution of the inter-event time for the cell shown in panel B. D - Frequency of spontaneous firing in TH-GFP cells under the indicated experimental conditions. CA cell attached, WC whole cell.

We studied the dopaminergic neurones under current- and voltage-clamp conditions to characterise the ionic currents underlying spontaneous firing. In voltage-clamped neurones, currents were elicited both by step and ramp depolarisations.

Depolarisation activates a complicated pattern of current flow, in which a variety of conductances coexist, the most prominent of which were a fast transient sodium current and a non-inactivating potassium current (Fig. 3A, B). We identified specific ionic currents present in the cells by measurements of their voltage-dependence and kinetics during step depolarisations, together with ionic substitution and blocking agents to isolate individual components of the currents. After block of the potassium currents, obtained by adding 20 mM TEA in the perfusing solution and by equimolar substitution of internal $K^+$ ions with $Cs^+$, a persistent inward current was observed after the fast transient inward current had completely subsided (Fig 3C, D). The amplitude of this persistent component, measured as the average of the current amplitude during the last 10 ms of the depolarising step, had a maximum amplitude of 223.3 $\pm$ 32.2 pA (n=21) at -20 mV, and could be separated in two components, sustained by sodium and calcium ions (see below).

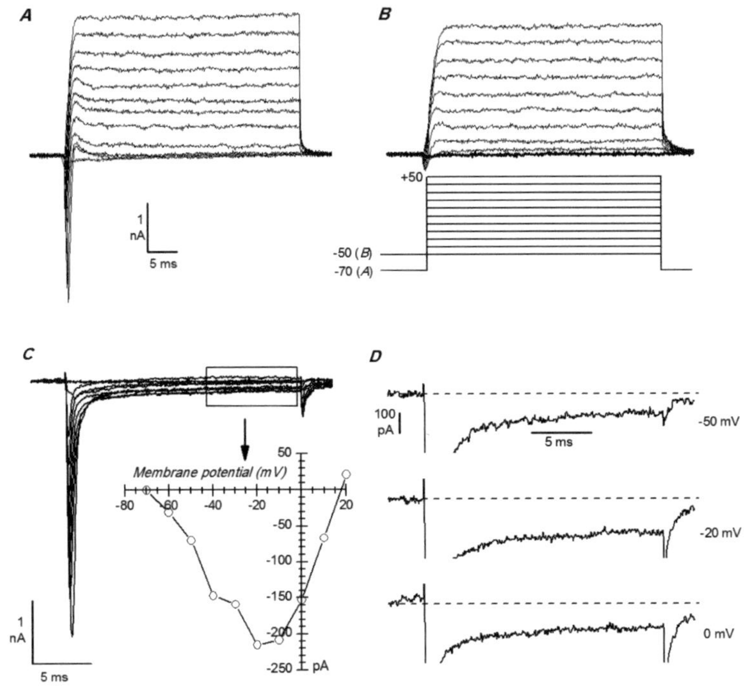


Fig. 3. Responses of DA neurones (PG cells) in thin slices to depolarising voltage steps under different conditions. A, B – Voltage-clamp recordings from the same cell, in normal saline, held at -70 mV (A) and at -50 mV (B), and depolarised to potentials ranging from -50 to +50 mV. C – Inward currents recorded under voltage-clamp conditions in response to depolarising steps ranging from -80 to +50 mV; holding potential was -100 mV. Potassium currents were suppressed by ionic substitution of intracellular $K^+$ ions with $Cs^+$, and addition of 20 mM TEA in the extracellular medium. The inset shows the current-voltage relationship of the persistent inward current, averaged at the times indicated by the box. D – Details of some of the traces shown in panel C, at higher magnification, to show the persistent inward current.

### 2.2 Fast transient Na current

The elimination of the concomitant currents was obtained by blocking the $Ca^{2+}$ current with 100 μM $Cd^+$, and by equimolar substitution of intracellular $K^+$ with $Cs^+$ or NMDG; in addition, the $K^+$ channels were blocked by adding 20 mM TEA in the perfusing solution (and occasionally also in the intracellular solution to complete the blockade). Under these conditions, depolarising voltage steps to potentials positive to -60 mV evoked a large, transient inward current, peaking in 0.4 ms at 0 mV which reached its maximum amplitude for steps near -30 mV (Fig. 4A). Its sensitivity to TTX (0.3 μM) at all voltages, and its abolition following removal of sodium ions from the perfusing medium indicate that it is a classical Na-current.

Although it was not always possible to exert an accurate control of membrane potential during the transient sodium current in DA cells in slice preparations (presumably because of currents generated at a distance from the soma on the axon or dendrites), an adequate space clamp and series resistance compensation could be achieved in 7 neurones in which we could obtain a complete series of recordings with and without TTX. The kinetic characterisation of the fast transient Na-current showed in Fig. 4 (and on which is based the numerical reconstruction of this current presented below), was carried out in a homogeneous group of 12 dissociated neurones, averaging 4.5 $\pm$ 0.12 pF, which were electrotonically compact and thus allowed for a more precise space clamp. The results were similar in the two cases, with I/V relationships showing a slightly larger maximum inward current in slices (3784 $\pm$ 369 pA, n=7) than in dissociated cells (3219 $\pm$ 223 pA, n=12), but with the same overall voltage dependence and kinetics.

The peak $I_{Na(F)}$ I-V relationship for a group of twelve dissociated neurones over a range of voltage pulses extending from -80 to +40 mV is shown in Fig. 4B. Reversal potentials for $I_{Na(F)}$ could not be measured directly in our experiments because of uncertainties regarding leakage correction in the presence of large non-specific outward currents. The Na equilibrium potential, evaluated indirectly from the positive limb of the I-V plot (Fig. 4B), is close to +40 mV, about 20 mV more negative than the value predicted by the Nernst equation for a pure Na potential.

The activation process is illustrated in Fig. 4 A-C and G. The fast Na-current develops following a third-order exponential; the activation time constant, $\tau_m$, studied in the -60 to +30 mV range, was computed from the least squares fit of a cubic exponential to the rising phase of the Na-current. In some cases the activation time constant was computed using the method proposed by Bonifazzi et al. (Bonifazzi et al.1988), allowing for the determination of $\tau_m$ from the time-to-peak ($t_p$) and the decay time constant, and consisting in the solution of the equation $t_p = \tau_m \ln(1+n \cdot \tau_h/\tau_m)$, where n is the order of the activation kinetics. Na-channels activate rapidly, with time constants extending from 0.66 to 0.14 ms in the -60 to +10 mV range. The continuous function describing the dependence of $\tau_m$ upon voltage in the range studied, is indicated in the legend of figure 4.

The open channel current as a function of voltage was obtained in a 12 neurones sample from the extrapolation at the time zero of the decaying phase of the current. From the obtained values, the open-channel Na conductance, $g_{Na(F)}$, was calculated using the equation $g_{Na(F)}(V) = I_{Na0}(V)/(V- E_{Na})$, where V is the membrane potential, $E_{Na}$ the sodium equilibrium potential and $I_{Na0}$ is the extrapolation at the zero time of the Na-current.

The conductance-voltage relationship, $g_{Na(F)}(V)$, was described by the Boltzmann equation exhibiting a threshold at about -60 mV, with a slope of 4.34 mV, midpoint at -39.9 mV and a maximum conductance $g_{Na(F)max}$ of 101 nS at -20 mV (Fig. 4C). Finally, the voltage-dependence of the steady-state activation parameter, $m_\infty$, was computed by extracting the

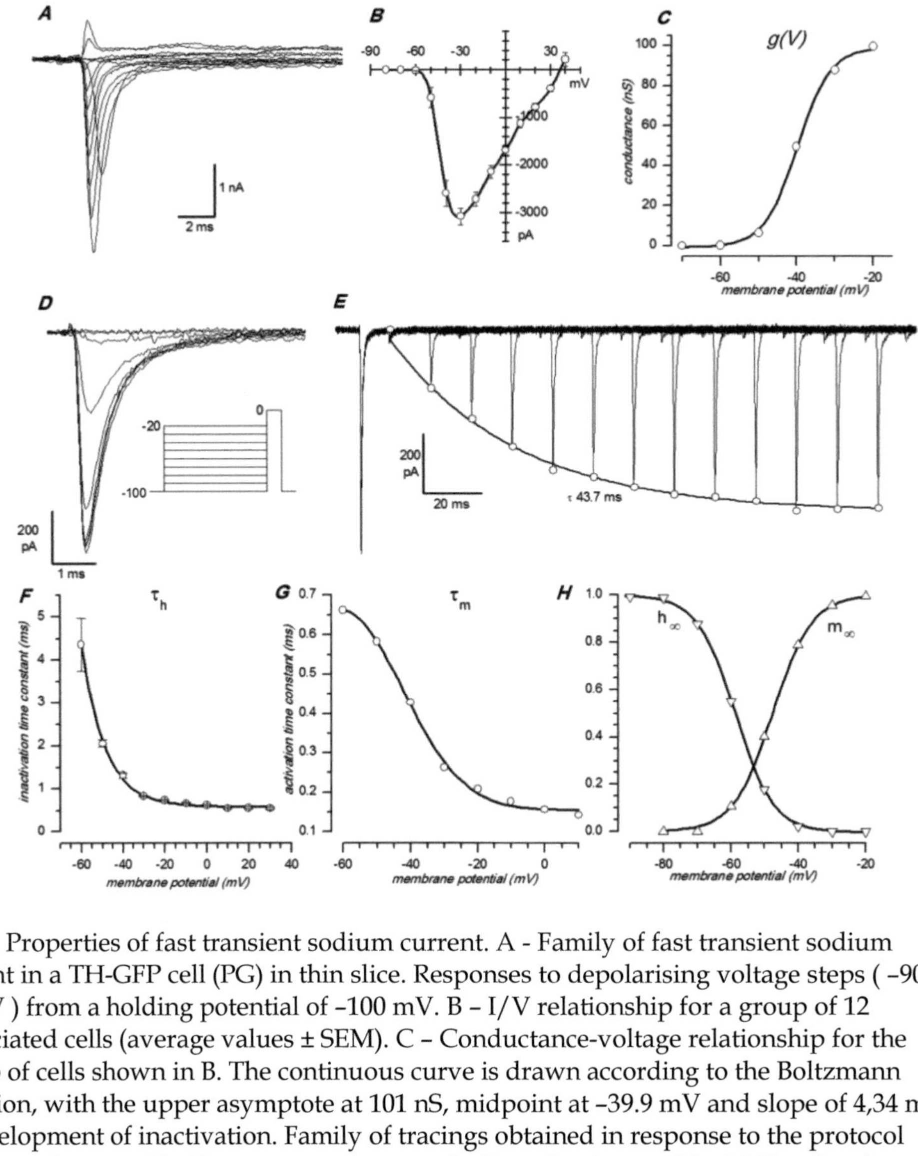


Fig. 4. Properties of fast transient sodium current. A - Family of fast transient sodium current in a TH-GFP cell (PG) in thin slice. Responses to depolarising voltage steps ( –90 to + 50 mV ) from a holding potential of –100 mV. B – I/V relationship for a group of 12 dissociated cells (average values ± SEM). C – Conductance-voltage relationship for the group of cells shown in B. The continuous curve is drawn according to the Boltzmann equation, with the upper asymptote at 101 nS, midpoint at –39.9 mV and slope of 4,34 mV. D - Development of inactivation. Family of tracings obtained in response to the protocol shown in the inset. E – Time course of removal of inactivation at –80 mV. Family of tracings obtained with a double-pulse protocol, consisting in two subsequent steps to –20 mV, the first from a holding potential of –100 mV, the second after a variable time at –80 mV. F – Voltage-dependence of inactivation time constant, measured from the decay of the current. The continuous curve, describing $\tau_h$ in the -60/+30 mV range, obeys the equation: $\tau_h(V) = .58 + .019 * \exp(-V / 11.3)$. G – Voltage-dependence of activation time constant, calculated as explained in the text in a 12 neurone sample. The continuous curve, describing $\tau_m$ in the –60/+10 mV range, obeys the equation: $\tau_m(V) = 0.155 + (23.2 / (36.4 * \sqrt{(\pi /2)})) * \exp(-2*((V+60.62) /36.4)^2)$ H – Steady-state values of activation and inactivation variables (m and h) of the fast sodium current. The continuous curves obey the equations: $m_\infty(V) = 1/(1+\exp((-47.6-V)/5.8))$, $h_\infty(V) = 1/(1+\exp((V+58.7)/4.5))$.

cubic root from the ratio $g_{Na}(V)$ / $g_{Na(F)max}$ (Fig 4H, upward triangles). The steady-state activation, $m_\infty(V)$, had a midpoint at -47.64 mV and a slope of 5.8 mV.

The steady-state voltage dependence of fast Na inactivation, $h_\infty$, was studied by evaluating the non-inactivated fraction of the Na current as a function of membrane potential (Hodgkin and Huxley1952)(Fig. 4D). The protocol used is illustrated in the inset of the same figure. $I_{Na(F)}$ was measured in each experiment at a constant test voltage of 0 mV after 200 ms preconditioning pulses to various potentials, and plotted after normalisation to the maximum current evoked with hyperpolarisation.

The 200 ms pre-pulse was sufficient to allow the inactivation variable to reach its steady-state value (see Fig. 4E). The steady-state inactivation curve $h_\infty(V)$ thus obtained from a twelve-neurone sample, shows a sigmoidal dependence on voltage which can be fitted by the equation: $h_\infty(V) = (1+\exp[(V-V_h)/k])^{-1}$, where $V_h$ (midpoint) is -58.7 mV and k (slope) is 4.5 mV (Fig. 4H, downward triangles). It should be noted that the inactivating fraction of $I_{Na(F)}$ falls virtually to zero at -30 mV, which is the potential at which $I_{Na(P)}$ reaches its maximum amplitude (Fig. 4B).

Fast sodium channels inactivate rapidly. The decay phase of the current, studied in the -60 to +30 mV range, could be adequately fitted with a single exponential. The continuous function describing the voltage-dependence of inactivation time constant, $\tau_h$, illustrated in Fig. 4F for a ten-neurone sample, can be approximated by the equation indicated in the figure, and has values spanning from 4.4 and 0.6 ms in the voltage range considered.

The rate of recovery from inactivation, was measured using the double-pulse protocol. Na-channel inactivation is removed over a course of a few tens of milliseconds, and the process is markedly voltage-dependent. This is illustrated in Fig. 4E for a typical neurone. The cell was maintained in normal saline at a holding potential of -100 mV, and stepped to -20 mV for 10 ms ($\tau_h$ is 0.74 ms at this potential). $I_{Na(F)}$ was then allowed to recover by applying a hyperpolarising pre-pulse of variable duration at different potentials.

Recovery was evaluated by measuring $I_{Na(F)}$ during a second test pulse to -20 mV. In Fig. 4E, a family of $I_{Na(F)}$ currents is shown for the conditioning potential of -80 mV. The current peak as a function of the conditioning pulse duration could be fitted by a simple exponential with a mean value of 42.1 $\pm$ 8.9 ms (n = 14) at -80 mV.

### 2.3 Delayed rectifier potassium current

A delayed rectifier-type potassium current was present in TH-GFP cells (e.g. Fig. 3B), and it has been kinetically characterised (Fig. 5). The current, isolated by blocking the sodium current with TTX, was calcium-dependent only for a small part (at 0 mV the fraction suppressed by $Cd^+$ 100 μM was about 10%), and thus it has been modelled as a single component. The equations describing the time- and voltage-dependence of the potassium current are shown in Fig. 5 and detailed in the relative legend.

### 2.4 Persistent sodium current

In DA cells, after the fast transient Na-current had completely subsided, a persistent inward current showing no sign of inactivation after 200 ms was observed.

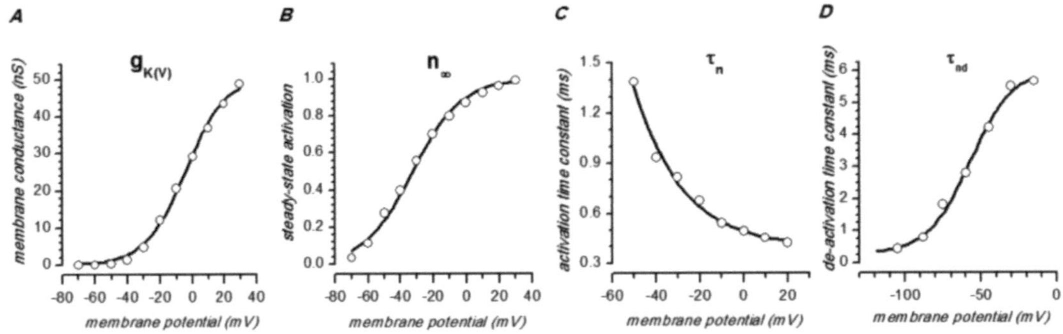


Fig. 5. Properties of delayed rectifier potassium current. A - Conductance-voltage relationship. The continuous curve is drawn according to the Boltzmann equation, with the upper asymptote (maximum conductance) at 50.5 nS, midpoint at -4.1 mV and slope of 12.5 mV. B - Steady-state values of activation (*n*) for the potassium current, obtained from the fourth root of the data shown in *A* after normalisation. The continuous curve obey the equations: $n_\infty(V) = 1/(1+\exp[(-32.2-V)/14.9])$. C - Voltage-dependence of activation time constant ($\tau_n$), obtained by fitting a fourth-order exponential to the rising phase of the current. The continuous curve obeys the equation: $\tau_n(V) = .42 + .097 * \exp(-V / 21.67)$. D - Voltage-dependence of de-activation time constant ($\tau_{nd}$). The continuous curve, describing $\tau_{nd}$ in the -105/-15 mV range, obeys the equation: $\tau_{nd} = 6.1 - 5.88/(1+\exp((V+57.6)/14.75))$. This parameter was calculated from the tail currents, independently from $\tau_n$.

We first applied TTX (0.3 to 1.2 μM), which did suppress a significant fraction of the persistent inward current, indicating it received a contribution from a non-inactivating, TTX-sensitive channels. This current-voltage relationship was virtually coincident with the residual persistent current measured after treatment with $Cd^{2+}$ 100 μM (see below), and therefore the data were pooled together. The current-voltage relationship of the fraction of current abolished by TTX or remaining after $Cd^{2+}$ treatment is shown in Fig. 6A.

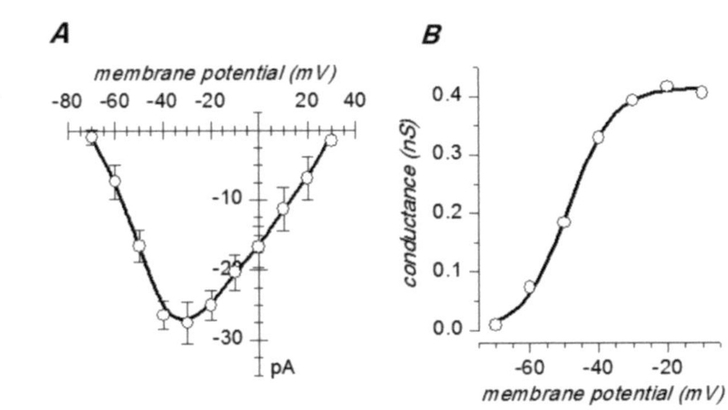


Fig. 6. Properties of persistent sodium current. A - I/V relationship. Pooled data obtained as fraction of non-inactivating current suppressed by TTX (n=12) and residual persistent current after $Cd^{2+}$ block (n=6). B - Conductance-voltage relationship of persistent sodium current, obtained from the average data shown in A. The continuous curve is the Boltzmann fit, with upper asymptote of 0.41 nS, midpoint at -48.8 mV and slope of 6.51 mV.

The persistent sodium current, $I_{Na(P)}$, was activated at potentials more negative than -70 mV, and reached a maximum amplitude of -27.5 $\pm$ 2.97 pA at -30 mV. The corresponding conductance-voltage relationship, calculated by dividing the current amplitude by the sodium driving force, could be fitted by a Boltzmann equation with a midpoint at -48.8 mV and a slope of 6.51 mV (Fig 6B). The maximum value of $g_{Na(P)}$ conductance was 0.41 nS, about 200 times smaller than that of the fast sodium current ($I_{Na(F)}$, see below), but contrary to the latter, this current is activated in the pacemaker range, showing an amplitude of -7.3 pA at -60 mV.

## 2.5 Calcium currents

After block of the TTX-sensitive component and suppression of the K-current by equimolar substitution of intracellular $K^+$ with $Cs^+$, a persistent inward current could be observed at the end of prolonged depolarising steps (Fig. 7A, upper trace). This residual fraction could be almost completely blocked by $Cd^{2+}$ or $Co^{2+}$ ions (Fig. 7A, lower traces), suggesting that this second component was sustained by calcium ions. The very small fraction of current remaining after TTX and $Cd^{2+}$ block has not been further investigated in the present study.

Using classical pharmacological tools, ionic substitutions and voltage-clamp protocols, we could dissect the voltage-dependent Ca currents, $Ca_v$, into several components.

The larger of these components, by its overall kinetics, its voltage-dependence and the absence of inactivation was identified as a possible L-type Ca-current. Its properties were studied in slices, after blockage of the Na-currents with 0.3 – 1.2 μM TTX and of the K-currents by equimolar substitution with $Cs^+$ in the pipette-filling solution and 20 mM TEA in the perfusing bath. The protocols used were either voltage steps or voltage ramps, giving virtually identical results. The I/V relationship of the Ca-current (Fig 7C), measured in a 10 neurones sample averaging the last 5 ms at the end of a 40 ms depolarising step, had a maximum amplitude of –108.7 ± 11.9 pA at –10 mV. The corresponding conductance-voltage relationship showed a maximum conductance of 2.3 nS, with a midpoint at -25.6 mV.

Equimolar substitution of $Ca^{2+}$ with $Ba^{2+}$ increased by a factor of about 3 the amplitude of this current (Fig. 7C), without changing the I/V relationship or the time constant of activation. On this current we tested the effects of two blockers of L-type calcium channels, nifedipine and calcicludine. The fraction of current blocked by the two drugs at different voltages was quantified by subtraction of I-V data acquired before and after treatment.

The effects of 10 μM nifedipine on peak $Ca^{2+}$ current amplitude was assessed in 6 PG cells (Fig. 7E and F). On average, the drug blocked 61.1 $\pm$ 14 % of the current measured at the point of its maximum amplitude (–10 mV).

A 60 aminoacid peptide isolated from the venom of the green mamba (*Dendroaspis augusticeps*), calcicludine (CaC) has been described to have a powerful effect on all type of high-voltage-activated Ca-channels (L-, N-, and P-type) (Schweitz et al.1994). Since one of the regions of the CNS presenting the highest densities of $^{125}$I-labeled CaC binding sites is the glomerular layer of the olfactory bulb (Schweitz et al.1994), we tested the ability of this toxin in suppressing the non-inactivating Ca-current found in the DA neurones. CaC (1 μM) was much more effective than nifedipine, with an inhibitory action averaging 72.7 $\pm$ 3.13 %.

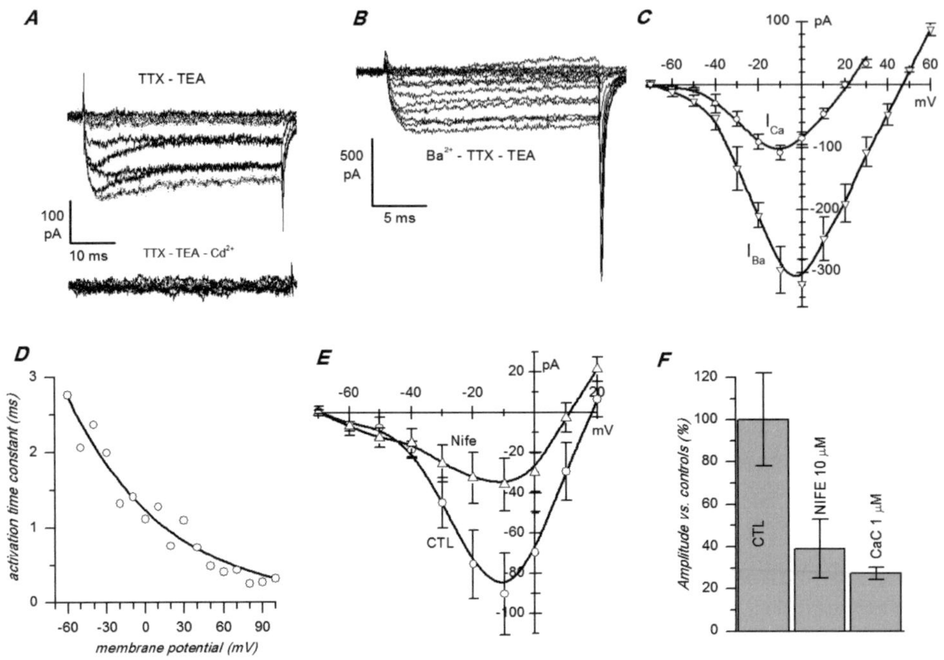


Fig. 7. Properties of HVA calcium currents. A – Calcium current recorded in response to depolarising voltage steps to potentials ranging from –70 to +50 mV from a holding potential of –100 mV. Above: tracings recorded in the presence of 1.2 μM TTX, 20 mM TEA in the extracellular solution, and with $Cs^+$ as a substitute for $K^+$ ions in the intracellular solution. Lower tracings were recorded in the same conditions after addition of 100 μM $Cd^{2+}$. B – Barium currents recorded in the same conditions described for A. C – I/V relationship of Ca and Ba currents in a 10 neurones sample from thin slices. D – Activation time constant, measured in a 10 neurones sample by fitting a single exponential to the rising phase of the current. The continuous line is described by the equation: $\tau_{Ca(L)} = 1.23 + \exp(-V/74.6)$. E – Effect of 10 μM nifedipine on calcium current in a group of six TH-GFP PG cells in slices. F - Histogram showing the effect of nifedipine (10 μM, cells shown in E) and calcicludine (1 μM, not shown, n=7) measured at –10 mV.

We also tried to define if other types of HVA neuronal $Ca_v$ channels (P/Q-, N-) were present in TH-GFP cells. Using classical blockers, like ω-conotoxin GVIA (0.82 μM) that blocks the N-type, or spider toxin ω-agatoxin IVA (10 nM) that blocks P/Q-type channels, we observed the suppression of a fraction of HVA Ca-current remaining after nifedipine block (at –10 mV 38% and 42%, respectively, not shown), suggesting the presence of limited amounts of the corresponding HVA Ca-channels.

Since the long-lasting HVA $Ca_v$ currents were not directly involved in the pacemaker process (see below), and for the dominance of L- over N- and P/Q-type current, for the purpose of the numerical reconstruction of the electrical activity of these cells (see below), they were kinetically modelled as a unique, non inactivating component. The rising phase of the current was fitted by a single exponential, with a time constant of 1.2 + 0.3 ms at 0 mV (n=10, see legend of figure 7D for further details).

Since *in situ* hybridisation experiments have localised the expression of two transcripts (α1G and α1I) of the T-type calcium channel in the glomerular layer of the olfactory bulb (Talley et al.1999; Klugbauer et al.1999), we checked for the presence of LVA Ca-current. Unfortunately several characteristics of these channels hampered their study in our preparation. First, contrary to the cardiac cells or transfected cells, in TH-GFP interneurones this current is small: we have calculated a maximum conductance of 0.35 nS, corresponding to a peak current of about 20 pA at -35 mV. The problem was further complicated by the fact that on one hand it was difficult to get accurate space clamping in slices, and on the other hand, in isolated cell preparations the current was difficult to resolve, probably because of the preferential localisation of these channels on the dendrites (Perez-Reyes2003). Second, the conductance of these channels cannot be significantly increased by substitution of $Ca^{2+}$ with $Ba^{2+}$ ions, as it can be done with HVA channels. Third, there are no effective pharmacological tools for the study of T-type Ca-channels, because they are relatively resistant to most organic calcium channel blockers, such as dihydropyridines, that block the L-type, or peptide toxins, such as ω-conotoxin or ω-agatoxin.

Despite these difficulties, we succeeded in isolating a T-type calcium current in dissociated cells (Fig. 8). The protocol used was a rapid ramp (7 V/s) from -100 to 40 mV, in the presence of TTX (1 μM) and after substitution of $Ca^{2+}$ with $Sr^{2+}$, which in known to have a slightly higher permeability than $Ca^{2+}$ in T-type Ca-channels (Takahashi et al.1991). Under these conditions, an inward inflection peaking at about -40 mV, distinct from the peak due to the L-type Ca-channels (Fig. 8A), could be seen. Nickel is a nonselective inhibitor of calcium channels, but transient low voltage-activated (LVA) T-type (Perchenet et al.2000; Wolfart and Roeper2002) Ca-channels are particularly sensitive ($IC_{50}$ < 50 μM; (Perez-Reyes et al.1998) whereas other HVA $Ca_v$ channels (L-, P/Q, and N-type) are less sensitive ($IC_{50}$ > 90 μM; (Zhang et al.1993; Randall1998). In fact Nickel did selectively eliminate the first peak, leaving the second unaltered. The difference, averaged in three cells, is shown in figure 8B, and the conductance, calculated assuming a $Ca^{2+}$ equilibrium potential of 45 mV, is illustrated in figure 8C. The current activates at potentials positive to -65 mV and peaks at about -35 mV, with a maximum conductance of 0.35 nS. The point of half activation is -45.3 mV, which is in line with the known values for this current (Perez-Reyes2003).

### 2.6 h-current

A likely candidate for the pacemaking process was the inward rectifier current ($I_h$). In a previous work (Pignatelli et al.2005), analysing the excitability profile of DA PG cells, we failed to detect any significant component activated by hyperpolarization (Fig. 9A). It was therefore with some disconcert that we observed that a drug blocking the h-current (ivabradine, 10 μM) did block the spontaneous activity (see below). We then switched to ionic settings known to enhance the amplitude of the h-current, i.e. high $[K^+]_o$, using an external saline where $[K^+]_o$ was 32.5 instead of 2.5 mM. In these conditions, we observed a measurable current activated by hyperpolarization (Fig. 9B), which could be separated in a classical inward rectifier (KIR) and a typical h-current (Fig. 9C). The h-current was suppressed by ivabradina 10 μM, ZD7288 30 μM and $Cs^+$ 1 mM (Fig. 9D).

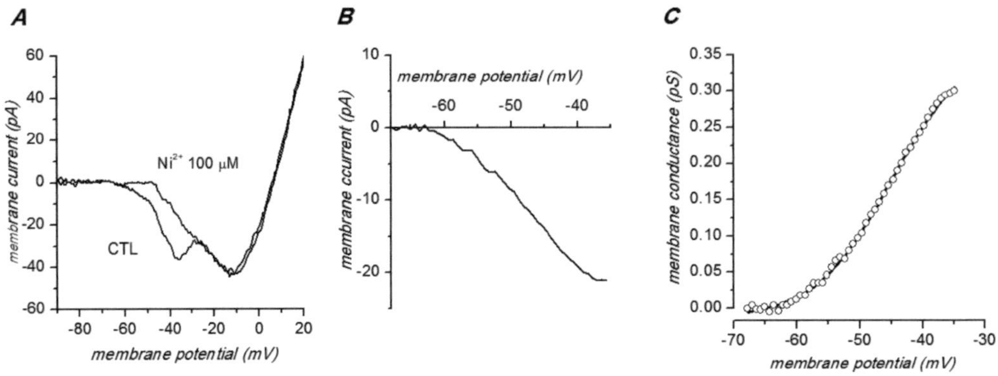


Fig. 8. Properties of the LVA calcium current. A – Voltage-clamp ramps were performed from –80 to +40 mV at a speed of 7 V/s in the presence of TTX (1 µM), and after substitution of $Sr^{2+}$ for $Ca^{2+}$; the traces were corrected for leakage. Under these conditions, a distinct bump can be seen preceding the HVA calcium current (here peaking at –10 mV), which is selectively suppressed by $Ni^{2+}$ 100 µM. B - Transient Ca-current generated using the protocol described in A calculated by subtracting the current-voltage curves in control and in the presence of 100 µM $Ni^{2+}$. The low-$Ni^{2+}$ sensitive current (average from three cells) is activated at membrane potentials more positive than –60 mV. C – Conductance-voltage relationship of the low-$Ni^{2+}$ sensitive current. The continuous line is a Boltzmann fit, with a midpoint at –45.3 mV and a maximum conductance of 0.35 nS. All recordings in this figure were performed from spontaneously bursting dissociated TH-GFP cells.

$I_h$ was evoked by a family of seven hyperpolarizing voltage steps (step amplitude -10 mV; step duration 3 s) from the holding potential of -40 to - 130 mV. The steps were applied in 7-s intervals. $I_h$ was calculated as the difference between the membrane current at the end of the voltage step ($I_{ss}$) and the instantaneous current ($I_{inst}$) measured after the settling of the capacitative transient. To determine $I_h$ voltage dependence, activation curves were constructed from $I_h$ tail currents, which were calculated by subtracting the pre-step holding current from the peak of the tail current. The activation curves were fitted by the Boltzmann function to estimate the potential of half-activation ($V_{50}$ , -91 mV) and the slope factor ($k$, 5 mV).

$I_h$ time dependence was studied by fitting current traces (from -100 to -130 mV) with a single exponential function. The activation time constant gave values ranging from 361 ± 112 ms at -100 mV to 155 ± 23 ms at -130 mV (n=10).

The reversal potential, calculated from the reversal of the tail currents (not shown) was -47 mV, from which the maximal conductance could be calculated, giving a value of 1.37 nS.

### 2.7 KIR current

KIR 2.1 channel subunits are highly expressed in the olfactory bulb, with the higher density in the glomerular layer (Prüss et al.2005), and KIR conductances are found in many dopaminergic systems, as in nucleus accumbens (Perez et al.2006) and substantia nigra (Bausch et al.1995). Here we describe a KIR conductance in the dopaminergic neurones of the olfactory bulb.

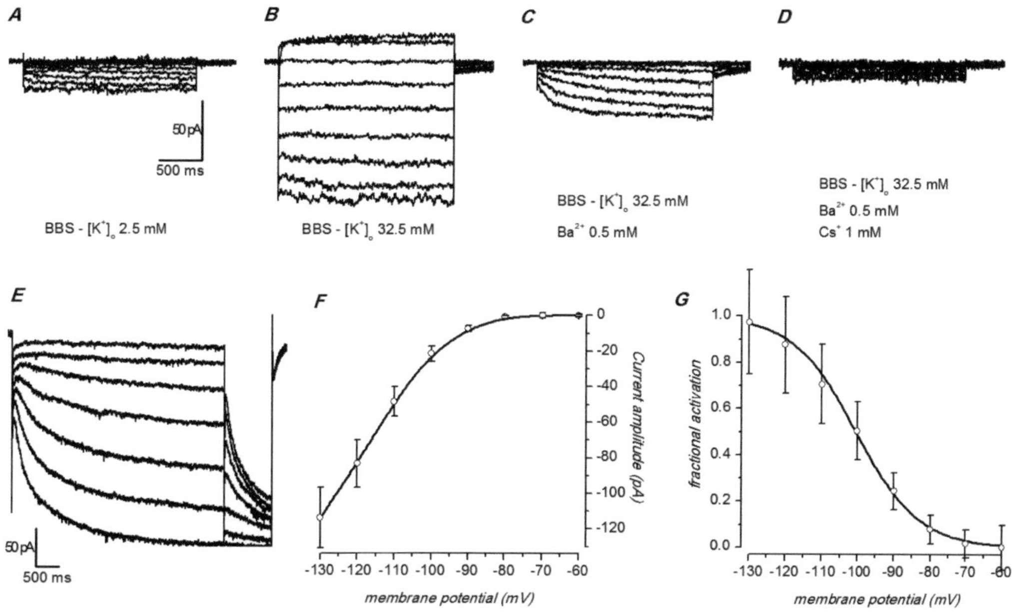


Fig. 9. Properties of the h-current. A,B – Currents activated by hyperpolarizing steps in normal saline and in high $K^+$, respectively. C – Currents activated by hyperpolarization in high $K^+$ and after blockage of the KIR component with $Ba^{2+}$ 0.5 mM. D – Same as C after addition of a blocker of the h-current ($Cs^+$ 1 mM) E – Representative current traces for the analysis of activation. The membrane was held at -40 mV, depolarised to test voltages from -60 to -130 mV in 10 mV increments. $I_h$ tails were elicited in response to a second pulse to −130 mV, following test voltages (see methods for explanation) F – I/V relationship of the h-current for a group of 15 cells. G – Fractional activation of the h-current as a function of voltage.

After block of the h-current with ivabradine 10 μMA, and using high concentration of $K^+$ in the external saline in order to enhance this KIR-current, a family of almost pure tracings could be evoked by hyperpolarising steps ranging from -50 to -130 mV in 10 mV increments, staring from a holding potential of -40 mV (Fig. 10A); the current could be rapidly and reversibly blocked by $Ba^{2+}$ 0.2 mM (Fig. 10B), and from the I/V curves (Fig. 10C) we calculated a reversal potential of -44 mV ($E_K$ -33 mV), giving conductance of 2 nS at the steady state.

### 2.8 Spontaneous activity

The presence of autorhythmic activity was the most salient feature of DA cells in the olfactory bulb, so the first efforts were aimed at elucidating the underlying mechanisms. We first tried to understand if the spontaneous activity was due to the presence of pacemaker currents or to synaptic mechanisms reverberating excitation from one cell to the other. Dissociated TH-GFP cells conserved their capacity of generating rhythmic activity, clearly indicating that this is an intrinsic property of these cells. Dissociated TH-GFP cells showed a spontaneous frequency of firing of 13.57 ± 1.79 (n=24) and 15.75 ± 3.12 (n=14) in whole-cell

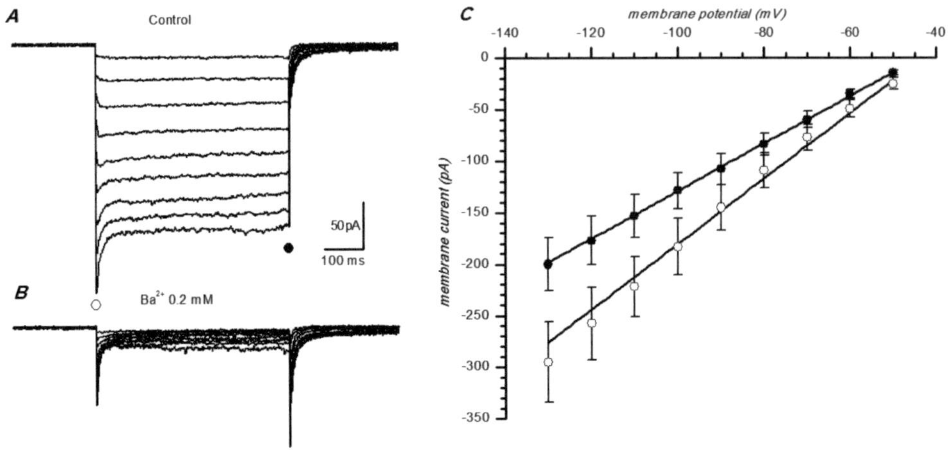


Fig. 10. Properties of the KIR current. A – Family of responses to hyperpolarizing steps from -50 to -130 mV in 10 mV increments from the holding potential of -40 mV. The h-current was blocked by ivabradine 10 μM, and the external saline was modified with high $K^+$ (32.5 mM) to enhance the KIR amplitude. B – Same as A, but with the addition of $Ba^{2+}$ 0.2 mM. C - I/V relationship of the KIR-current measured at the onset (open circle) and at the steady state (filled circle), at the time points marked in A by the relative symbols; average values ± SE from 11 cells. The reversal potential, calculated from the intercept of the x-axis, was -44 mV, not too far from the $E_K$, which was -33 mV.

and cell-attached modes respectively (Fig. 2D). This frequency was about double the corresponding value observed in thin slices, suggesting the existence in semi-intact tissue of some inhibitory control, possibly autoinhibition, which has not been further investigated in this study.

### 2.9 The pacemaker currents

We next tried to elucidate the ionic basis of the pacemaker current underlying the spontaneous firing.

The presence of the h-current, typically associated with the pacemaking process in a large number of autorhythmic cell (see (Wahl-Schott and Biel2009) for a review) has suggested that it could play its archetypal role also in bulbar DA neurons. The $I_h$ blockade with ivabradine did break the spontaneous activity, but this effect was associated to a prominent hyperpolarization (Fig. 11A). It was therefore necessary to clarify if this block was the demonstration of a direct role of the h-current in the pacemaker mechanism, or only a secondary effect, due to the hyperpolarization. If, in the presence of ivabradine block, the membrane was depolarised to the original resting potential, then the spontaneous activity resumed immediately (Fig. 11B), clearly showing that the h-current had no direct role in it.

We next analysed the role of the Ca-current. $Ca^{2+}$ is involved in the pacemaker process, as $Cd^{2+}$ 100 μM completely and reversibly blocked the spontaneous firing (Fig 12B). Then, using a panel of different $Ca_v$ channels inhibitors, we tried to define which types of neuronal $Ca_v$ channels (L-, P/Q-, N-, R-, and T-type) contributed to the pacemaker current.

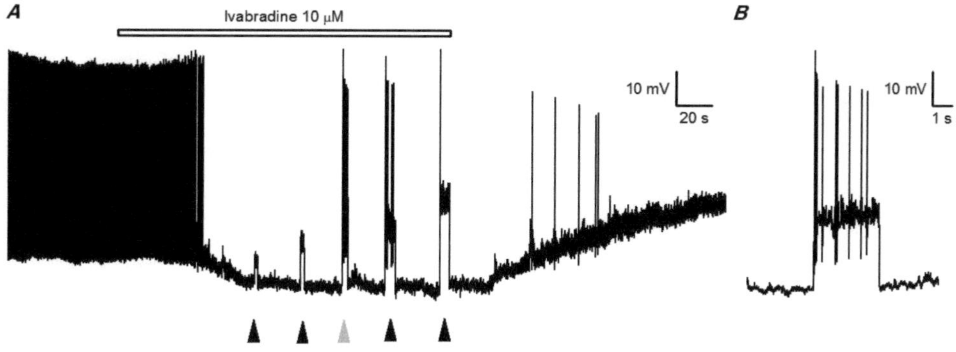


Fig. 11. Effect of blockers of h-channels on spontaneous firing. A – Ivabradine (10 μM, bar) block of spontaneous activity; note the large hyperpolarization. At the times indicated by arrowheads, depolarising currents of increasing amplitudes were delivered. B - Enlargement of the response to the third injection of depolarising current (grey arrowhead) to show that the block of the h-current does not impairs the spontaneous activity, provided that the membrane is brought back to resting values.

The classical selective L-type Ca-channel antagonist nifedipine (10 μM), which blocked the long-lasting Ca-current by about two thirds (Fig. 7E and F), had no effect at all in the spontaneous firing frequency, either in cell-attached mode (Fig. 12C) or in whole-cell configuration, in a total of 6 cells recorded in slices. Also calcicludine (1 μM), a powerful although less selective HVA channel blocker (Schweitz et al.1994), which inhibited the long-lasting Ca-channel component (73%, Fig. 7F), was equally ineffective, even after very long periods of application (Fig. 12E). Analogous results were obtained using other classical blockers of HVA Ca-channels, like ω-conotoxin GVIA (0.82 μM), which blocks the N-type, or spider toxin ω-agatoxin IVA (10 nM) which blocks P/Q-type channels. Both did suppress a fraction of the residual HVA Ca-current after nifedipine block (at –10 mV 38% and 42%, respectively), suggesting the presence of the corresponding types of HVA Ca-channels, but none of them affected the spontaneous firing (not shown).

Among the remaining candidates for a role in pacemaking was the LVA, T-type. Mibefradil, an anti-hypertensive drug, has been reported to inhibit T-type calcium channel current in cerebellar granule cells (Randall and Tsien1997), sensory neurones (Todorovic and Lingle1998) and spinal motor neurones (Viana et al.1997).

We therefore tried this drug, which proved to be considerably powerful in blocking the spontaneous activity of PG DA neurones, both in cell attached (Fig. 13A) and in whole-cell mode (Fig. 13B). Mibefradil (5 to 10 μM) completely and reversibly blocks the spontaneous activity, inducing an evident hyperpolarisation that on average amounted to about 15 mV (Fig. 13B). Nickel 100 μM, that we have shown to be a selective blocker of T-type calcium current in these cells (Fig. 8A), induced a reversible block of spontaneous firing, also accompanied by a hyperpolarisation of 10-15 mV (Fig. 13C), an effect almost superimposable to that observed with mibefradil, further confirming a role of $I_{Ca(T)}$ in the pacemaking process.

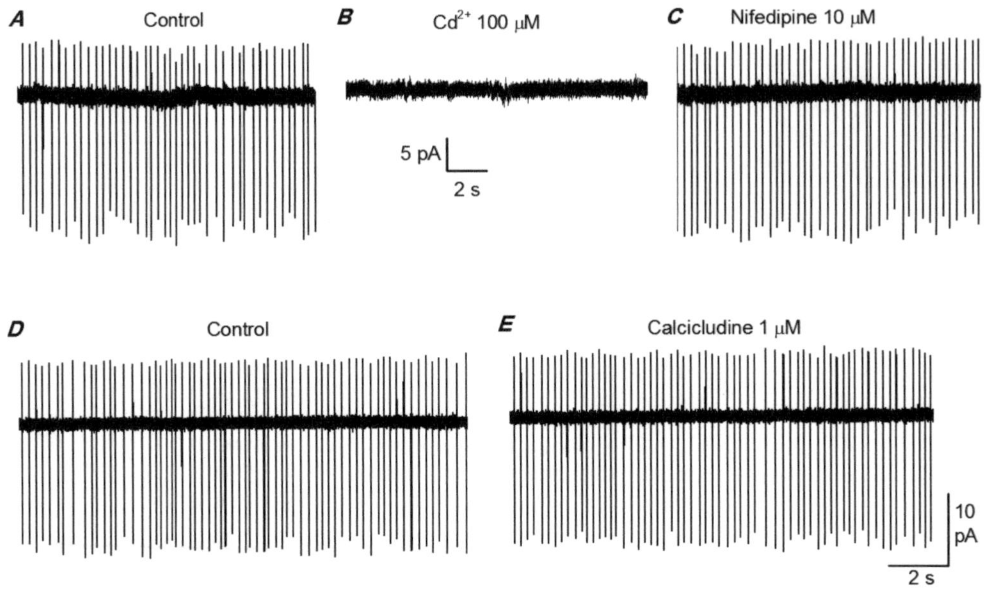


Fig. 12. Effect of blockers of HVA Ca-channels on spontaneous firing. A-B – Effect of the $Cd^{2+}$ (100 μM) on action currents recorded in cell attached mode. C – Effect of L-type Ca-channel antagonist, nifedipine (10 μM). D-E – Effect of L-type Ca-channel antagonist calcicludine (1 μM), recorded 15 min after application.

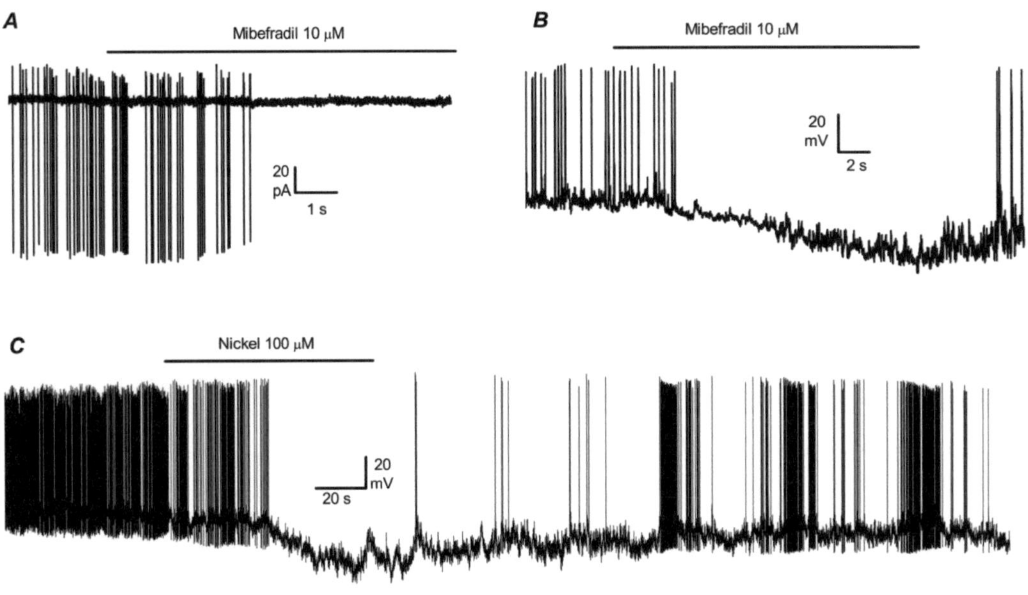


Fig. 13. Effect of blockers of LVA Ca-channels on spontaneous firing. A – Effect of the T-type Ca-channel blocker mibefradil (10 μM) on action currents recorded in cell attached mode. B – Effect of mibefradil in a different TH-GFP cell, recorded in whole-cell configuration. C – Effect of nickel 100 μM on spontaneous firing.

Finally, we investigated the role of the KIR-current on spontaneous activity. The block of the KIR channels with $Ba^{2+}$ 1 mM induced a large depolarization (on average 12 mV), accompanied by a complete stopover of the spontaneous firing.

The effect is illustrated in Fig. 14: a progressive depolarization leads to a complete break of spontaneous activity with a stop at a very depolarised potential (-30 mV in the example shown in figure). In these conditions, the injection of hyperpolarizing currents allows a complete recovery of spontaneous firing, suggesting that the KIR currents plays a relevant role in determining the resting membrane potential, but not in the pacemaking process.

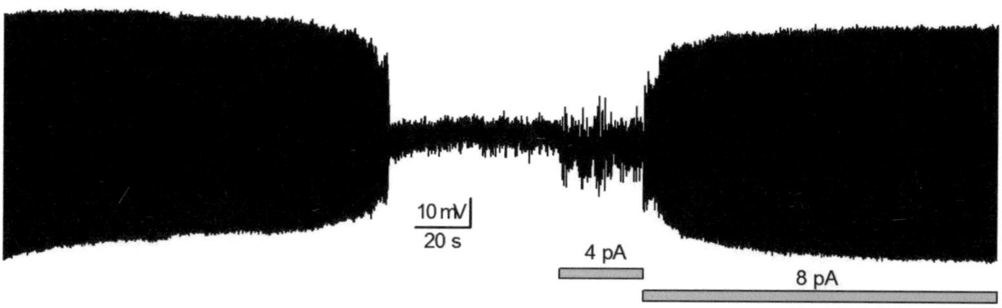


Fig. 14. Effect of blockers of KIR-channels on spontaneous firing. $Ba^{2+}$ (0.5 mM) was applied in the bath 60 s before the beginning of the record; note the progressive depolarization and the stop of any activity in a depolarised state. In this condition, a hyperpolarizing current of 8 pA restores the resting potential, restarting the spontaneous activity.

### 2.10 Modelling the natural burst firing in bulbar DA neurones

Finally, we have modelled the bulbar DA neurones in Hodgkin-Huxley terms (Hodgkin and Huxley1952), considering the cell as a single electrical and spatial compartment. As for the conductances considered, we incorporated the two sodium currents (fast transient and persistent), the L-type Ca-current, the delayed rectifier K-current, all according to the experimental data presented above, and the T-type calcium current. Since our characterisation of this current was incomplete (and because of the difficulty in obtaining a complete kinetic description of this current), in our model we have integrated our data with others derived from the literature (Wang et al.1996; Perez-Reyes2003), and consistent with our experimental data.

All the equations and parameters used, as well as the assumptions made, are listed in the appendix. The solution of the set of differential equations describing the kinetics of the currents considered lead to the tracings reported in Fig. 15. The model we set up shows intrinsic spiking capabilities with full-size action potentials at the same frequencies observed in TH-GFP cells. The model behaves much like the cells studied: each action potential is followed by a slow depolarisation which brings the model cell at the fast sodium channel threshold, and initiating a new Hodgkin cycle.

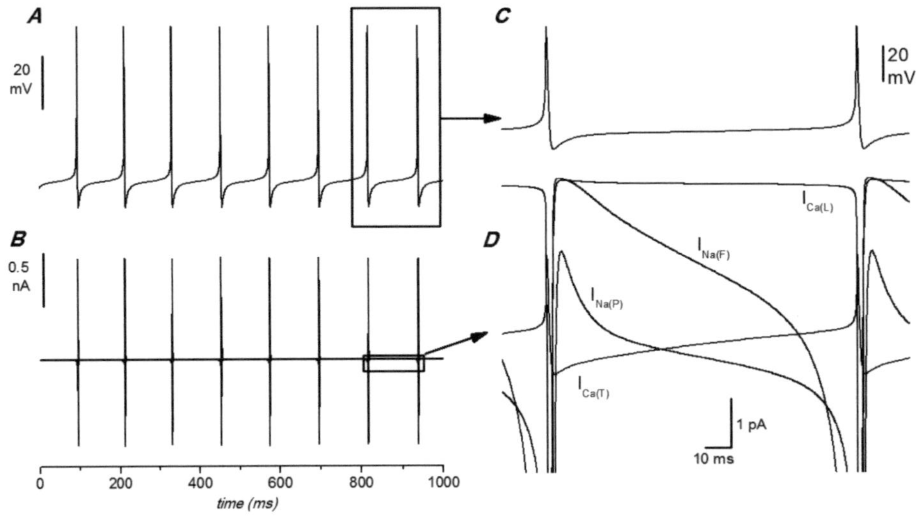


Fig. 15. Numerical reconstitution of spontaneous activity in TH-GFP PG cells. A - Voltage tracings. B - Current tracings including the five conductances: $I_{Na(F)}$, $I_{Na(P)}$, $I_{Ca(T)}$, $I_{Ca(L)}$, $I_{K(V)}$. C, D - Enlargement of the last two events of panels A-B to show the pacemaking process. In D the outward current has been omitted, and the inward currents have been amplified by a factor of about 500 with respect to panel B.

The model is effective to verify the accuracy of the kinetics calculated, and it is particularly useful to understand the details of the interplay of the currents underlying the pacemaking process. The main findings provided by the numerical simulations can be summarised as follows.

First, during the interspike interval, the currents present which cause the progressive depolarisation of the cell are, in order, the T-type calcium current, and then the persistent sodium current. These currents are amazingly small in amplitude (max 4 pA) compared with fast transient sodium and delayed rectifier potassium currents associated to the action potential (about 1 nA), but nevertheless they are sufficient to depolarise these cells, due to their rather high input resistance (about 700 MΩ).

Second, both $I_{Na(P)}$ and $I_{Ca(T)}$ are necessary to sustain spontaneous firing as the selective block of one or both abolish spontaneous activity: the model cell is still capable of responding with a single action potential to the injection of a depolarising current pulse, but it fails to fire repetitively.

Third, the model suggests that it is the T-type calcium current which sets in motion the depolarising process: although essential to the rhythm generation, $I_{Na(P)}$ replaces $I_{Ca(T)}$ only in the second half of the depolarising phase. The T-type calcium conductance amplitude is critical in determining the firing frequency: small changes in its value (from 0.35 to 0.4 nS) are sufficient to drive the intrinsic spiking from 8 Hz to 16 Hz.

Fourth, the HVA calcium currents are unnecessary for the pacemaking process, and their suppression has no consequence on the frequency of spontaneous firing, exactly as in living TH-GFP cells.

Fifth, small changes in the parameters of $I_{Na(F)}$ and of $I_{K(V)}$, such as the half activation point shift of a few millivolts, were sufficient to arrest spontaneous firing but did not affect the capacity to respond with single action potentials to depolarising stimuli. This proves that the pacemaking process is due to an interplay of conductances which are in a delicate and precise equilibrium. Furthermore it confirms the model is capable of capturing the essential features of the excitability profile of these cells.

The model thus confirms that, in addition to $I_{Na(P)}$, another component is necessary to sustain repetitive firing, a T-type calcium current. Together with the experimental finding that treatments which block $I_{Ca(T)}$, such as mibefradil and nickel at micromolar concentrations, are both capable of preventing repetitive firing. Therefore, it appears that such current is an essential component of the pacemaking process.

## 3. Discussion

This study aims at providing a description as comprehensive as possible of the functional properties of DA neurones in the mammalian olfactory bulb. The animal model used for these experiments, a strain of transgenic mice expressing a reporter protein under the TH promoter (Sawamoto et al.2001; Matsushita et al.2002), allows an easy identification of DA neurones both in thin slices and dissociated cells, proving to be a superb tool for targeting live DA neurones in electrophysiological studies. The main results obtained are the demonstration that DA neurones in the OB are autorhythmic, and the description of the interplay of subthreshold currents underlying intrinsic spiking.

### 3.1 Distribution and general properties of DA neurones

Neurones expressing high levels of the reporter protein were found in the glomerular layer, as expected from abundant literature, indicating that this is the only region of the main olfactory bulb where TH is expressed (Halász1990; Kratskin and Belluzzi2003). A previous study in the same mice strain has demonstrated an overlapping expression of the fluorescent reporter and TH protein in olfactory bulb only in those DA neurons that received afferent stimulation from receptor cells (Baker et al.2003).

DA neurones in the mice OB have a complement of voltage-dependent currents, which have been kinetically characterised in our study. Among these, the persistent Na current deserves some comment. Many neurones in the mammalian CNS have a non-inactivating component of the TTX-sensitive sodium current (Crill1996). Although its magnitude in bulbar DA neurones is about 0.5 % of the transient sodium current, $I_{Na(P)}$ appears to have an important functional significance because it is activated at potentials 8-10 mV more negative than the transient sodium current. At this potential few voltage-gated channels are activated and the neuron input resistance is high. The conductance-voltage relationship for $g_{Na(P)}$ in TH-GFP DA neurones has a half-activation point at -47.7 mV, very close to the values found in hippocampal CA1 neurones (French et al.1990), and pyramidal neurones of the neocortex (Brown et al.1994). Although this current might appear small, 7.3 pA at -60 mV (Fig. 6A), it suffices to depolarise the cell membrane of these cells, which have an average input resistance of 700 MΩ, by about 5 mV.

We have considered the possibility that $I_{Na(P)}$ is in fact a window current, the steady current predicted by the HH model and arising from overlap of the steady-state activation and inactivation curves for sodium conductance (Attwell et al.1979; Colatsky1982). Based on the kinetic analysis of the fast Na-current described in the previous paragraph (Fig. 4H), we calculated the window current at different potentials. The numerical simulation indicates this current does provide a measurable contribution to the TTX-sensitive persistent inward current. However, this contribution, which is maximum at -55 mV, becomes virtually zero at -30 mV (Fig. 4H), the potential at which the persistent sodium current displays its maximum amplitude (Fig. 6A). In other words, $I_{Na(P)}$ and the window current of $I_{Na(F)}$ develop at different potentials, and therefore are distinct currents.

### 3.2 Interaction of ionic currents to produce spontaneous firing

The pharmacological treatments, ion substitution experiments, kinetic analysis and numerical simulations allow a rather precise understanding of mechanisms underlying spontaneous firing in TH-GFP cells. The analysis indicates that the slow depolarisation between spikes results from an interplay between the persistent, tetrodotoxin-sensitive sodium current and the T-type calcium current.

The role of a calcium current in rhythm generation is revealed by the rapid and reversible block of the spontaneous firing by $Cd^{2+}$, both in slices and in dissociated cells (Fig. 12B). However, among the many HVA Ca-channels present in the DA neurones of the olfactory bulb (a large L-, and smaller N- and P/Q types), none proved to be effective in the control of spontaneous firing. On the contrary, conditions which are known to block the LVA T-type Ca-channels (mibefradil and nickel in the micromolar range) did break off the spontaneous activity.

We developed a numerical HH-type model (Hodgkin and Huxley1952), based on the kinetic characterisation of the voltage-dependent currents described above, which appears to be capable of reproducing fairly well the behaviour of TH-GFP cells. The model was designed in order to verify the accuracy of our kinetic analysis, and, moreover, in order to understand the mechanisms underlying the intrinsic spiking.

Our model reproduces the properties of real neurones, and clearly indicates that the rhythm generation requires the presence of both $I_{Na(P)}$ and $I_{Ca(T)}$: in the absence of any of the two currents, the model can respond with a single action potential to a depolarising pulse, but is unable to produce repetitive firing.

The model shows that the current which sets in motion the spontaneous spiking is the T-type calcium current, which in turn brings into play the persistent sodium current. In spite of the limits inherent to this type of models, we note that small changes in the kinetic parameters lead to the loss of intrinsic spiking but not of the capacity of the cell to respond with a single action potential to the "injection" of a short depolarising current step, thus suggesting that the model has captured the essential features of the real cell.

### 3.3 The role of hyperpolarization-activated currents

Our results exclude a direct contribution of the h-current to the spontaneous firing and, although less conclusively, also for the KIR current. However, it is of great interest that, as we show, both currents exert a powerful control on the resting membrane potential, the first depolarising, the second hyperpolarising the membrane at rest. The resting membrane potential, therefore, whose influence on the interplay of pacemaker currents can be well understood with the numerical model proposed, can be adjusted in either directions by a modulation of the two hyperpolarization-activated currents. Both currents can be modulated by a variety of neurotransmitters (see (Biel et al.2009) and (Hibino et al.2010) for recent reviews on h-current and KIR, respectively). Interestingly, some intracellular pathway, like AC/cAMP, can act on both $I_h$ and KIR, enhancing the first and hampering the second (Podda et al.2010); the contrary effect is also observed, e.g. in the rat substantia nigra neurones, where bath application of noradrenaline or dopamine both inhibit $I_h$ and increase the KIR conductance (Cathala and Paupardin-Tritsch1999). Elucidating these interactions will be a critical step in order to understand the functioning of these cells and, in a longer perspective, the still elusive role of dopaminergic neurones in signal processing in the olfactory bulb.

### 3.4 Significance to olfactory function

Our results, and especially the indication that DA neurones in the glomerular layer are autorhythmic, open the field to many speculations.

It is known that the glomerular neuropile, far from being a homogeneous structure, shows a complex subcompartimental organisation: within a single glomerulus, olfactory nerve (ON) islets delimit areas in which dendritic branches receive sensory input from ON terminals, and are well separated from non-ON zones, from which ON terminals are excluded (Chao et al.1997; Kasowski et al.1999; Toida et al.2000). Some TH-immunoreactive PG cells arborise on the ON islets, others in the non-ON zone (Kosaka et al.1997). Although it has been reported that in some mouse strains TH positive cells are not in contact with ON terminals (Weruaga et al.2000), in the strain used for these experiments - C57BL/6J, one of the most commons - such contacts have been demonstrated (T. Kosaka and K. Kosaka, personal communication).

The glomerular compartmentalisation supports the hypothesis that information processing is subdivided regionally within the mammalian glomerulus (Kasowski et al.1999). DA neurones establishing contacts in ON- or in non-ON zones, possibly play different roles. Within the ON zones, dendrites of DA neurones receive excitatory synapses from ON axon terminals (Chao et al.1997; Kasowski et al.1999; Toida et al.2000). It has been reported that D2 dopaminergic receptors are located in ON terminals (Levey et al.1993; Coronas et al.1997), and electrophysiological studies have shown that their activation can reduce the probability of glutamate release, and hence the excitation of projection neurones (Duchamp-Viret et al.1997; Hsia et al.1999; Berkowicz and Trombley2000; Ennis et al.2001). In fact, the most significant impact of DA neurones is expected at the level of the synaptic triad formed by the ON and the dendrites of mitral/tufted (MT) cells and PG cells (Bardoni et al.1996), where DA neurones directly control the input of projection neurones from receptor cell axons (Brünig et al.1999). Since the ON islets appear to be further segregated from the rest of the glomerular neuropile due to the presence of "glial wraps" (Kasowski et al.1999), the spontaneous activity of DA neurones (which implies continuous release of dopamine within a restricted space), would create a condition of tonic inhibition of the ON.

In addition, DA neurones send their dendrites also in non-ON zones, where they contact dendrites of projection neurones and interneurons, and centrifugal axons. Projection neurones express D1 and D2 receptors (Brünig et al.1999; Davila et al.2003) , and it has been shown that dopamine exerts a complex modulatory action between them and interneurons (*ibidem*), an effect that also in this case would be amplified by the restricted space of the glomerular neuropile. Within this framework, dopamine might play a central role in the processing of olfactory information by acting at two levels: it would control the input of the sensory signal, and it would modulate the mechanism of GABAergic inhibition (Brünig et al.1999; Davila et al.2003).

It remains to be explained why DA neurones in the glomerular region of the OB are among the very few in the mammalian CNS which are generated also in adulthood. On one end this brings up series of questions concerning the mechanisms controlling their migration and differentiation, and, on the other end, it opens interesting perspectives for the exploitation of the olfactory bulb as a source of undifferentiated DA cells that could be expanded *ex vivo* and used for transplants in neurodegenerative diseases.

## 4. Acknowledgements

This work was supported by grants from MURST (PRIN 2009) and from Programma Medicina Rigenerativa Regione E.R. - Università, 2007–2009.

## 5. References

Attwell D, Cohen I, Eisner D, Ohba M, Ojeda C (1979): The steady state TTX-sensitive ("window") sodium current in cardiac Purkinje fibres. *Pflugers Arch* 379:137-142.

Baker H, Kawano T, Margolis FL, Joh TH (1983): Transneuronal regulation of tyrosine hydroxylase expression in olfactory bulb of mouse and rat. *J Neurosci* 3:69-78.

Baker H, Kobayashi K, Okano H, Saino-Saito S (2003): Cortical and striatal expression of tyrosine hydroxylase mRNA in neonatal and adult mice. *Cell Mol Neurobiol* 23:507-518.

Baker H, Liu N, Chun HS, Saino S, Berlin R, Volpe B, *et al* (2001): Phenotypic differentiation during migration of dopaminergic progenitor cells to the olfactory bulb. *J Neurosci* 21:8505-8513.

Bardoni R, Magherini PC, Belluzzi O (1996): Excitatory synapses in the glomerular triad of frog olfactory bulb *in vitro*. *Neuroreport* 7:1851-1855.

Bausch SB, Patterson TA, Ehrengruber MU, Lester HA, Davidson N, Chavkin C (1995): Colocalization of mu opioid receptors with GIRK1 potassium channels in the rat brain: an immunocytochemical study. *Receptors Channels* 3:221-241.

Berkowicz DA, Trombley PQ (2000): Dopaminergic modulation at the olfactory nerve synapse. *Brain Res* 855:90-99.

Betarbet R, Zigova T, Bakay RA, Luskin MB (1996): Dopaminergic and GABAergic interneurons of the olfactory bulb are derived from the neonatal subventricular zone. *Int J Dev Neurosci* 14:921-930.

Biel M, Wahl-Schott C, Michalakis S, Zong X (2009): Hyperpolarization-activated cation channels: from genes to function. *Physiol Rev* 89:847-885.

Bonifazzi C, Belluzzi O, Sacchi O (1988): Kinetic analysis of incomplete current tracings according to the Hodgkin-Huxley model. *J Theor Biol* 130:183-190.

Brown AM, Schwindt PC, Crill WE (1994): Different voltage dependence of transient and persistent $Na^+$ currents is compatible with modal-gating hypothesis for sodium channels. *J Neurophysiol* 71:2562-2565.

Brünig I, Sommer M, Hatt H, Bormann J (1999): Dopamine receptor subtypes modulate olfactory bulb gamma-aminobutyric acid type A receptors. *Proc Natl Acad Sci USA* 96:2456-2460.

Cathala L, Paupardin-Tritsch D (1999): Effect of catecholamines on the hyperpolarization-activated cationic Ih and the inwardly rectifying potassium I(Kir) currents in the rat substantia nigra pars compacta. *Eur J Neurosci* 11:398-406.

Chao TI, Kasa P, Wolff JR (1997): Distribution of astroglia in glomeruli of the rat main olfactory bulb: exclusion from the sensory subcompartment of neuropil. *J Comp Neurol* 388:191-210.

Colatsky TJ (1982): Mechanisms of action of lidocaine and quinidine on action potential duration in rabbit cardiac Purkinje fibers. An effect on steady state sodium currents? *Circ Res* 50:17-27.

Coronas V, Srivastava LK, Liang JJ, Jourdan F, Moyse E (1997): Identification and localization of dopamine receptor subtypes in rat olfactory mucosa and bulb: a combined in situ hybridization and ligand binding radioautographic approach. *J Chem Neuroanat* 12:243-257.

Crill WE (1996): Persistent sodium current in mammalian central neurons. *Annu Rev Physiol* 58:349-362.

Davila NG, Blakemore LJ, Trombley PQ (2003): Dopamine modulates synaptic transmission between rat olfactory bulb neurons in culture. *J Neurophysiol* 90:395-404.

Doty RL, Risser JM (1989): Influence of the D-2 dopamine receptor agonist quinpirole on the odor detection performance of rats before and after spiperone administration. *Psychopharmacology (Berl)* 98:310-315.

Duchamp-Viret P, Coronas V, Delaleu JC, Moyse E, Duchamp A (1997): Dopaminergic modulation of mitral cell activity in the frog olfactory bulb: A combined radioligand binding electrophysiological study. *Neuroscience* 79:203-216.

Ennis M, Zhou FM, Ciombor KJ, Aroniadou-Anderjaska V, Hayar A, Borrelli E, *et al* (2001): Dopamine D2 receptor-mediated presynaptic inhibition of olfactory nerve terminals. *J Neurophysiol* 86:2986-2997.

Feigenspan A, Gustincich S, Bean BP, Raviola E (1998): Spontaneous activity of solitary dopaminergic cells of the retina. *J Neurosci* 18:6776-6789.

French CR, Sah P, Buckett KJ, Gage PW (1990): A voltage-dependent persistent sodium current in mammalian hippocampal neurons. *J Gen Physiol* 95:1139-1157.

Gall CM, Hendry SH, Seroogy KB, Jones EG, Haycock JW (1987): Evidence for coexistence of GABA and dopamine in neurons of the rat olfactory bulb. *J Comp Neurol* 266:307-318.

Grace AA, Onn SP (1989): Morphology and electrophysiological properties of immunocytochemically identified rat dopamine neurons recorded in vitro. *J Neurosci* 9:3463-3481.

Gross CG (2000): Neurogenesis in the adult brain: death of a dogma. *Nat Rev Neurosci* 1:67-73.

Gustincich S, Feigenspan A, Wu DK, Koopman LJ, Raviola E (1997): Control of dopamine release in the retina: a transgenic approach to neural networks. *Neuron* 18:723-736.

Guthrie KM, Pullara JM, Marshall JF, Leon M (1991): Olfactory deprivation increases dopamine D2 receptor density in the rat olfactory bulb. *Synapse* 8:61-70.

Hainsworth AH, Roper J, Kapoor R, Ashcroft FM (1991): Identification and electrophysiology of isolated pars compacta neurons from guinea-pig substantia nigra. *Neuroscience* 43:81-93.

Halász N (1990): *The vertebrate olfactory system: chemical neuroanatomy, function and development.* Budapest: Académiai Kiadó.

Halász N, Hökfelt T, Ljungdahl A, Johansson O, Goldstein M (1977): Dopamine neurons in the olfactory bulb. *Adv Biochem Psychopharmacol* 16:169-177.

Hibino H, Inanobe A, Furutani K, Murakami S, Findlay I, Kurachi Y (2010): Inwardly rectifying potassium channels: their structure, function, and physiological roles. *Physiol Rev* 90:291-366.

Hodgkin AL, Huxley AF (1952): A quantitative description of membrane currents and its application to conduction and excitation in nerve. *J Physiol (Lond )* 117:500-544.

Hsia AY, Vincent JD, Lledo PM (1999): Dopamine depresses synaptic inputs into the olfactory bulb. *J Neurophysiol* 82:1082-1085.

Kasowski HJ, Kim H, Greer CA (1999): Compartmental organization of the olfactory bulb glomerulus. *J Comp Neurol* 407:261-274.

Klugbauer N, Marais E, Lacinova L, Hofmann F (1999): A T-type calcium channel from mouse brain. *Pflugers Arch* 437:710-715.

Kosaka K, Toida K, Margolis FL, Kosaka T (1997): Chemically defined neuron groups and their subpopulations in the glomerular layer of the rat main olfactory bulb .2. Prominent differences in the intraglomerular dendritic arborization and their relationship to olfactory nerve terminals. *Neuroscience* 76:775-786.

Kosaka T, Hataguchi Y, Hama K, Nagatsu I, Wu JY (1985): Coexistence of immunoreactivities for glutamate decarboxylase and tyrosine hydroxylase in some neurons in the periglomerular region of the rat main olfactory bulb: possible coexistence of gamma-aminobutyric acid (GABA) and dopamine. *Brain Res* 343:166-171.

Kratskin I, Belluzzi O (2003): Anatomy and neurochemistry of the olfactory bulb. In: Doty RL, editor. *Handbook of Olfaction and Gustation*, 2nd ed. New York - Basel: Marcel Dekker, pp 139-164.

Levey AI, Hersch SM, Rye DB, Sunahara RK, Niznik HB, Kitt CA, *et al* (1993): Localization of D1 and D2 dopamine receptors in brain with subtype-specific antibodies. *Proc Natl Acad Sci U S A* 90:8861-8865.

Matsushita N, Okada H, Yasoshima Y, Takahashi K, Kiuchi K, Kobayashi K (2002): Dynamics of tyrosine hydroxylase promoter activity during midbrain dopaminergic neuron development. *J Neurochem* 82:295-304.

McLean JH, Shipley MT (1988): Postmitotic, postmigrational expression of tyrosine hydroxylase in olfactory bulb dopaminergic neurons. *J Neurosci* 8:3658-3669.

Neuhoff H, Neu A, Liss B, Roeper J (2002): I(h) channels contribute to the different functional properties of identified dopaminergic subpopulations in the midbrain. *J Neurosci* 22:1290-1302.

Nowycky MC, Halász N, Shepherd GM (1983): Evoked field potential analysis of dopaminergic mechanisms in the isolated turtle olfactory bulb. *Neuroscience* 8:717-722.

Perchenet L, Benardeau A, Ertel EA (2000): Pharmacological properties of Ca(V)3.2, a low voltage-activated $Ca^{2+}$ channel cloned from human heart. *Naunyn Schmiedebergs Arch Pharmacol* 361:590-599.

Perez MF, White FJ, Hu XT (2006): Dopamine D(2) receptor modulation of K(+) channel activity regulates excitability of nucleus accumbens neurons at different membrane potentials. *J Neurophysiol* 96:2217-2228.

Perez-Reyes E (2003): Molecular physiology of low-voltage-activated t-type calcium channels. *Physiol Rev* 83:117-161.

Perez-Reyes E, Cribbs LL, Daud A, Lacerda AE, Barclay J, Williamson MP, *et al* (1998): Molecular characterization of a neuronal low-voltage-activated T-type calcium channel. *Nature* 391:896-900.

Pignatelli A, Kobayashi K, Okano H, Belluzzi O (2005): Functional properties of dopaminergic neurones in the mouse olfactory bulb. *J Physiol* 564:501-514.

Podda MV, Riccardi E, D'Ascenzo M, Azzena GB, Grassi C (2010): Dopamine D1-like receptor activation depolarizes medium spiny neurons of the mouse nucleus accumbens by inhibiting inwardly rectifying $K^+$ currents through a cAMP-dependent protein kinase A-independent mechanism. *Neuroscience* 167:678-690.

Prüss H, Derst C, Lommel R, Veh RW (2005): Differential distribution of individual subunits of strongly inwardly rectifying potassium channels (Kir2 family) in rat brain. *Brain Res Mol Brain Res* 139:63-79.

Randall AD (1998): The molecular basis of voltage-gated $Ca^{2+}$ channel diversity: is it time for T? *J Membr Biol* 161:207-213.

Randall AD, Tsien RW (1997): Contrasting biophysical and pharmacological properties of T-type and R-type calcium channels. *Neuropharmacology* 36:879-893.

Sawamoto K, Nakao N, Kobayashi K, Matsushita N, Takahashi H, Kakishita K, *et al* (2001): Visualization, direct isolation, and transplantation of midbrain dopaminergic neurons. *Proc Natl Acad Sci U S A* 98:6423-6428.

Schweitz H, Heurteaux C, Bois P, Moinier D, Romey G, Lazdunski M (1994): Calcicludine, a venom peptide of the Kunitz-type protease inhibitor family, is a potent blocker of high-threshold $Ca^{2+}$ channels with a high affinity for L-type channels in cerebellar granule neurons. *Proc Natl Acad Sci U S A* 91:878-882.

Takahashi K, Ueno S, Akaike N (1991): Kinetic properties of T-type $Ca^{2+}$ currents in isolated rat hippocampal CA1 pyramidal neurons, 65 ed, pp 148-155.

Talley EM, Cribbs LL, Lee JH, Daud A, Perez-Reyes E, Bayliss DA (1999): Differential distribution of three members of a gene family encoding low voltage-activated (T-type) calcium channels. *J Neurosci* 19:1895-1911.

Todorovic SM, Lingle CJ (1998): Pharmacological properties of T-type $Ca^{2+}$ current in adult rat sensory neurons: effects of anticonvulsant and anesthetic agents. *J Neurophysiol* 79:240-252.

Toida K, Kosaka K, Aika Y, Kosaka T (2000): Chemically defined neuron groups and their subpopulations in the glomerular layer of the rat main olfactory bulb. IV. Intraglomerular synapses of tyrosine hydroxylase-immunoreactive neurons. *Neuroscience* 101:11-17.

Viana F, Van den BL, Missiaen L, Vandenberghe W, Droogmans G, Nilius B, *et al* (1997): Mibefradil (Ro 40-5967) blocks multiple types of voltage-gated calcium channels in cultured rat spinal motoneurones. *Cell Calcium* 22:299-311.

Wahl-Schott C, Biel M (2009): HCN channels: structure, cellular regulation and physiological function. *Cell Mol Life Sci* 66:470-494.

Wang X, Mckenzie JS, Kemm RE (1996): Whole cell calcium currents in acutely isolated olfactory bulb output neurons of the rat. *J Neurophysiol* 75:1138-1151.

Weruaga E, Brinon JG, Porteros A, Arevalo R, Aijon J, Alonso JR (2000): Expression of neuronal nitric oxide synthase/NADPH-diaphorase during olfactory deafferentation and regeneration. *Eur J Neurosci* 12:1177-1193.

Wolfart J, Roeper J (2002): Selective coupling of T-type calcium channels to SK potassium channels prevents intrinsic bursting in dopaminergic midbrain neurons. *J Neurosci* 22:3404-3413.

Yung WH, Hausser MA, Jack JJ (1991): Electrophysiology of dopaminergic and non-dopaminergic neurones of the guinea-pig substantia nigra pars compacta in vitro. *J Physiol* 436:643-667.

Zhang JF, Randall AD, Ellinor PT, Horne WA, Sather WA, Tanabe T, *et al* (1993): Distinctive pharmacology and kinetics of cloned neuronal $Ca^{2+}$ channels and their possible counterparts in mammalian CNS neurons. *Neuropharmacology* 32:1075-1088.

# 3

# Hippocampal Slices and Their Electrophysiogy in the Study of Brain Energy Metabolism

Avital Schurr
*Department of Anesthesiology & Perioperative Medicine, University of Louisville School of Medicine, Louisville, KY, USA*

## 1. Introduction

Dorland's Illustrated Medical Dictionary in its 24th Edition (1965), describes the term "Electrophysiology" as "The Science of physiology in its relations to electricity; the study of the electric reactions of the body in health." The ability of scientists to observe and record physiology's electrical phenomena long preceded the understanding of the membranous ionic processes that are responsible for them. Consequently, for a while, electrophysiology has been considered a subfield of physiology, aiming at improving our understanding of cellular, organ and bodily functions. With the advances made in molecular biology, genetics and neuroscience, the role of electrophysiology has shifted, where today it is being employed as one of the best, most accurate and least expensive real-time monitoring tools in basic science research and clinical studies and practice alike.

The discovery in the early 1950s that brain slices can sustain certain electrophysiological characteristics typical of the intact brain opened a wide range of possibilities for studying cerebral tissue and its electrophysiology *in vitro*. Obviously, the brain slice preparation affords the experimenter both the control and manipulation of the environmental conditions under which the neural tissue is maintained. Employing electrophysiological techniques allows a continuous monitoring/recording of the neural tissue's viability, its functions and its responses to environmental and other changes brought about by the experimenter's chosen manipulations.

Thousands of papers and several books have been published over the past 30 years, where brain slices were the topic itself or where studies employed them in combination with various techniques, including electrophysiological ones. The present chapter describes some important advances made over the past three decades using brain slices and their electrophysiology in our laboratory, advances that provided us with a better understanding of cerebral energy metabolism. All the experiments detailed herewith employed the rat hippocampal slice preparation, using a continuous extracellular, real-time monitoring of the electrically-evoked CA1 population spike (PS).

Of the different brain slice preparations available, the rat hippocampal slice preparation is without a doubt the most studied. Henry McIlwain and colleagues were the first to use thin brain sections for metabolic studies (McIlwain et al., 1951; McIlwain & Buddle, 1953;

Rodnight & McIlwain, 1954). McIlwain's laboratory was also the first to demonstrate that neurons in brain slices were in a healthy state, as was evidenced by the investigators' ability to record resting membrane potentials in slices that were more negative than -60 mV (Li and McIlwain, 1957). By the mid 1960s they have established that brain slices maintain their synaptic potential, exhibit synaptic plasticity and are capable of recovering their synaptic function following drug-induced depolarization (Gibson & McIlwain, 1965; Yamamoto & McIlwain, 1966).

## 2. Preparation of rat hippocampal slices, their maintenance and their electrophysiology

### 2.1 The preparation and its maintenance

In all the experiments described in this chapter, adult (200-350 g) male Sprague-Dawley rats were used. For each experiment one rat was decapitated and its brain rapidly removed, rinsed with cold (6-8°C) artificial cerebrospinal fluid (aSCF) of the following composition (in mM): NaCl, 124; KCl, 5; $NaH_2PO_4$, 3; $CaCl_2$, 2.5; $MgSO_4$, 2.4; $NaHCO_3$, 23; glucose, 10 or as indicated. Then, the hippocampi were dissected out and were sliced transversely at 400 μm with a McIlwain tissue chopper. The resulting slices were transferred to a dual linear-flow interface chamber (Schurr et al., 1985). Twelve to 15 slices were placed in each compartment of the dual chamber. Each compartment had its own supply of aCSF via a two-channel peristaltic pump (40 ml/h) and a humidified gas mixture of 95% $O_2$/5% $CO_2$, which was circulated above the slices that were supported on a nylon mesh. The temperature in the incubation chamber was maintained at 34±0.5°C. For each experiment, the slices in one compartment were used as 'control', while those in the other as 'experimental'. The great advantage of this *in vitro* system is the ability of the experimenter to control and change the environmental conditions under which the slices are maintained, including the concentration of any of the aCSF components, the supplied gas atmosphere composition and the incubation temperature. Moreover, additional chemicals can be added either to the aCSF or to the gas mixture.

### 2.2 Electrophysiological measurements

Continuous extracellular recording of evoked population responses in the stratum pyramidale of the hippocampal CA1 region were made from one slice in each compartment of the dual incubation chamber using borosilicate micropipettes filled with aCSF (impedance = 2-5 MΩ). A bipolar stimulating electrode was placed in the Schaffer collaterals (orthodromic stimulation) in one slice in each compartment from which the recording was made. Stimulus pulses of 0.1 ms in duration and amplitude of 8-10 V were applied once per minute. A two-channel preamplifier (x 100) and two field-effect transistor head-stages were used and their output was fed into a waveform analysis program to determine the amplitude of the evoked response. Although only the electrophysiological response from one slice in each compartment was recorded continuously throughout any given experiment, all slices were tested for the presence of such response i.e., a population spike (PS) amplitude of $\geq$3 mV (neuronal function) prior to the beginning of the experiment. Slices exhibiting a population spike amplitude <3 mV were discarded. Recordings were begun 90 min after the preparation of the slices, allowing them to fully recover from the process. At the end of each experiment all the remaining slices in both compartments of the chamber were tested again for the presence of neuronal function. Those slices exhibiting a PS amplitude <3 mV were considered non-functional due to the experimental manipulation(s). Figure 1 is an illustration of a rat hippocampal slice showing the neuronal circuits within it and the synaptic connections between axons of one neuronal population and dendrites of another.

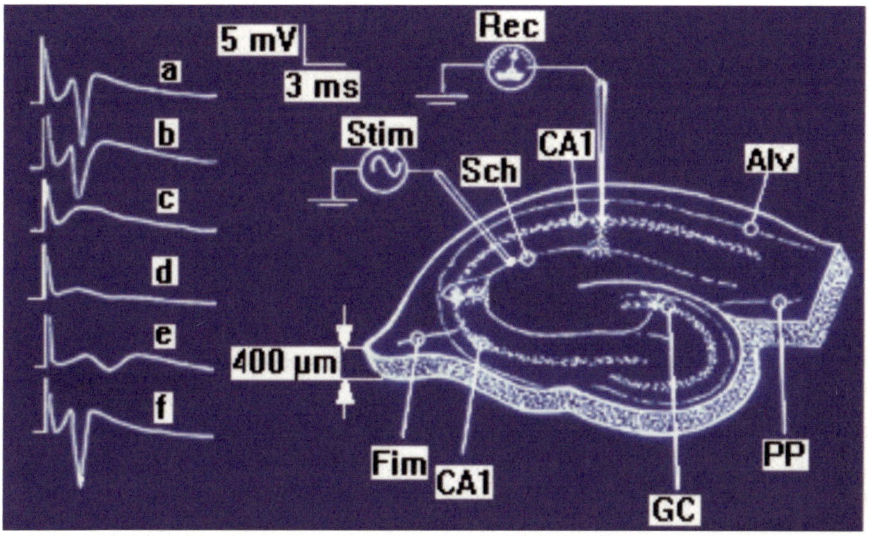


Fig. 1. A schematic illustration of a rat hippocampal slice. Shown are the typical positions where a stimulating (Stim) and a recording (Rec) electrodes were placed and a series of representative records (a-f) produced by stimulating the Schaffer (Sch) collaterals (orthodromic stimulation) to evoke a PS (neuronal function) in the CA1 region. When a given condition, which is necessary for normal maintenance of neuronal function, is removed and then replenished, the disappearance of the PS (b-c) and its recovery (d-f), respectively, is apparent. Similarly, the addition of a toxin and its removal may lead to the disappearance and the reappearance of the PS, respectively. Scales of amplitude (mV) and time (ms) are also shown. Additional abbreviations: CA1, cornu ammonis 1; CA3, cornu ammonis 3; Alv, alveus; PP, perforant path; GC, granule cells of the dentate gyrus; Fim, fimbria.

The presence of neuronal function (an orthodromically-evoked, CA1 PS) has been used as a sensitive and responsive signal to indicate both tissue viability and stability over time. Histological and morphological studies of hippocampal slices from which electrophysiological recordings were taken over time, confirmed that the tissue function was correlated with its structural integrity (Schurr et al., 1984). Hence, throughout all the experiments described in this chapter this neuronal function (PS amplitude $\geq$3 mV) was used to differentiate between functional (viable) and nonfunctional (damaged) hippocampal slices.

### 2.3 Statistical analysis

Each data point in every experiment described in this chapter was repeated at least three times. Values shown in the figures are mean ± either SD (standard deviation of the mean) or

SEM (standard error of the mean). Statistical analysis for significant differences was performed using either the paired *t* test or the $\chi^2$ test. A $P \leq 0.05$ was considered to be statistically significant.

## 3. A major dogma of ischemic brain damage sheds new light on brain energy metabolism

The 1981 inaugural issue of the Journal of Cerebral Blood Flow and Metabolism includes a review paper written by B.K. Siesjö, at the time, one of the leading researchers in the field of cerebral ischemia who studied the cellular and biochemical mechanisms of ischemic brain damage. Although Siesjö's article was, according to its title, "a speculative synthesis," it became one of the most cited papers in the field ever, receiving over 1,500 citations so far. This speculative synthesis was based, among others, on two research papers from Siesjö's own laboratory published in that very issue of the journal (Rehncrona et al., 1981; Kalimo et al., 1981). With the use of biochemical, neurophysiological and histopathological methodologies, Siesjö all but concluded that lactic acidosis is a major culprit in cerebral ischemia, responsible for the well-documented delayed neuronal damage observed post-ischemia. Quickly, the lactic acidosis hypothesis had immerged as the leading hypothesis in the field, highlighted in many other research papers, review articles, specialized books and textbooks. The hypothesis was accepted unopposed by almost all investigators in the field as the most plausible cellular mechanism that explains ischemic delayed neuronal damage. Although Siesjö's group was interested in the relationship between cerebral ischemic damage and acidosis for some years prior to the 1981 publications, a study by Myers and Yamaguchi (1977) was a major impetus for the formulation of Siesjö's speculative synthesis. Myers and Yamaguchi (1977) discovered that pre-ischemic hyperglycemia aggravates cerebral ischemia delayed neuronal damage, a finding that nestled nicely within the idea of 'higher blood [glucose] pre-ischemia = higher brain [lactic acid] during cerebral ischemia.' Consequently, to establish the hippocampal slice preparation as an adequate *in vitro* model for studying cerebral ischemia, we aimed to demonstrate that increased [glucose] in the aCSF prior to *in vitro* ischemia aggravates ischemic neuronal damage post-ischemia. Similarly, we also attempted to demonstrate that lactic acidosis aggravates ischemic neuronal damage in this model system, an approach difficult to duplicate *in vivo*. It is worth emphasizing that Siesjö's hypothesis was so entrenched in the annals of the field that hardly anyone questioned the paradoxical effect of elevated glucose concentration; why the only energy substrate the neural tissue is able to utilize in the absence of oxygen and which would avert ischemic damage, appears instead to increase the ischemic damage? Fittingly, this phenomenon has been thus termed "the glucose paradox of cerebral ischemia."

### 3.1 The effect of oxygen or glucose deprivation on neuronal function in hippocampal slices

Glucose is an essential component of the aCSF without which slices cannot survive. Early slicers have standardized an aCSF glucose concentration of 10 mM, twice the level considered to be isoglycemic *in vivo*. Since the slice preparation's supply of nutrients is dependent entirely on simple diffusion, this relatively high level of glucose in the aCSF was established to assure ample supply of this energy substrate. Thus, when we first tested the sensitivity of neuronal function in hippocampal slices to $O_2$ deprivation (*in vitro* ischemia/hypoxia) we used the standard, 10 mM glucose in the aCSF. Oxygen deprivation or hypoxia in the slice preparation is achieved by simply replacing the supply of 95% $O_2$/5% $CO_2$ with 95% $N_2$/5% $CO_2$. Similarly, by exposing slices to aCSF depleted of glucose (0 mM glucose) an *in vitro* 'hypoglycemia' can be achieved. Fig. 2 shows the percentage of slices that exhibited recovery of neuronal function 30 min after depriving them for different durations of either $O_2$ or glucose (see also Schurr et al., 1989a). Neuronal function is clearly a sensitive measure of the effect of nutrient deprivation on the tissue. While $O_2$ was entirely depleted within 2 to 3 min from the moment it was replaced with $N_2$, an average 40-min was required for a complete depletion of glucose from the aCSF. Hence, the time slices were exposed to 0 mM glucose as shown in Fig. 2 is 40 + X min. It is obvious from the results shown in Fig. 2 that hippocampal slices are significantly more sensitive to 'hypoxia' than to 'hypoglycemia.' The data compiled in Fig. 2 are the percentages of slices that exhibited the presence of neuronal function after 30-min recovery period. A typical response of the PS continuously recorded from one slice during the experiment can be seen in Fig. 1, traces a-f. These traces represent normal neuronal function prior to $O_2$ deprivation (a), neuronal function at 3-min $O_2$ deprivation (b), at 5-min $O_2$ deprivation (c), at 10-min $O_2$ deprivation (d) at 10-min re-oxygenation (e) and at 30-min re-oxygenation. The results indicate that the hippocampal slice preparation is responsive to changes in both oxygen and glucose concentrations and was ready for its ultimate test that should establish whether or not this preparation is a worthy *in vitro* model of cerebral ischemia. Such a model should exhibit an aggravation of 'ischemic' neuronal damage with the elevation in [glucose] and a similar aggravation with increasing [lactic acid, pH]. These were our expectations based on the leading hypotheses of the time.

### 3.2 The effect of changing [glucose] on neuronal function in hippocampal slices post-hypoxia

In a series of experiments we then tested the effect of several glucose levels on the ability of hippocampal slices to recover their neuronal function from 10-, 15- or 20-min hypoxia. The results are shown in Fig. 3 (see also Schurr et al., 1987, 1989a). It is clear from these results that the higher the [glucose] in the aCSF, the longer the hypoxic period hippocampal slices tolerate. Weather the hypoxic period was short or long, elevating [glucose] had a neuroprotective effect against hypoxic damage, an effect completely opposite to the one expected and reported *in vivo* (Myers & Yamaguchi, 1977). Although understandably, we had some doubts about the slice preparation's suitability as an *in vitro* model of cerebral ischemia, at least from a biochemical stand point, increased [glucose] during hypoxia, when anaerobic glycolysis is the only metabolic pathway available for significant adenosine triphosphate (ATP) synthesis, should afford the tissue a longer survival time under such conditions. After all, an increase in glucose consumption under anaerobic conditions (Pasture's Effect) suggests that the higher the glucose concentration, the longer the time it would last under anaerobic conditions. In light of this unexpected outcome, we were anxious to find out what would be the effect of lactic acidosis on neuronal function post-hypoxia.

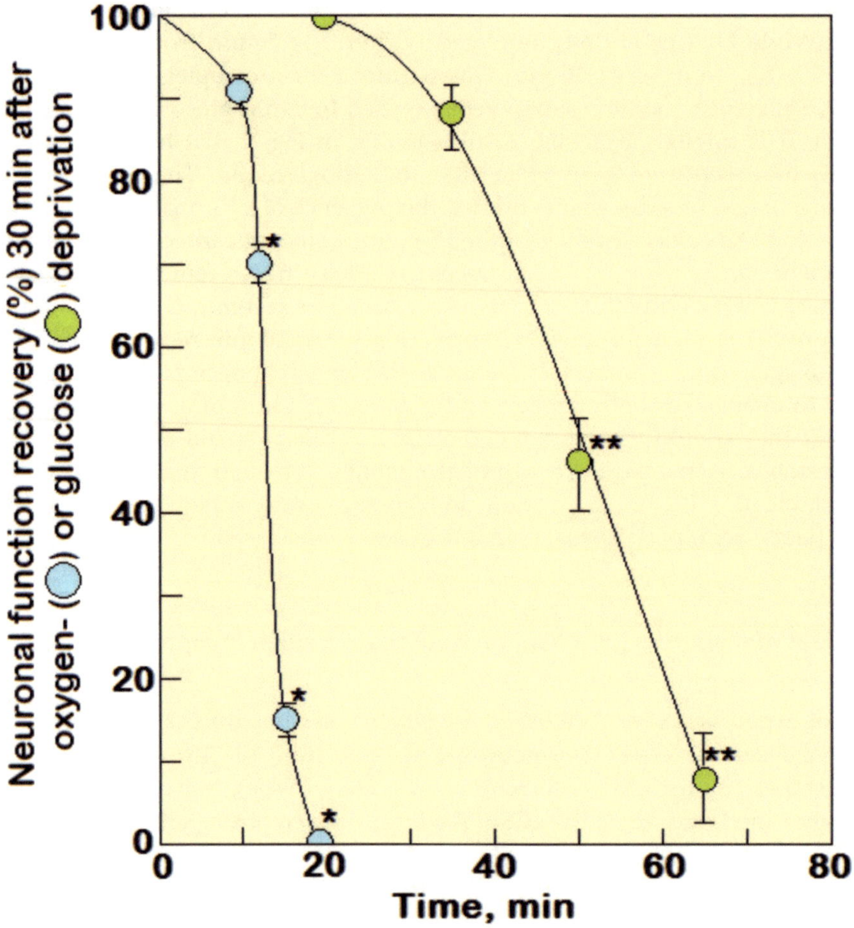


Fig. 2. The effects of different durations of $O_2$ or glucose deprivation on the recovery of neuronal function 30 min after the end of either deprivation in rat hippocampal slices. Neuronal function is much more tolerant to lack of glucose than to lack of oxygen (hypoxia). Data points are mean ± SD; *significantly different from 10-min hypoxia ($P < 0.0005$); **significantly different from 20-min glucose deprivation ($P < 0.005$).

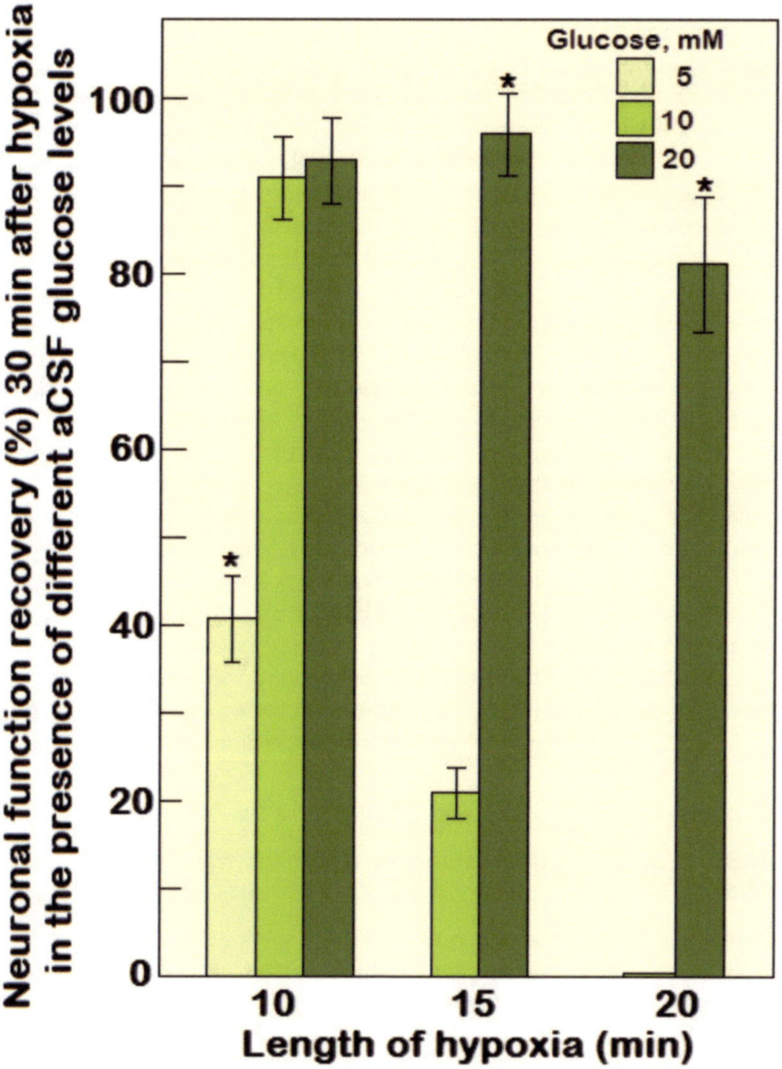


Fig. 3. The effect of elevated aCSF glucose levels during hypoxia on the ability of hippocampal slices to recover neuronal function 30-min post-hypoxia. The higher the glucose level during hypoxia, the better the recovery rate of neuronal function post-hypoxia. Data points are mean ± SD; *significantly different from 10 mM glucose ($P < 0.0005$).

### 3.3 The effect of lactic acid on the recovery of neuronal function in hippocampal slices post-hypoxia

Hippcampal slices were first exposed to either 10 mM or 20 mM lactic acid for 30 min. The pH of the aCSF in each compartment of the dual chamber was measured shortly before slices were exposed to hypoxia (10, 12 or 15 min) in the presence of lactic acid. At the end of the hypoxic period, re-oxygenation ensued and the lactic acid aCSF was replaced with normal, glucose (10 mM) containing aCSF of physiological pH. At the end of a 30-min post-hypoxic period, all slices were tested for the presence of neuronal function. The outcome of these experiments is summarized in Fig. 4. Surprisingly, lactic acidosis, at least at moderate pH values, appeared to be neuroprotective against hypoxic neuronal damage. Weather the hypoxic period was shorter (10 min) or longer (12 or 15 min), slices exposed to 30-min lactic acidosis (10 mM lactic acid, pH 6.8-6.9) prior to and during hypoxia, exhibited a decrease in the degree of neuronal damage compared to control slices (no lactic acid, 10 mM glucose, pH 7.30-7.34) or slices that were exposed to 20 mM lactic acid (pH 5.53-5.75). Thus, our *in vitro* model system of cerebral ischemia/hypoxia failed to demonstrate a detrimental effect of lactic acidosis on cerebral ischemic (hypoxic) neuronal damage (see also Schurr et al., 1988a). High lactic acid concentration (20 mM) seemed to only slightly worsen the post-hypoxic outcome when combined with 10-min hypoxia. Thus, at least where the lactic acidosis hypothesis of cerebral ischemic neuronal damage is concerned, the outcome of these experiments was unexpected. Also unexpected, although more plausible, were the results showing the beneficial effect of elevated glucose levels (section 3.2). In light of these results, we had to reevaluate not only the premise of the lactic acidosis hypothesis of cerebral ischemic damage, but also the usefulness of our *in vitro* system as a model of cerebral ischemia. The intriguing possibility that lactic acid is being utilized by neurons upon re-oxygenation, and thus, improved neuronal survival post-hypoxia, as the results in Fig. 4 suggested, led us to reconsider the fundamental principle of energy metabolism namely, that lactic acid (lactate) is an end-product of anaerobic glycolysis with no other function in energy metabolism (Huckabee, 1958). Consequently, our research branched into two avenues: one aiming at re-examining the role of lactate in cerebral energy metabolism, the branch with which this chapter deals, the other attempting to better understand the roles both glucose and lactate play in cerebral ischemic damage, if any.

### 3.4 Cerebral lactate – from a useless end product to a useful energy substrate

#### 3.4.1 Hippocampal slices can utilize lactate as a sole energy substrate to support neuronal function

The results shown in Fig. 4, although hinting at the possibility that lactic acid could be utilized as an oxidative energy substrate, also indicate that an acidic pH is not optimal for such utilization. Thus, in all the experiments described henceforth, when indicated, Na-lactate, rather than lactic acid, was used as a component of the aCSF, while maintaining physiological pH (7.30-7.35). If neural tissue is capable of utilizing lactate as an energy substrate, the hippocampal slice preparation is probably one of the most suitable systems to test such capability. Fig. 5 illustrates a set of experiments performed with rat hippocampal slices, where their supply of normal, glucose-containing aCSF (10 mM glucose) was replaced with 0 mM glucose aCSF supplemented with 0, 1, 2, 5, 10 or 20 mM lactate. The osmolality of the aCSF was kept at 330 mOsm by adjusting the NaCl concentration. A lactate supplementation of 2 mM or higher was enough to maintain normal neuronal function in a great majority of the slices. This breakthrough demonstration that neural tissue is capable of maintaining normal function when lactate is the sole energy substrate, was published in detail almost a quarter of century ago (Schurr et al. 1988b). In that publication it was also demonstrated that oxidative lactate utilization by hippocampal slices is insensitive to the glycolytic inhibitor iodoacetic acid, which indicates that lactate enters the mitochondrial tricarboxylic acid (TCA) cycle directly via its conversion to pyruvate by lactate dehydrogenase, not through the glycolytic pathway. Needless to say, these findings have

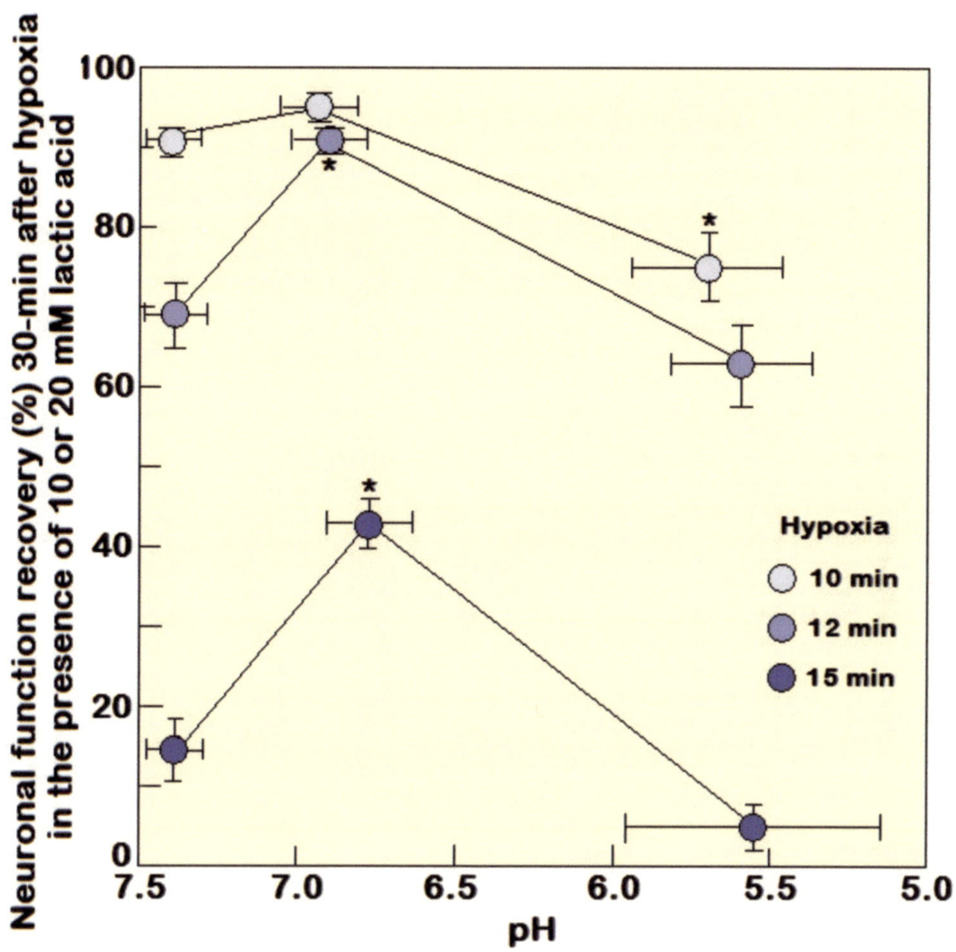


Fig. 4. The effects of lactic acidosis combined with hypoxia on the ability of hippocampal slices to recover their neuronal function 30 min post-hypoxia. At pH values approaching those found in the ischemic brain *in vivo* i.e., 6.5-6.9, lactic acidosis significantly improve the recovery of neuronal function at 12- and 15-min hypoxic durations. At lower pH values, values that are rarely reached *in vivo* (5.5-5.7) some aggravation of neuronal damage was observed, but only with the shorter (10 min) hypoxic period. Bars are means ± SD; *significantly different from control slices supplied with normal, glucose-containing aCSF, pH 7.3-7.35 ($P < 0.0005$).

challenged the long-established dogma of lactate's fate in energy metabolism and thus have faced much skepticism and even ridicule. Clarke & Sokoloff (1994) actually recognized the ability of brain slices, homogenates or cell-free fractions to utilize lactate, pyruvate and other compounds as energy substrates, but have listed several reasons why they cannot be considered to be significant alternatives to glucose *in vivo*. Consequently, the prevailing notion at the time among the majority of scientists in the field had been that lactate utilization by brain slices is an *in vitro* oddity without any significant ramifications for the *in vivo* situation. Obviously, our findings were not, in any way, meant to challenge the leading role glucose plays in normal aerobic energy metabolism.

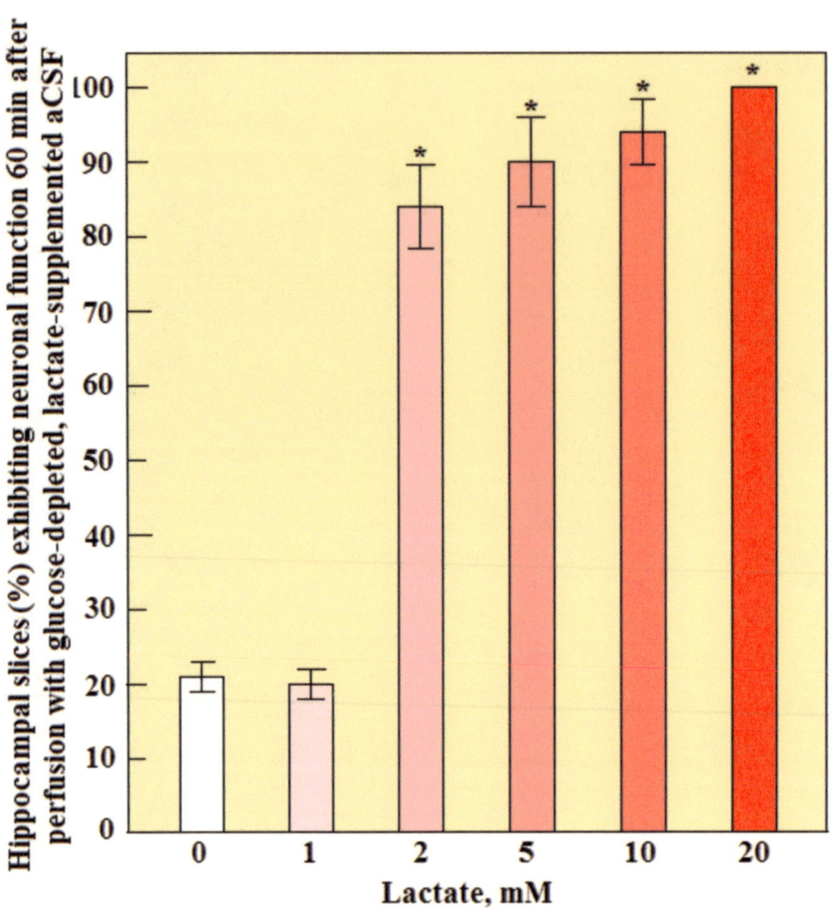


Fig. 5. The ability of hippocampal slices to maintain neuronal function in glucose-depleted, lactate-supplemented aCSF over a period of 60 min. Twenty percent of the slices supplemented with 0 or 1 mM lactate-aCSF still exhibited neuronal function after 60 min, but could not maintained it for an additional 30 min. Bars are means ± SD; *significantly different from 0 mM lactate-aCSF ($P < 0.0005$).

### 3.4.2 Lactate utilization post-hypoxia is crucial and obligatory for recovery of neuronal function

The demonstration that neural tissue is capable of utilizing lactate aerobically, invited a look into the possible role that this monocarboxylate plays in the brain under conditions where glucose is limited or unavailable. One such possible condition is the utilization of lactate accumulating in cerebral tissue during hypoxia/ischemia, upon re-oxygenation, when tissue glucose and ATP levels are very low. The hippocampal slice preparation again proved itself to be a most adept system, allowing manipulations that are impossible *in vivo* to test the role lactate plays in the recovery of neuronal function upon re-oxygenation post-hypoxia. The picture that emerged from this set of experimental paradigms also confirmed the original finding that neural tissue can function normally when lactate is the sole energy

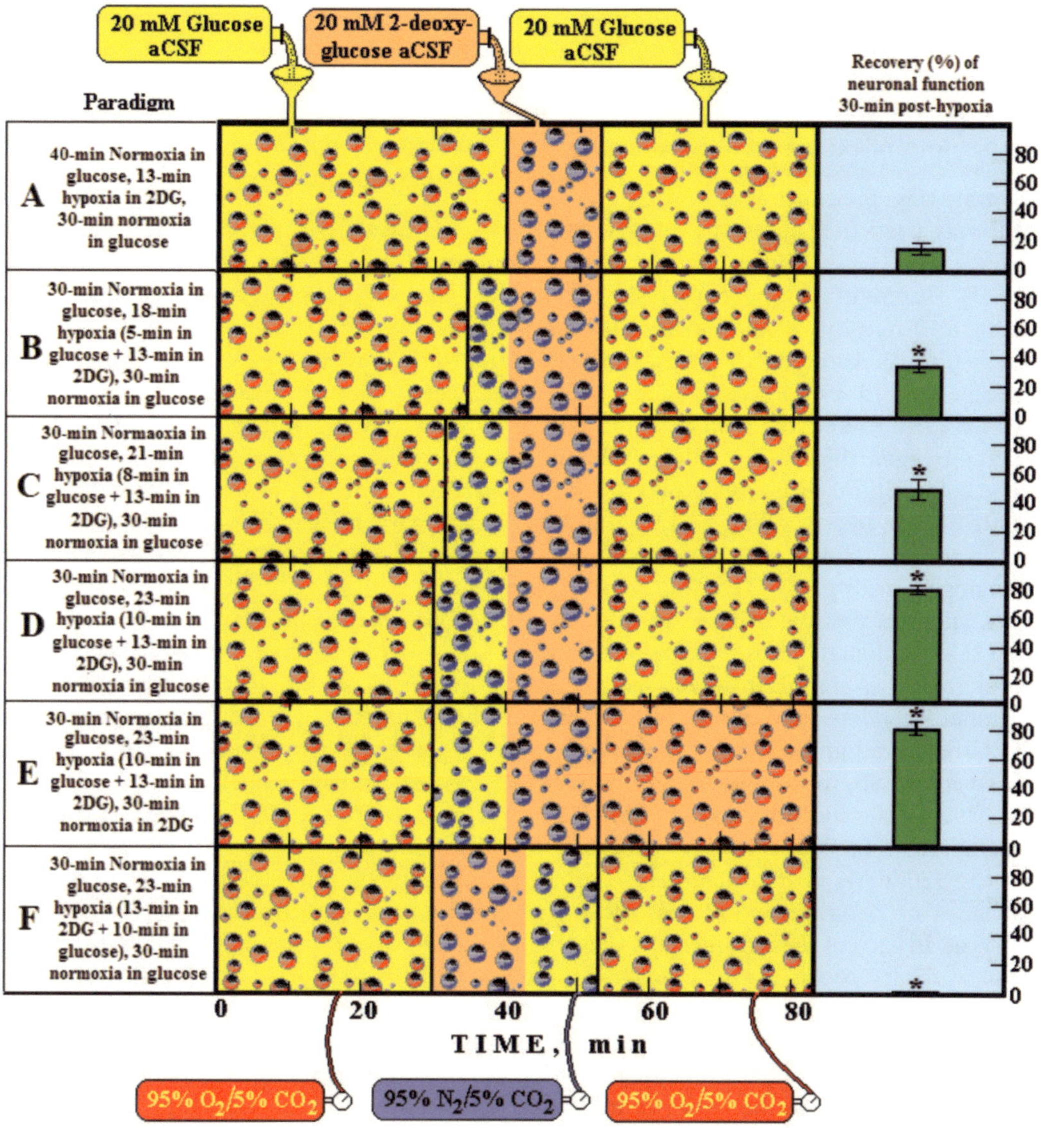


Fig. 6. A schematic representation of six different experimental paradigms using rat hippocampal slices and electrophysiological recording of CA1 evoked population spikes (PS, neuronal function). In each experimental paradigm, slices were supplied either with 20 mM glucose-aCSF (yellow bottle) or 20 mM 2-deoxy glucose (2DG)-aCSF (orange bottle) and the gas mixture bubbled through the dual incubation chamber and the aCSF was either 95% $O_2$/5% $CO_2$ (normoxia, red bubbles) or 95% $N_2$/5% $CO_2$ (hypoxia, blue bubbles). At the end of each experimental paradigm, all slices in each compartment of the dual chamber were tested for the presence of neuronal function. Functional slices are shown as percentage of the total number of slices present (green histograms on the right). Accordingly, by following the timeline from left to right, paradigm A is a protocol in which slices were incubated under normoxic conditions for 40 min, followed by 13-min hypoxia in the presence of 2DG and

then re-oxygenated for 30 min in the presence of glucose. Under these conditions less than 20% of the slices recovered their neuronal function at the end of the 80-min protocol. Similarly, each of the remaining paradigms (B-F) describes its corresponding protocol and its outcome in terms of percentage of slices exhibiting neuronal function. Bars are means ± SD; *significantly different from paradigm A ($P < 0.0005$).

substrate (Fig. 5; Schurr et al., 1988b). In all six paradigms a relatively high glucose level (20 mM) was used that allowed a long enough hypoxic insult without causing a significant damage to the tissue (Fig. 3) yet, had produced measureable levels of anaerobic tissue lactate (Fig. 7). Supplying hippocampal slices with the glucose analog 2-deoxy glucose (2DG) during a 13-min hypoxia, an insult that slices incubated in 20 mM glucose aCSF can easily handle (Fig. 3), resulted in a dismal recovery of neuronal function (<20%, paradigm A). Such outcome would be expected, since the tissue was unable to produce glycolytic ATP anaerobically from 2DG, which meant that slices were actually suffering from a combined glucose-oxygen deprivation, an insult much harsher than the deprivation of one or the other. In addition, slices treated according to paradigm A were not able to produce much lactate during hypoxia (Fig. 7). In paradigm B slices were exposed to 18-min hypoxia, the first 5 min of which was continued to be supplied with 20 mM glucose aCSF before changing that supply to 20 mM 2DG aCSF for the remaining 13 min of the hypoxic period. Thus, slices in paradigm B produced lactate for 5 min before the replacement of glucose with 2DG. Although slices in paradigm B were exposed to hypoxia 38% longer than those in paradigm A, a significantly higher percentage of slices in the former recovered their neuronal function at the end of the 30-min re-oxygenation period than in the latter. Similarly, paradigms C and D included even longer hypoxic periods than the hypoxic period in paradigms A and B, yet, the recovery rate of neuronal function in paradigms C and D was significantly higher than that seen in paradigms A or B. Based on earlier experiments (Fig. 3) it would be expected that slices supplied with relatively high level of glucose (20 mM) would tolerate 20-min hypoxia almost unscathed. Considering the outcomes of paradigms B-D it is clear that most of the recovery of neuronal function observed in each of these paradigms was due to the ability of the incubated slices to produce lactate during hypoxia via the glycolytic pathway, which was utilized aerobically during the re-oxygenation period to bring about recovery of neuronal function. Moreover, the longer glucose-supplied slices were allowed to produce lactate during hypoxia, the higher was the recovery rate of neuronal function post-hypoxia. Thus, doubling the time slices were exposed to hypoxia in the presence of 20 mM glucose from 5 min (paradigm B) to 10 min (paradigm D) more than doubled the recovery rate of neuronal function, from 35% to 80%, respectively. The outcome in slices treated according to paradigm E demonstrates that even when glucose supply during re-oxygenation was not renewed (2DG supplementation continued throughout the re-oxygenation period), recovery of function was possible solely on lactate produced during the first 10 min of hypoxia. When the production of lactate was blocked by 2DG supplementation at the onset of hypoxia, none of the slices could recover neuronal function upon re-oxygenation (Paradigm F). Hence, the outcome of the above described experiments (Fig. 6) strongly suggests that, during hypoxia, anaerobic lactate production is crucial for the recovery of neuronal function post-hypoxia. While glucose is clearly an obligatory energy substrate during periods of oxygen deprivation, as glycolysis is the only pathway available for the production of enough ATP to assure the survival of ischemic/hypoxic neural tissue for at least a few minutes, the experiments above show that the oxidative utilization upon re-oxygenation of the anaerobically produced lactate is obligatory for the recovery of the tissue post-hypoxia (Schurr et al., 1997a, b). On one hand, paradigm F in Fig. 6 clearly indicated that without glucose present during the initial stages of hypoxia, the neural tissue suffered a fatal damage and could not recover its neuronal function even when glucose was present during the latter part of the hypoxic period and the re-oxygenation period. On the other hand, paradigm E in Fig. 6 indicated that the presence of glucose during hypoxia in relatively high levels protected neural tissue from fatal damage, while the lactate produced during hypoxia allowed almost a full recovery of neuronal function in the absence of glucose during the re-oxygenation period. These conclusions are supported by results of lactate content analysis in hippocampal slices at several time points during their exposure to normoxic and hypoxic conditions in the presence of glucose or 2DG. Fig. 7 illustrates that the level of lactate produced in hippocampal slices during normoxia is minimal, but steady and similar to the *in vivo* situation. However, upon the initiation of hypoxia, the levels of tissue lactate immediately begin to rise as long as glucose is available, increasing more than 5-fold within 10 min (paradigm D). In the presence of 2DG, the rise in lactate level was insignificant (paradigm F). Concomitantly with the suggestion that lactate is an obligatory energy substrate for recovery of neuronal function post-hypoxia, we also postulated that following a severe hypoxic period that would completely exhaust glucose and ATP supplies, functional recovery would be entirely dependent on ATP that can be produced via a pathway that bypasses glycolysis, since glycolysis is a metabolic pathway that requires ATP investment if glucose is to be utilized. Lactate aerobic utilization via its conversion to pyruvate by lactate dehydrogenase (LDH) allows a direct entry of pyruvate into the mitochondrial tricarboxylic acid (TCA) cycle. This process does not require any ATP investment and can be resumed instantaneously upon re-oxygenation in the presence of lactate. As effective as 2DG was in blocking glucose utilization (Figs. 6 & 7), 2DG is ineffective in blocking or affecting in anyway the utilization of lactate. To expand our investigation into the possible role lactate may play in other cerebral functions, a "blocker" of lactate utilization was needed. The lactate transporter inhibitor, α-cyano-4-hydroxycinamate (4-CIN) is one such blocker (Halestrap & Denton (1975). Lactate and other monocarboxylates, such as pyruvate and β-hydroxybutyrate, are known to be transported via a facilitated diffusion process, similar to the one glucose is being transported across biological membranes. Although these processes always proceeds along the concentration gradient, they do involve the mediation of specific transporters and in the case of lactate a monocarboxylate transporter (MCT), of which several types have been identified (Garcia et al., 1994; Garcia et al., 1995; Gerhart et al., 1997; Broer et al., 1997; Volk et al., 1997). First, 4-CIN was able to block lactate-supplemented slices from exhibiting evoked CA1 population spike without affecting neuronal function of glucose-supported slices (Fig. 8). This simple experiment demonstrated the potential of 4-CIN in blocking the MCT responsible for transporting lactate into cells that utilize it aerobically for the production of ATP. Clearly, blockade of MCT does not interfere with glucose transport or its utilization, including any lactate that may be produced during glucose metabolism. This important ability of 4-CIN to discriminate between glucose and lactate utilization provided not only a great experimental tool, but also helped us in sorting several mechanistic issues, as will be discussed later. First, to assess 4-CIN potential in a familiar paradigm, slices were treated with the blocker in a set of experiments where hypoxia was used to induce accumulation of lactate, which we have shown to be used preferentially post-hypoxia. Fig. 9 illustrates the effects of 4-CIN on both the ability of hippocampal slices to recover their neuronal function after 10-min hypoxia

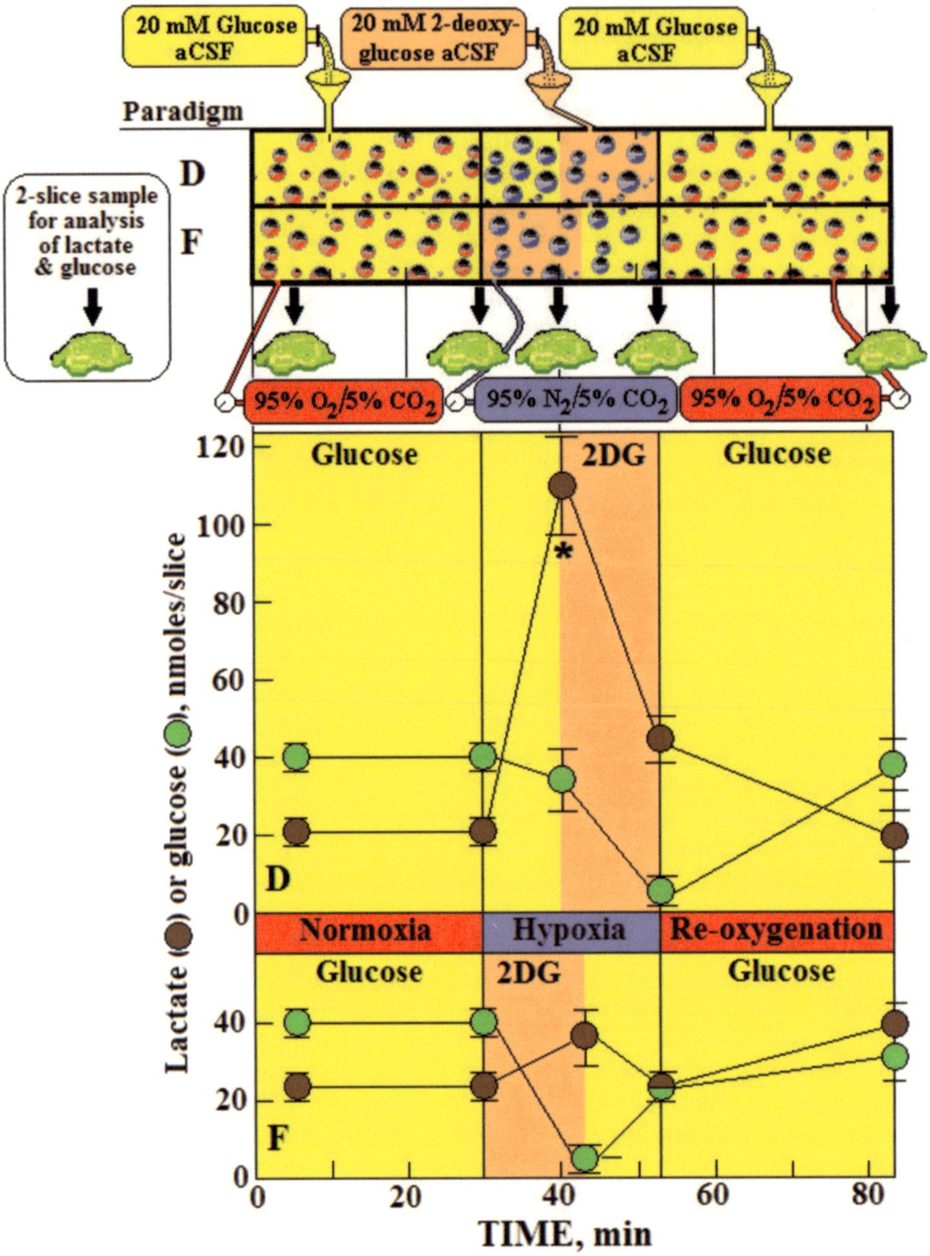


Fig. 7. The levels of lactate and glucose (nmoles/slice), as determined by using enzymatic kits (Schurr et al., 1997a), during the experimental paradigms D and F detailed in Fig. 6. Allowing slices to utilize glucose anaerobically during the first 10 min of a 23-min hypoxia resulted in an over 5-fold increase in tissue lactate content. Changing the supply of glucose to 2DG at the very beginning of a 23-min hypoxia blocked the ability of hippocampal slices to produce lactate via anaerobic glycolysis. Bars are means ± SD; *significantly different from normoxic lactate level ($P<0.05$).

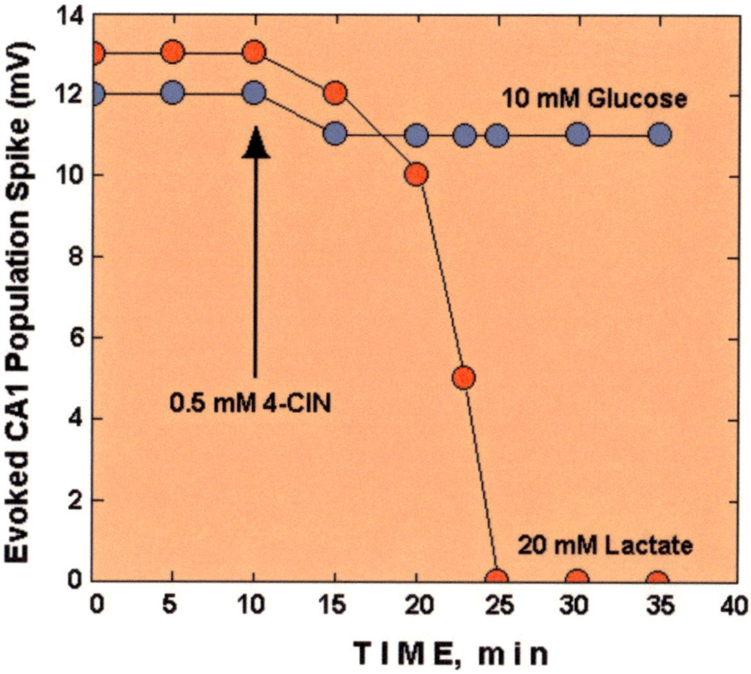


Fig. 8. The effect of adding 0.5 mM α-cyano-4-hydroxycinnamate (4-CIN) to the aCSF in which hippocampal slices were incubated on their ability to exhibit an evoked CA1 population spike. Slices incubated in 10 mM glucose aCSF were unaffected by 4-CIN. Slices incubated in 20 mM lactate could not maintain their evoked response in the presence of 4-CIN, as the inhibitor blocked the transport of lactate into neurons and/or out of astrocytes.

and on tissue levels of lactate and glucose at several time points during the experimental protocol. The inhibition of lactate transport by 4-CIN significantly attenuated the recovery of neuronal function post-hypoxia, most likely by blocking the entry of lactate, which accumulated during the hypoxic period, into cells and possibly mitochondria upon re-oxygenation. This blockade is evident in the post-hypoxic period by the higher lactate tissue content measured in slices treated with 4-CIN. The transporter blocker had no effect on the levels of tissue glucose at any time during the experimental protocol in comparison to control conditions (lack of 4-CIN). Although not shown, a CA1 evoked population spike was completely abolished, as expected, during the hypoxic period. Considering the results shown in both Fig. 8 and Fig. 9, it was concluded that 4-CIN could be used as a chemical tool in the investigation of additional possible roles lactate may play in neural tissue by potentially interfering with any cellular process that requires this monocarboxylate. In 1994, Pellerin & Magistretti hypothesized that the excitation of neurons by the excitatory neurotransmitter, glutamate (Glu), is coupled to its uptake by astrocytes, an uptake that induces aerobic glycolysis, which is responsible for the observed increase in glucose consumption during brain activation. They further hypothesized that the product of this elevated aerobic glycolysis in astrocytes is lactate, which is shuttled from astrocytes to neurons where it is aerobically consumed. This hypothesized transfer of lactate from the former to the latter was named the astrocytic-neuronal lactate shuttle hypothesis or ANLSH

(Pellerin & Magistretti, 1994). The hippocampal slice preparation is an excellent model system for testing the premise of the ANLSH.

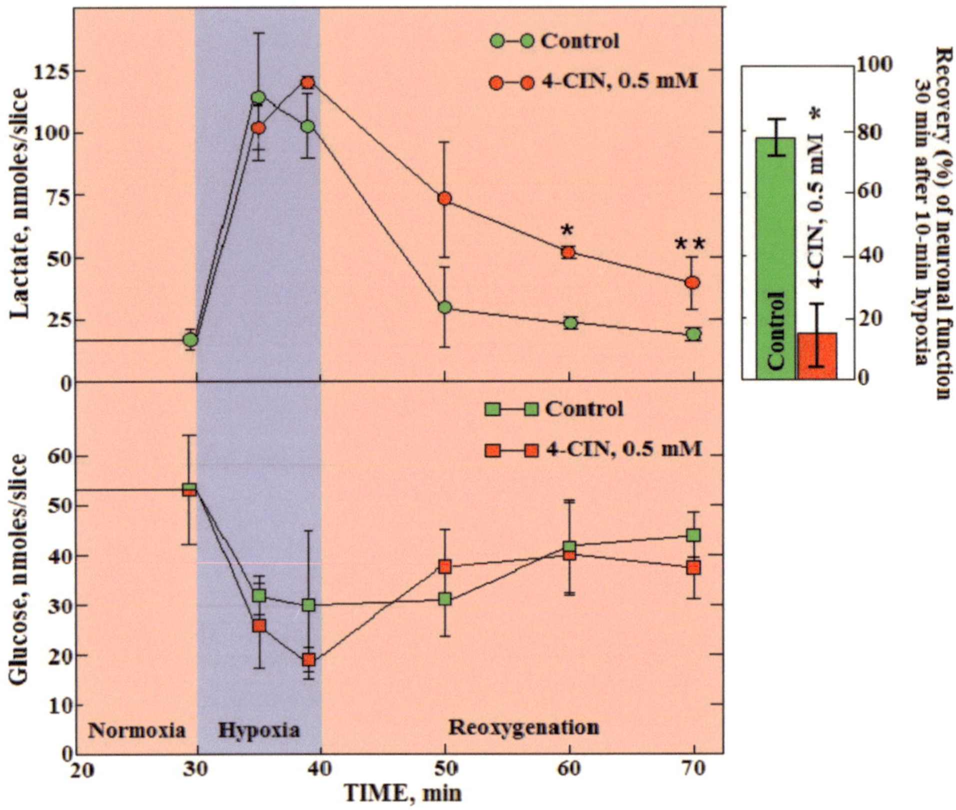


Fig. 9. The effects of α-cyano-4-hydroxycinnamate (4-CIN) on the recovery of neuronal function post-hypoxia in hippocampal slices and the levels of lactate and glucose in these slices at several times points along the experimental protocol. Glucose concentration in the aCSF was 10 mM. Normoxia was achieved by supplying slices with 95% $O_2$/5% $CO_2$. Hypoxia was created by replacing the normoxic atmosphere with 95% $N_2$/5% $CO_2$. Bars are means ± SD; *significantly different from control ($P < 0.0005$); **significantly different from control ($P < 0.05$).

### 3.4.3 Lactate as an aerobic energy substrate for excited neurons

In testing the potential role of lactate in neuronal activation by glutamate, only relatively small changes were made in the experimental paradigms that already proved themselves useful when hypoxia was the insult applied to neurons (Figs 6, 7, 9). Supplying hippocampal slices with aCSF containing high, excitotoxic concentrations of Glu is similar in its detrimental effect on neurons to that of hypoxia. Actually, Glu's excitotoxicity has been suggested to be part of the hypoxic/ischemic mechanism of neuronal damage (Olney, 1969, 1990; Novelli et al., 1988, Choi, 1988; Siesjö, 1988; Schurr & Rigor, 1989; Henneberry, 1989; Cox et al., 1989; Choi & Rothman, 1990). Figure 10 summarizes the results of two sets of

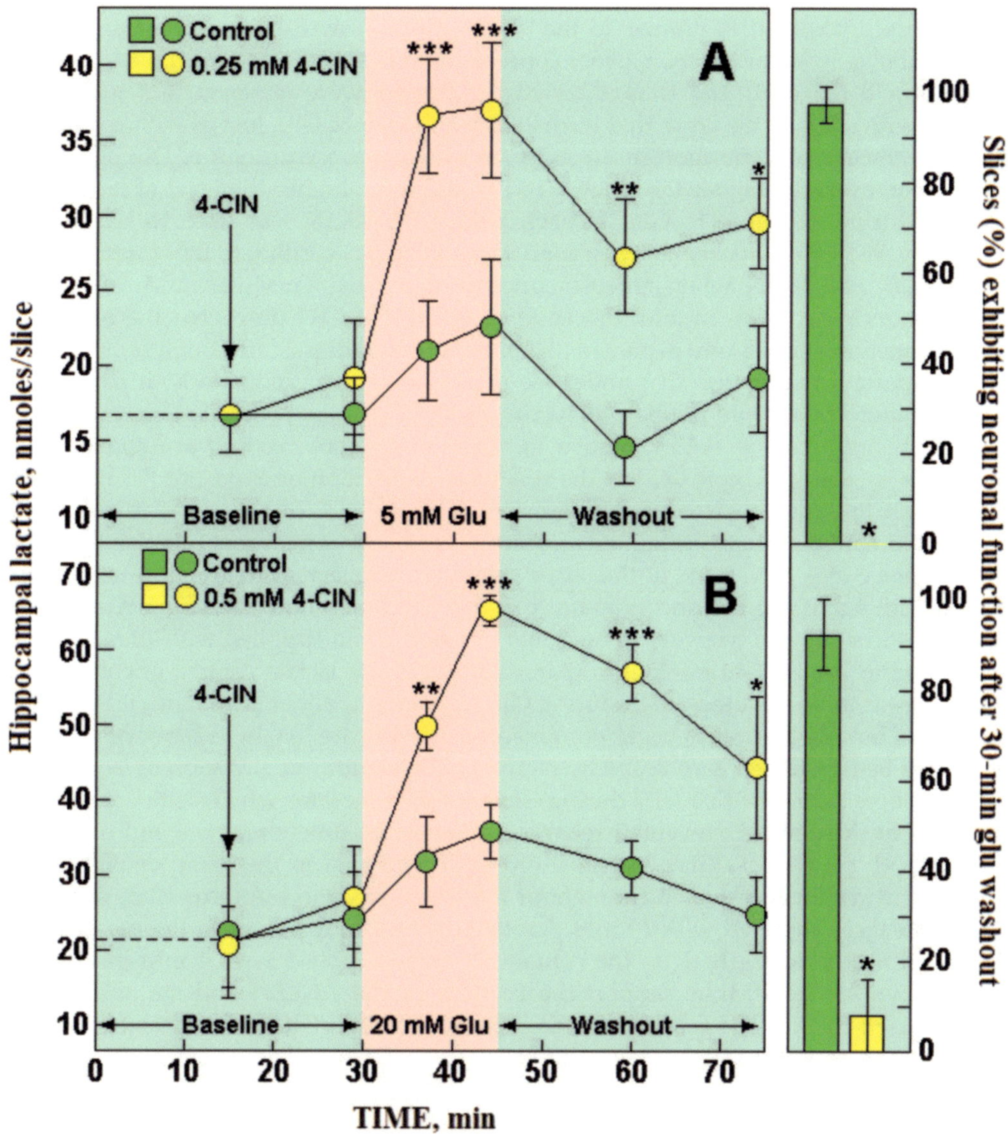


Fig. 10. The effect of 15-min exposure to glutamate (Glu) on the ability of hippocampal slices to recover their neuronal function following a 30-min Glu washout and on the content of tissue lactate at several time points during the two experimental paradigms used: (A) Perfusion of slices with 4 mM glucose aCSF for 30 min, followed by a 15-min exposure to 5 mM Glu, followed by a 30-min washout with 4 mM glucose aCSF, either in the presence of 0.25 mM 4-CIN (yellow symbols) or in the absence of 4-CIN (green symbols); (B) perfusion of slices with 10 mM glucose aCSF, followed by a 15-min exposure to 20 mM Glu, followed by a 30-min washout with 10 mM glucose aCSF in the presence of 0.5 mM 4-CIN (yellow symbols) or in the absence of 4-CIN (green symbols). Bars are means ± SD; significantly different from control (*$P < 0.003$; **$P < 0.01$; ***$P < 0.004$).

experimental paradigms in which exposure to Glu for a given period of time was used as an excitatory/excitotoxic event similar to the way hypoxia was used in earlier experiments described above. In paradigm A, glucose concentration in the aCSF (4 mM) was lower than in paradigm B (10 mM) and thus slices in the former were exposed to 5 mM Glu as compared with slices in the latter that were exposed to 20 mM Glu. Just as with hypoxia, the higher the glucose concentration in the aCSF, the higher concentration of Glu slices could tolerate. Moreover, the higher the glucose in the aCSF, the higher the level of lactate slices produced during exposure to Glu. In each paradigm, 4-CIN was used to block lactate transport by MCT. The blocker concentration was adjusted according to the concentration of glucose; 0.25 mM 4-CIN when glucose concentration was 4 mM, 0.5 mM 4-CIN when glucose concentration was 10 mM. Blockade of MCT by 4-CIN prevented the recovery of neuronal function after 15-min exposure to Glu in both paradigms. Although not seen in Fig. 10, it is important to mention that under the experimental conditions in both paradigms a CA1 population spike could not be evoked during the 15-min exposure to Glu regardless of the presence or absence of 4-CIN, similar to when slices were exposed to hypoxia. Glu at these levels is clearly excitotoxic, but the relatively short time of exposure (15 min) is not long enough to cause an irreversible damage, as over 90% of the slices under control conditions in both paradigms exhibited almost full recovery of neuronal function. However, in the presence of 4-CIN, none of the slices exhibited recovery of neuronal function when supplied with 4 mM glucose and exposed to 5 mM Glu for 15 min (Paradigm A). Less than 10% of the slices showed recovery of neuronal function when supplied with 10 mM glucose and exposed to 20 mM Glu for 15 min (paradigm B). While lactate content of control slices did not appear to be elevated much during Glu exposure in either paradigm, it is probably indicative of how fast lactate is being produced upon exposure to Glu in astrocytes and how quickly it is being utilized aerobically by neurons. The significant elevation in lactate tissue content of slices treated with 4-CIN during Glu exposure explains why lactate unavailability to neurons in these slices prevented recovery of neuronal function at the end of washout period in both paradigms. Since lactate could not be utilized in the presence of 4-CIN, its tissue content remained elevated throughout the washout period. As expected, the content of lactate in slices supplied with 10 mM glucose during Glu exposure in the presence of 4-CIN was almost twice as high as the content in slices supplied with 4 mM glucose. The results shown in Fig. 10 thus support the premise of the ANLSH and are schematically summarized in Fig. 11. The outcome of the experiments with Glu above (see also Schurr et al., 1999a, b) strongly indicates that the activation of neural tissue with an excitatory neurotransmitter increases the utilization of glucose via aerobic glycolysis and a large elevation in lactate production. The only difference between the effects of Glu and hypoxia on neural tissue is that in the former, lactate is produced in the presence of oxygen, while in the latter it is produced in the absence of oxygen. In both cases, glycolysis is the main pathway to provide the extra energy required to assure survival of the neural tissue during either insult. Moreover, as indicated by the effects of 4-CIN in the presence of Glu or hypoxia, the glycolytic product, lactate, is the oxidative energy substrate that secures the recovery of neuronal function post-Glu activation or post-hypoxia. In the debate that has ensued after Pellerin & Magistretti (1994) proposed the ANLSH (Tsacopoulos & Magistretti, 1996; Magistretti, 1999, 2000; Magistretti et al., 1999; Pellerin & Magistretti, 2003, 2004a, b; Chih & Roberts, 2003; Hertz, 2004; Schurr, 2006) the skeptics have tended to reject the hypothesis mainly on its premise that lactate is postulated to be a major oxidative energy substrate, not on the proposed lactate shuttle *per se*. The debate is not limited to the ANLSH;

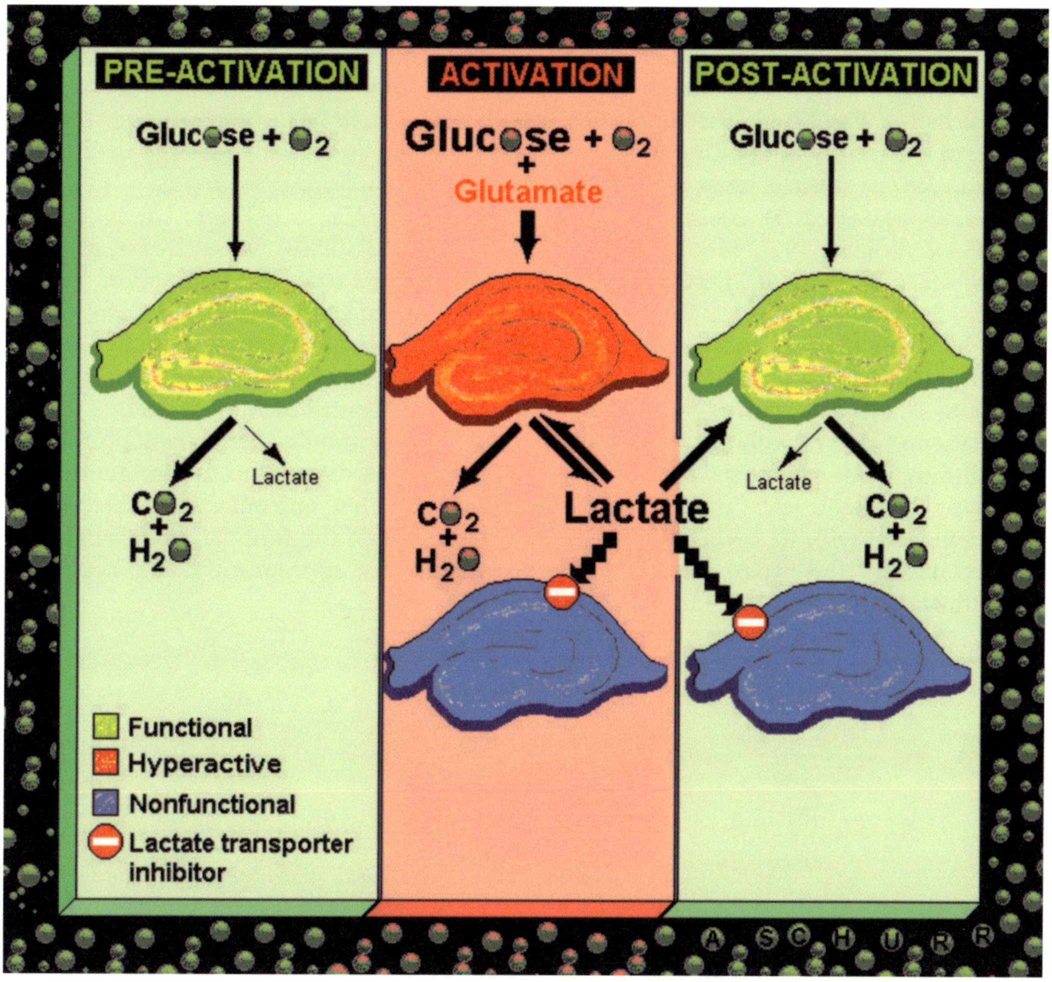


Fig. 11. A schematic representation of the biochemical events that took place in the experiments shown in Fig. 10. The first panel on the left (green) depicts a neuronally functional hippocampal slice (green-yellow) under resting baseline conditions, supplied with glucose and oxygen and produces mainly $CO_2$, $H_2O$ and a minimal amount of lactate. The middle panel (red) depicts the same hippocampal slice when exposed to Glu (red), which increases aerobic glucose utilization and lactate production. When this hippocampal slice is also treated with a monocarboxylate transporter inhibitor that prevents lactate from being transported from astrocytes to neurons, the slice cannot remain functional (blue). The panel on the right (green) depicts the hippocampal slice (green-yellow) of the upper middle panel from which Glu has been washed out, allowing its neuronal function to recover and its energy production to return to baseline conditions. Also shown is a slice (blue) that was treated with a monocarboxylate transporter inhibitor during the exposure to Glu and thus could not recover its neuronal function despite Glu washout.

it is still raging about a similar hypothesis of lactate shuttles in other tissues, which preceded the ANLSH and for the same reason (see Gladden, 2004, for review). The objection to the idea of a major role for lactate in energy metabolism beyond just being a waste product or, at best, a minor player, is understandable. The dogma of glucose's obligatory role in energy metabolism in all tissues, organs and most aerobic organisms is an inseparable part of our understanding and acceptance of this process as formulated during the first half of the 20th century. However, experimental data have emerged over the past quarter of a century, all pointing to a major role for lactate in oxidative energy metabolism in brain, skeletal muscle, heart and probably many other mammalian tissues. These data (Brooks, 1985, 1998, 2000, 2002a, b; Schurr et al., 1988b, 1997a, b, 1999a, b; Larrabee, 1995, 1996; Hu & Wilson, 1997; Brooks et al., 1999; Mangia et al., 2003; Kassischke et al., 2004; Ivanov et al., 2011) in addition to several forgotten studies from the first half of the 20th century (Ashford & Holmes, 1929, 1931; Holmes, 1930; Holmes & Ashford, 1930; Flock et al., 1938), impelled me to hypothesize that lactate is the ultimate cerebral oxidative energy substrate in the brain (Schurr, 2006) and possibly in other organs and tissues. The electrophysiological experiments described here have contributed enormously to the formulation of this hypothesis. The ability to continuously monitor the function of neural tissue throughout each experiment and its many replications allowed us to confidently state what we understood to be the meaning of these experiments' outcome. The other studies cited here, each with its own methodology, only strengthen the foundation on which the interpretation of the experimental results was made and, consequently, the hypothesis herewith was postulated.

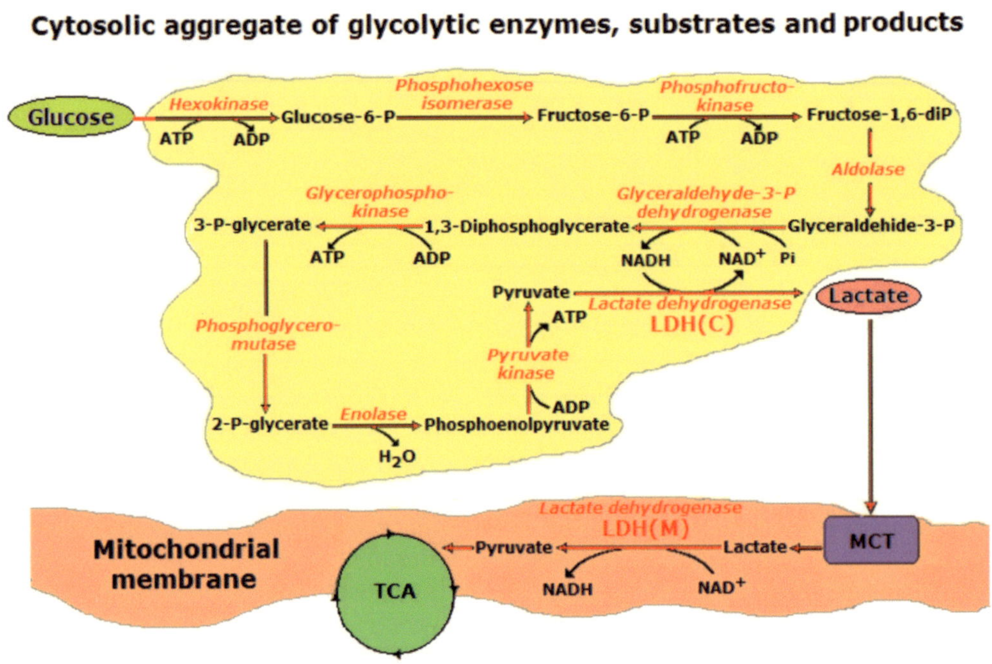


Fig. 12. A schematic illustration of a hypothesis first presented elsewhere (Schurr, 2006), postulating lactate, not pyruvate, to be the end product of aerobic glycolysis. This hypothesis is founded on thermodynamic and other considerations, including data from many studies spanning almost eight decades of research by scientists in laboratories all around the world. The illustration shows the glycolytic apparatus as an aggregate of the glycolytic enzymes, all in close proximity to each other, as required by such a pathway for a

maximized efficient output, with the entry of glucose into this pathway on the upper left side and an exit of lactate from the pathway on the right side through the action of cytosolic lactate dehydrogenase [LDH(C)]. Lactate is shuttled via an intracellular shuttle to the mitochondrial membrane, where it is converted back into pyruvate via mitochondrial lactate dehydrogenase [LDH(M)] and into the tricarboxylic acid (TCA) cycle.

### 3.4.4 Lactate, not pyruvate, is neuronal aerobic glycolysis end-product

Although the role of lactate in energy metabolism, both in the adult brain and other organs and tissues is controversial, more and more studies have produced an increasing amount of data in support of such a role, especially under certain conditions. Over the twenty odd years of using the hippocampal slice preparation and its electrophysiology and in consideration of the accumulated data from other studies during that period, the concept of lactate as a major player in brain energy metabolism seems to gather steam; not only under certain conditions, such as post-hypoxia or during neural activation, but as an integral intermediate of the normal cellular process of glucose conversion to ATP i.e., aerobic glycolysis and oxidative phosphorylation. Therefore, a hypothesis was put forward according to which in the brain (and possibly in other organs and tissues) lactate is the principal product of both aerobic and anaerobic glycolysis (Schurr, 2006). This hypothesis is schematically illustrated in Fig. 12. Additional evidence to support it could be provided by an efficient and specific lactate dehydrogenase inhibitor(s). The availability of enzymatic inhibitors in the study of the roles of enzymes, their substrates and products in any given metabolic pathway is paramount for the elucidation and understanding of these roles. For years, the absence of specific and efficient inhibitors for the two LDH-catalyzed reactions, the conversion of pyruvate to lactate in the cytosol by LDH(C), and the conversion of lactate to pyruvate by the mitochondrial form of the enzyme, LDH(M), has greatly impeded the assessment of lactate's role in energy metabolism. According to the prevailing dogma, pyruvate is the main end product of aerobic glycolysis. If specific and efficient LDH inhibitors exist, [X inhibitor for LDH(C) and Y inhibitor for LDH(M)], one could predict that, according to the prevailing dogma, glucose-supported neuronal function in a fully oxygenated hippocampal slice preparation would not be affected by either inhibitor, since LDH (either C or M form) does not participate in the conversion of glucose to pyruvate. However, if lactate, according to the above-mentioned hypothesis (Fig. 12), is the end product of aerobic glycolysis or if it is supplied exogenously as the sole energy substrate, neuronal function would be suppressed by inhibitor Y, but not by inhibitor X. Although the latter would inhibit lactate formation from glucose, it should not prevent glucose conversion to pyruvate and therefore, its utilization by mitochondria. Practically, all known LDH inhibitors, inefficient as they may be, exhibit both X and Y inhibitory capabilities, although with different potencies toward one reaction or the other. Hence, an inhibitor showing stronger Y than X inhibitory capability should be innocuous in inhibiting pyruvate-supported neuronal function yet, be able to suppress lactate-supported neuronal function. Moreover, if lactate is the end product of aerobic glycolysis, as the hypothesis postulates, then, glucose-supported neuronal function should be suppressed by an LDH inhibitor with Y>X inhibitory capability to the same degree that it would suppress lactate-supported neuronal function, since it should inhibit the LDH(M) form. However, because such an inhibitor can also inhibit the LDH(C) form, although to a lesser and slower extent, one could expect that, after a while, pyruvate would begin to accumulate, becoming the main product of glycolysis. Consequently, over time, pyruvate would, essentially, become the main glycolytic product and therefore the main substrate for the mitochondrial TCA cycle, an occurrence that should fully or partially relieve the initial suppression of neuronal function. Hence, the availability of a specific, efficient LDH inhibitor would clarify lactate's role in cerebral aerobic energy metabolism. Recently, malonate, a known competitive inhibitor of succinate dehydrogenase, has been shown to inhibit the conversion of lactate to pyruvate (Saad et al., 2006). Malonate is a dicarboxylate that is transported into neurons, astrocytes and mitochondria via the same transporter that tranports succinate (Yodoya et al., 2006; Aliverdieva et al., 2006). With the availability of malonate we were able to perform a series of electrophysiological experiments aimed at testing the hypothesis that the end product of aerobic glycolysis in cerebral tissue is lactate (Schurr & Payne, 2007). In this set of experiments, we used much lower concentrations of the different energy substrates, as compared to other experiments described above, although sufficient for sustenance of normal neuronal function. It was verified by a separate set of experiments that 2.5 mM glucose, 5 mM lactate and 5 mM pyruvate (equicaloric concentrations) were all able to sustain similar and healthy evoked population spike (PS) amplitudes (data not shown). These "low" concentrations of the energy substrates that are closer to their *in vivo* levels were chosen in order to "sensitize" the hippocampal slice preparation to the effects of both malonate and Glu, while allowing also the use of relatively low malonate (10 mM) and Glu (2.5 mM) concentrations. As can be seen from Fig. 13, malonate (M) drastically attenuated the amplitude of lactate-supported evoked hippocampal CA1 PS, as can be seen from the two representative traces before (L) and after 75-min exposure to malonate (L + M). As predicted, lactate-supplemented slices were clearly susceptible to malonate, exhibiting a time-dependent diminishment in PS amplitude, while malonate was innocuous when slices were supplemented with pyruvate (P, P + M). Thus malonate appears to be an efficient inhibitor of the LDH(M) form, inhibition that slow down significantly the conversion of lactate to pyruvate, resulting in the suppression of neuronal function. Since pyruvate can directly enter the mitochondrial TCA cycle, as it is transported by the same transporter of lactate (MCT), pyruvate-supported neuronal function is unaffected by malonate. Furthermore, initially, glucose-supplemented slices, exhibited suppression of neuronal function by malonate (45′, G + M), a suppression that was relieved later on (75′, G + M). This outcome is the very scenario that was predicted above; malonate, being an LDH inhibitor with stronger inhibitory potency toward LDH(M) than toward LDH(C), would initially block mainly the conversion of lactate to pyruvate, strongly suggesting that lactate is eventually the end product of aerobic glycolysis, as expressed by the partial suppression of neuronal function (45′, G + M). However, being also an inhibitor of LDH(C), over time, malonate would also inhibit that form of the enzyme, blocking the conversion of pyruvate to lactate in the glycolytic pathway, bringing about the accumulation of pyruvate and its utilization by the mitochondrial TCA cycle, as expressed by the recovery of neuronal function (75′, G + M). Hence, these results support the hypothesis that postulates lactate to be the end product of cerebral aerobic glycolysis. These results also confirm that, for lactate to be utilized aerobically, it must first be converted to pyruvate via the LDH(M). One additional set of experiments was performed (Schurr & Payne, 2007), which provided further support for the major role lactate plays in cerebral energy metabolism (Fig. 14). This set tested the combined effect of Glu and malonate and emphasized the importance of lactate as a mitochondrial energy substrate for the maintenance of neuronal function during neural activation, whether lactate originates in neurons or astrocytes. That malonate is

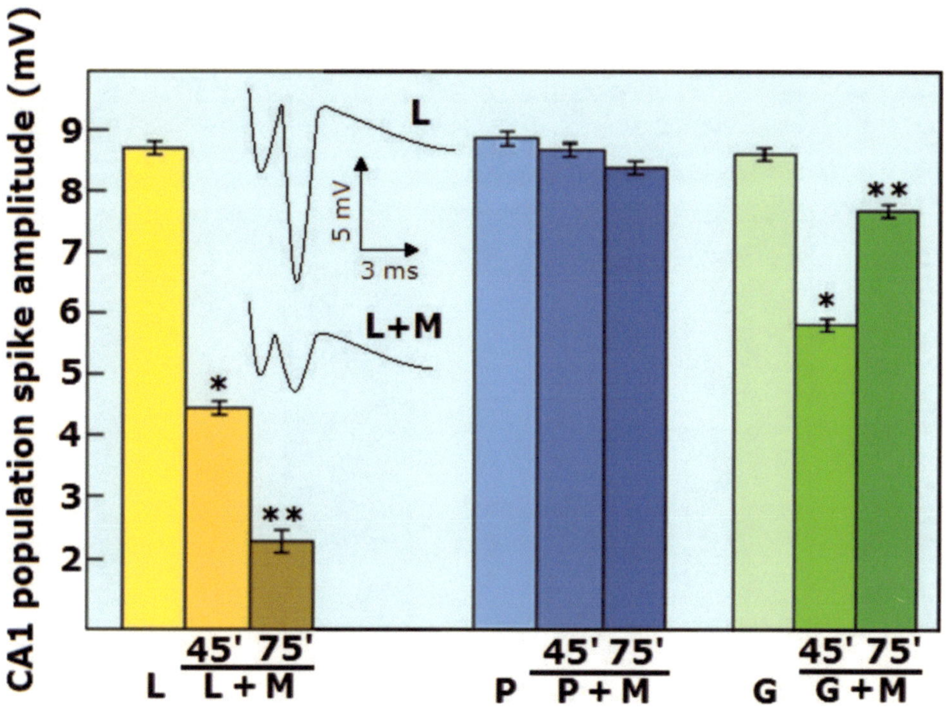


Fig. 13. The effect of the LDH inhibitor, malonate (M, 10 mM) on the evoked CA1 population spike amplitude (neuronal function) of rat hippocampal slices maintained in aCSF containing either lactate (L, 5 mM), pyruvate (P, 5 mM) or glucose (G, 2.5 mM). Malonate progressively inhibited lactate-supported neuronal function over time and was innocuous against pyruvate-supported neuronal function. Malonate initially inhibited glucose-supported neuronal function, inhibition that was later mostly relieved. Bars are means ± SEM; * significantly different from energy substrate alone; **significantly different from energy substrate or energy substrate + malonate at 45 min ($P$<0.0001).

detrimental to neuronal viability of glutamate-activated, glucose-supported hippocampal slices is apparent from the partial recovery (50%) of the energy-dependent PS amplitude (Fig. 14). This outcome indicates that lactate, whether neuronal or astrocytic in origin, is crucial for neuronal viability upon excitation. Alternatively, the outcome of these experiments may be explained by postulating an increase in astrocytic glucose consumption and lactate production in response to glutamate uptake, whereupon lactate becomes a major neuronal energy substrate (Pellerin & magistretti, 1994; Schurr et al., 1999). Any interference with neuronal utilization of astrocytic lactate under this scenario i.e., LDH inhibition by malonate, would suppress normal neuronal function. However, such suppression should be overcome if astrocytes, while incapable of producing lactate in the presence of malonate, would produce enough pyruvate, which would be sufficient, upon Glu washout, to fuel neuronal function recovery, as observed in slices supplied with exogenous pyruvate (Fig. 14). Nevertheless, such recovery did not occur, indicating that astrocytic pyruvate, if it had been produced during exposure to Glu and malonate, is not readily available to neurons, in contrast to astrocytic lactate and neuronal pyruvate. Why is 2.5 mM glucose, in contrast to

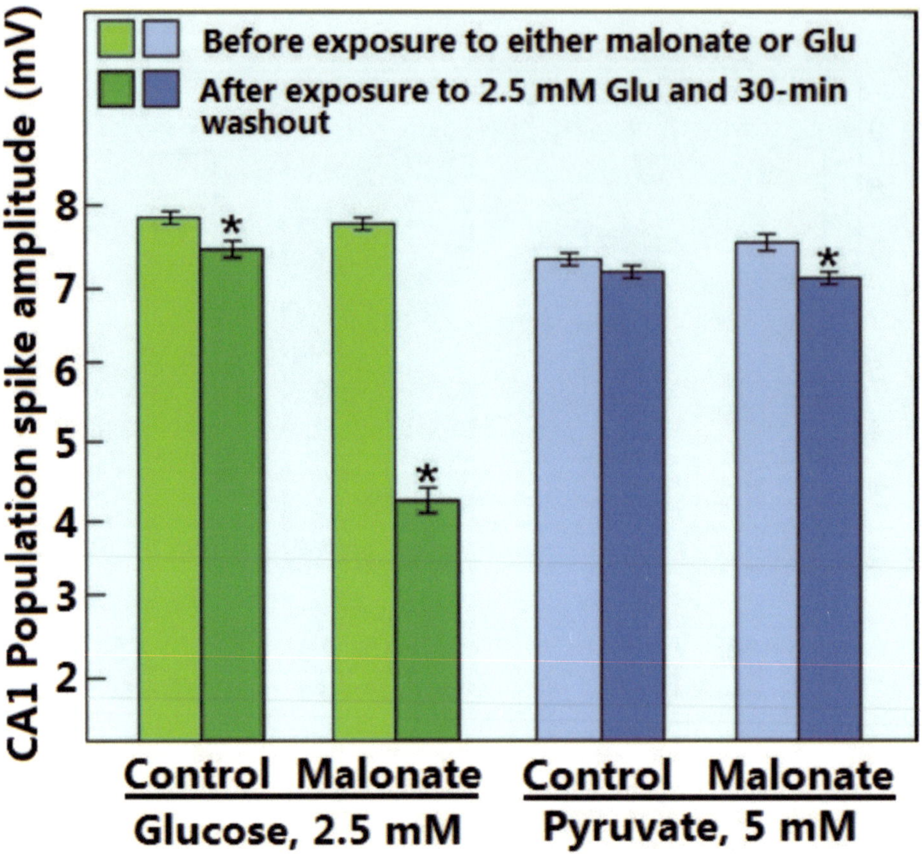


Fig. 14. The effect of 20-min exposure to glutamate (Glu, 2.5 mM) on hippocampal CA1 evoked population spike (PS, neuronal function) in the absence or presence of the LDH inhibitor, malonate (10 mM) when either glucose (2.5 mM) or pyruvate (5 mM) was the sole energy substrate. Slices maintained in glucose-aCSF could not recover their PS amplitude following Glu washout in the presence of malonate as compared to those maintained in the absence of malonate or those maintained with pyruvate wether malonate was absent or present. Bars are means ± SEM; *significantly different from the mean values before exposure to either malonate or Glu ($P<0.01$).

5 mM pyruvate, was unable to sustain neuronal viability in slices treated both with malonate and Glu? It is possible that not all the available glucose is converted to pyruvate under these conditions. However, a more compelling possibility is that glucose cannot increase the rate of mitochondrial respiration under aerobic conditions, while lactate, and most likely pyruvate, can. Levasseur et al. (2006) have demonstrated that glucose sustains mitochondrial respiration at low, "fixed" rate, since, despite increasing the glucose concentration nearly 100-fold, oxygen consumption was not up-regulated. In contrast, an increase in lactate concentration did elevate mitochondrial oxygen consumption, plausibly allowing mitochondria to meet heightened energy demands. Consequently, glucose-supplemented and oxygenated hippocampal slices are incapable of increasing their mitochondrial respiration rate in response to activation by Glu, since they are unable to up-

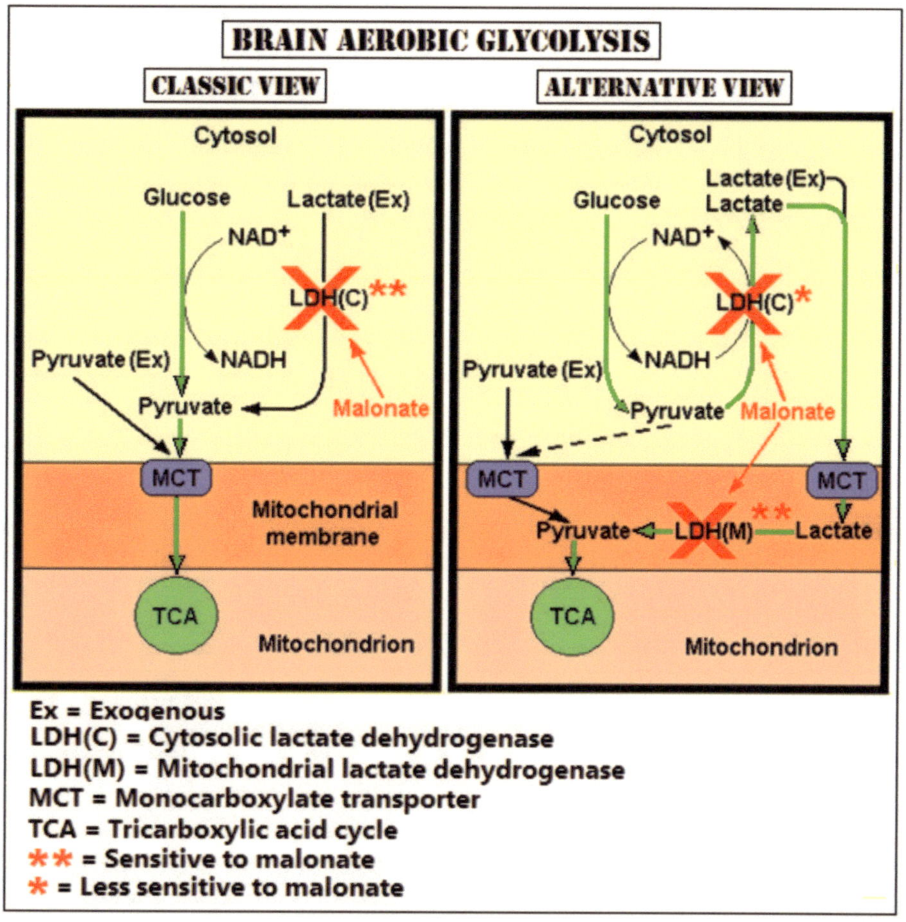


Fig. 15. Two views of aerobic glycolysis. The classic view depicts pyruvate as the glycolytic pathway's end product (green arrows, left panel) and thus as the pathway that should not be affected by an LDH inhibitor such as malonate in supplying pyruvate to mitochondria. The results shown in Figs. 13 & 14 cannot be explained by this view. The alternative view of the aerobic glycolytic pathway postulates lactate to be its end product (green arrows, right panel, Schurr, 2006). Since glycolytically-produced lactate must be converted to pyruvate to allow the latter to enter the TCA cycle, this alternative view explains the ability of malonate to interfere with glucose-supported neuronal function as shown in Fig. 13 (right side histograms). However, over time, malonate's weaker inhibiting activity of the conversion of pyruvate to lactate will shift the glycolytic conversion of glucose from lactate to pyruvate, at which time, the latter could become the main glycolytic end product and the mitochondrial substrate (broken arrow, right panel), relieving the suppression of neuronal function observed earlier when glucose is the energy substrate (Fig. 13).

regulate their glycolytic flux. More recently, Ivanov et al. (2011) have demonstrated that lactate can cover the energy needs of activated neonatal hippocampal slices and that lactate utilization augmented oxidative phosphorylation. Normally, both neuronal and astrocytic lactate produced from glucose would overcome this limitation (see Fig. 14, control glucose,

2.5 mM), but in the presence of malonate this avenue is unavailable (Fig. 14, malonate, glucose, 2.5 mM). Obviously, exogenous lactate would be useless in the presence of malonate, which is the reason why results with lactate-supported slices are not shown. Nonetheless, the results of the experiments that combined Glu and malonate in slices supplemented with 2.5 mM glucose (Fig. 14) suggest that under this condition there is an augmented shortfall in lactate (or pyruvate) supply. This outcome emphasizes the importance of lactate both at rest and during neural activation. These results (Fig. 14) cannot be explained by the classic depiction of aerobic glycolysis (Fig. 15, left panel) however, the hypothesis that lactate is the end product of aerobic glycolysis (schurr, 2006) could be a suitable explanation (Fig. 15, right panel). Therefore, it was concluded that the results, as shown in Figs. 13 & 14, support this hypothesis and signal that lactate is the most plausible mitochondrial energy substrate in the brain (and possibly in other organs and tissues), especially under neural activation.

## 4. Conclusion

The original intent of employing the rat hippocampal slice preparation and its electrophysiology in our laboratory was to establish an *in vitro* model system of cerebral ischemia/hypoxia. It has proved itself to be an excellent model system for that purpose. However, some key experiments have yielded unexpected results that have challenged conventional dogmas and "common knowledge." These unexpected results, a repeating theme throughout the history of science and its major discoveries, have spurred debates and reexamination of those dogmas.

The present chapter describes the more provocative of those results, dealing with cerebral energy metabolism and the role lactate plays in these most important and basic cellular pathways. As important, considering the purpose of the book of which this chapter is a part, the electrophysiology of the hippocampal slice preparation has been its most important aspect in making it one of the most versatile *in vitro* systems in neuroscience today. The experiments described in this chapter demonstrate this versatility. The continuous electrophysiological monitoring of neuronal function offered an immediate assessment of the influence of experimental manipulations and the determination of the final outcome of each of these manipulations. Our journey began taking the necessary steps to establish this *in vitro* model adequacy for the purpose of answering outstanding questions in the field of cerebral ischemia/hypoxia. Naturally, the intention for any model is to produce the expected outcome based on the most established, yet current information that exists in the field. A failure to produce the expected outcome may question the usefulness of the model. In this respect, the hippocampal slice preparation had not always produced what was expected. Although where the study of cerebral ischemia/hypoxia has been concerned, the hippocampal slice preparation has led to some of the more important findings in this field, it has been the unexpected results produced by this system that have propelled it to its high place among all *in vitro* systems. The sheer number of papers and books written in which the brain slice preparation was used or where the preparation had been the topic described and discussed, attests to its scientific success. Nevertheless, without its electrophysiology, the preparation would have never inherited the place it occupies today in neuroscience research. The list below is a summary of the experiments described in this chapter, their outcome and their possible contribution to our understanding of cerebral energy metabolism:

1. Hyperglycemia does not worsen ischemic/hypoxic neuronal damage beyond the damage seen in isoglycemia, contrary to the perception advanced among researchers in the field in the last two decades of the 20th century. Moreover, increased tissue glucose concentration provided an increased tolerance against oxygen deprivation (Fig. 3). These experiments have led to the reexamination of the *in vivo* studies that reported glucose's detrimental effect (Myers & Yamaguchi, 1977), reexamination that found the interpretation of those results questionable (Schurr, 2001; Schurr et al., 2001; Payne et al., 2003).
2. Lactic acidosis, a hypothesized culprit in the worsening ischemic/hypoxic neuronal damage by hyperglycemia was found to be not only innocuous in this respect, but, just as it was shown for elevated glucose levels, lactic acid, too, was found to provide neuroprotection against the ischemic/hypoxic insult (Fig. 4). This unexpected outcome has presented strong evidence to refute the lactic acidosis hypothesis of cerebral ischemic damage and has been the driving force behind the renewed interest and active research in the field of cerebral energy metabolism.
3. Demonstrating that lactate is an excellent oxidative energy substrate for neural tissue has been a breakthrough discovery that can be specifically attributed to the employment of the hippocampal slice preparation and its electrophysiology in these experiments (Fig. 5). It took an additional six years for the published results (Schurr et al., 1988b) to receive significant confirmation (Pellerin & Magistretti, 1994). Since then, a large number of studies have been published that contain growing body of evidence in support of the original discovery.
4. Questioning the importance of neural tissue's ability to utilize lactate as the sole oxidative energy substrate to support its neuronal function, some have dismissed it as an *in vitro* aberration (Clarke & Sokoloff, 1994). Nevertheless, in a series of experiments (Figs. 6-11), while employing the glucose analog 2DG or the MCT inhibitor 4-CIN, the crucial role of endogenously-produced lactate in the recovery and/or sustenance of neuronal function post-hypoxia or during and after neuronal excitation has been demonstrated.
5. Lastly, a hypothesis was offered (Schurr, 2006) based on the experimental results described here and on many findings by others, according to which lactate, not pyruvate, is the end product of aerobic glycolysis (Fig. 12). The hypothesis was put to the test in a set of experiments illustrated in Figs. 13-15, using a newly discovered lactate dehydrogenase (LDH) inhibitor, malonate. The outcome of these experiments has provided support for the premise of this hypothesis (Schurr & Payne, 2007).

## 5. References


Aliverdieva, D.A., Manaev, D.V., Bondarenko, D.I., and Sholtz, K.F. (2006) Properties of yeast *Saccharomyces cerevisiae* plasma membrane dicarboxylate transporter. *Biochemistry (Mosc)*, 71, 1161-1169

Ashford, C.A., and Holmes, E.G. (1929) LXXXV. Contributions to the study of brain metabolism. V. Role of phosphates in lactic acid production. *Biochem J*, 23, 748-759.

Ashford, C.A., and Holmes, E.G (1931) CCXXI. Further observations on the oxidation of lactic acid by brain tissue. *Biochem J*, 25, 2028-2049.

Bröer, S., Rahman, B., Pellegri G., Pellerin L., Martin, J-L., Verleysdonk, S., Hamprecht, B., and magistretti, P.J. (1997) Comparison of lactate transport in astroglial cells and monocarboxylate transporter 1 (MCT 1) expressing *Xenopus laevis* oocytes. *J Biol Chem*, 272, 30096-30102

Brooks, G.A. (1985) Lactate: glycolytic product and oxidative substrate during sustained exercise in mammals – 'the lactate shuttle'. In: *Comparative physiology and biochemistry – currecnt topics and trends* Vol A. *Respiration-Metabolism-Circulation*, Gilles, R., Editor, 208-218. Springer-Verlag, Berlin.

Brooks, G.A. (1998) Mammalian fuel utilization during sustained exercise. *Comp Biochem Physiol B Biochem Mol Biol*, 120, 89-107

Brooks, G.A. (2000) Intra- and extra-cellular lactate shuttles. *Med Sci Sports Exerc*, 32, 790-799

Brooks, G.A. (2002a) Lactate shuttle – between but not within cells? *J Physiol*, 541, 333

Brooks, G.A. (2002b) Lactate shuttles in nature. *Biochem Soc Trans*, 30, 258-264

Brooks, G.A., Dubouchaud, H., Brown, M., Sicurello, J.P., and Butz, C.E. (1999) Role of mitochondrial lactate dehydrogenase and lactate oxidation in the intracellular lactate shuttle. *Proc Natl Acad Sci USA*, 96, 1129-1134

Chih, C-P., and Roberts, E.L., Jr. (2003) Energy substrates for neurons during neural activity: a critical review of the astrocyte-neuron lactate shuttle hypothesis. *J Cereb Blood Flow metab*, 23, 1263-1281.

Choi, D.W. (1988) Glutamate neurotoxicity and diseases of the nervous system. *Neuron*, 1, 623-634.

Choi, D.W., and Rothman, S.M. (1990) The role of glutamate neurotoxicity in hypoxic-ischemic neuronal death. *Annu Rev Neurosci*, 13, 171-182.

Clarke, D.D., and Sokoloff, L (1994) Chapter 31, Circulation and energy metabolism of the brain, in: *Basic Neurochemistry*, Siegel, G.J., Agranoff, B.W., Albers, R.W., Molinoff, P.B., pp 645-680, Raven Press.

Cox, J.A., Lysko, P.G., and Henneberry R.C. (1989) Excitatory amino acid neurotoxicity at the N-methyl-D-aspartate receptor in cultured neurons: role of the voltage-dependent magnesium block. *Brain Res*, 499, 267-272.

Dorland's Illustrated Medical Dictionary (1965) 24th Edition, p. 474, W.B. Saunders Company Press, Philadelphia and London.

Flock, E., Bollman, J.L., Mann, D.C. (1938) The utilization of pyruvic acid by the dog. *J Biol Chem*, 125, 49-56.

Garcia, C.K., Goldstein, J.L., Pathak, R.K., Anderson, R.G.W., and Brown, M.S. (1994) Molecular characterization of the membrane transporter for lactate, pyruvate and other monocarboxylates: implications for the Cori cycle. *Cell*, 76, 865-873.

Garcia, C.K., Brown, M.S., Pathak, R.K., and Goldstein, R.K. (1995) cDNA cloning of MCT2, a second monocarboxylate transporter expressed in different cells than MCT1. *J Biol Chem*, 270, 1843-1849.

Gerhart, D.Z., Enerson, B.E., Zhdankina, O.Y., Leino, R.L., and Drewes, L.R. (1997) Expression of monocarboxylate transporter MCT1 by brain endothelium and glia in adult and suckling rats. *Am J Physiol*, E207-E213.

Gibson, I.M., & McIlwain, H. (1965) Continuous recording of changes in membrane potential in mammalian cerebral tissues in vitro; recovery after depolarization by added substances. *J Physiol*, Vol. 176, 261-283.

Gladden, L.B. (2004) Lactate metabolism: a new paradigm for the third millennium. *J Physiol*, 558, 5-30.

Halestrap, A.P. and Denton, R.M. (1975) The specificity and metabolic implications of the inhibition of pyruvate transport in isolated mitochondria and intact tissue preparations by α-cyano-4-hydroxycinnamate and related compounds. *Biochem J*, 148, 97-106.

Henneberry, R.C. (1989) The role of neuronal energy in the neurotoxicity of excitatory amino acids. *Neurobiol Aging* 10, 611-613.

Hertz, L. (2004) The astrocyte-neuron lactate shuttle: a challenge of a challenge. *J Cereb Blood Flow metab*, 24, 1241-1248.

Holmes, E.G. (1930) CL. Oxidations in central and peripheral nervous tissue. *Biochem J*, 24, 914-925.

Holmes E.G., and Ashford, C.A. (1930) CXXVII. Lactic acid oxidation in brain with reference to the 'Myerhof cycle'. *Biochem J*, 24, 1119-1127.

Hu, Y., and Wilson G.S. (1997) A temporary local energy pool coupled to neuronal activity: fluctuations of extracellular lactate levels in rat brain monitored with rapid-response enzymae-based sensor. *J Neurochem*, 69, 1484-1490

Huckabee, W.E. (1958) Relationship of pyruvate and lactate during anaerobic metabolism. I. Effects of infusion of pyruvate or glucose and of hyperventilation. *J Clin Invest*, 37, 244-254.

Ivanov, A., Mukhtarov, M., Bregestovski, P., and Zilberter, Y. (2011) Lactate effectively covers energy demands during neuronal network activity in neonatal hippocampal slices. *Front Neuroenerg*, 3:2. doi: 10.3389/fnene.2011.00002

Kalimo, H., Rehncrona, S., Soderfeldt, B., Olsson, Y., Siesjö, B.K (1981) Brain lactic acidosis and ischemic cell-damage. 2. Histopathology. *J Cereb Blood flow Metab*, Vol.1, No. 3, 313-327.

Kasischke, K.A., Vishwasrao, H.D., Fisher, P.J., Zipfel, W.R., and Webb, W.W. (2004) Neural activity triggers neuronal oxidative metabolism followed by astrocytic glycolysis. *Science*, 305, 99-103

Larrabee, M.G. (1995) Lactate metabolism and its effects on glucose metabolism in the excised neural tissue. *J Neurochem* 64, 1734-41

Larrabee, M.G. (1996) Partitioning of $CO_2$ production between glucose and lactate in excised sympathetic ganglia, with implications for brain. *J Neurochem* 67, 1726-1734

Levasseur, J.E., Alessandri, B., Reinert, M., Clausen, T., Zhou, Z., Altememi, N., and Bullock, M.R. (2006) Lactate, not glucose, up-regulates mitochondrial oxygen consumption both in sham and lateral fluid percussed rat brains. *Neurosurgery*, 59, 1122-1131.

Li, C.-L., and McIlwain, H. (1957) Maintenance of resting membrane potentials in slices of mammalian cerebral cortex and other tissues in vitro. *J Physiol*, 139,178-190.

Magistretti, P.J. (1999) Cellular mechanisms of brain energy metabolism and their relevance to functional brain imaging. *Philos Tarns R Soc Lond B Biol Sc*, 354, 1155-1163.

Magistretti, P.J. (2000) Cellular bases of functional brain imaging: insights from neuron-glia metabolic coupling. *Brain Res*, 886, 108-112.

Magistretti, P.J., Pellerin, L., Rothman, D.L., Shulamn, R.G. (1999) Energy on demand. *Science*, 283, 496-497.

Mangia, S., Garreffa, G., Bianciardi, M., Giove, F., Di Salle, F., and Maraviglia, B. (2003) The aerobic brain: lactate decrease at the onset of neural activity. *Neuroscience*, 118, 7-10

McIlwain, H., Buchel, L., & Cheshire, J.D. (1951). The inorganic phosphate and phosphocreatine of brain especially during metabolism in vitro. *Biochem J*, Vol. 48, 12-20.

McIlwan, H., & Buddle, H.L., (1953). Techniques in tissue metabolism. 1. A mechanical chopper, *Biochem J*, Vol. 53, 412-420.

Myers, R.E., and Yamaguchi, S.I. (1977) Nervous-system effects of cardiac-arrest in monkeys - Preservation of vision. *Arch Neurol*, Vol. 34, No. 2, 65-74.

Novelli, A., Reilly, J.A., Lysko, P.G., and Henneberry, R.C. (1988) Glutamate becomes neurotoxic via the N-methyl-D-aspartate receptor when intracellular energy levels are reduced. *Brain Res*, 451,205-212.

Olney, J.W. (1969) Brain lesion, obesity and other disturbances in mice treated with sodium monoglutamate. *Science*, 164, 719-721.

Olney, J.W. (1990) Excitotoxic amino acids and neuropsychiatric disorders. *Annu Rev Pharmacol Toxicol*, 30, 47-71.

Payne, R.S., Tseng, M.T., and Schurr, A. (2003) The glucose paradox of cerebral ischemia: evidence for corticosterone involvement. *Brain Res* 971, 9-17.

Pellerin, L., and Magistretti, P.J. (1994) Glutamate uptake into astrocytes stimulates aerobic glycolysis: a mechanism coupling neuronal activity to clucose utilization. *Proc Natl Acad Sci USA*, 91, 10625-10629.

Pellerin, L., and Magistretti, P.J. (2003) Food for thought: challenging the dogmas. *J Cereb Blood Flow Metab*, 23, 1282-1286.

Pellerin, L., and Magistretti, P.J. (2004a) Let there be (NADH) light. *Science*, 305, 50-52.

Pellerin, L., and Magistretti, P.J. (2004b) Empiricism and rationalism: two paths toward the same goal. *J Cereb Blood Flow metab*, 24, 1240-1241.

Rehncrona, S., Rosen, I., Seisjö, B.K. (1981) Brain lactic acidosis and ischemic cell-damage. 1. Biochemistry and neurophysiology. *J Cereb Blood flow Metab*, Vol. 1, No. 3, 297-311.

Rodnight, R., & McIlwain, H. (1954). Techniques in tissue metabolism, *Biochem J*, Vol. 57, 649-661.

Saad, L.O., Mirandola, S.R., Maciel, E.N. and Castiho, R.F. (2006) Lactate dehydrogenase activity is inhibited by methyl malonate in vitro. *Neurochem Res*, 31, 541-548.

Schurr, A. (2001) Glucose and the ischemic brain: a sour grape or a sweet treat? *Curr Opin Clin Nutri Metab Care* 4, 287-292.

Schurr, A. (2006) Lactate: the ultimate cerebral oxidative energy substrate? *J Cereb Blood Flow metab*, 26, 142-152.

Schurr, A., Reid, K.H.., Tseng, M.T., and Edmonds Jr., H.L. (1984) The stability of the hippocampal slice Preparation: an electrophysiological and ultrastructural analysis. *Brain Res*, 297, 357-362.

Schurr, A. Reid, K.H.., Tseng, M.T., Edmonds Jr., H.L., and Rigor, B.M. (1985) A dual chamber for comparative studies using the brain slice preparation. *Comp Biochem Physiol,* 82A, 701-704.

Schurr, A., West, C.A., Reid, K.H., Tseng, M.T., Reiss, S.J. and Rigor, B.M. (1987) Increased glucose improves recovery of neuronal function after cerebral hypoxia in vitro. *Brain Res,* 421, 135-139.

Schurr, A., Dong, W-Q., Reid, K.H., West, C.A., and Rigor, B.M. (1988a) Lactic acidosis and recovery of neuronal function following cerebral hypoxia in vitro. *Brain Res.* 438, 311-314.

Schurr, A., West, C.A., and Rigor, B.M. (1988b) Lactate-supported synaptic function in the rat hippocampal slice preparation. *Science* 240, 1326-1328.

Schurr, A., West, C.A., and Rigor, B.M. (1989) Electrophysiology of energy metabolism and neuronal function in the hippocampal slice preparation. *J Neurosci meth,* 28, 7-13.

Schurr, A., and Rigor, B.M. (1989) Cerebral ischemia revisited: New insights as revealed using in vitro brain slice preparations. *Experientia,* 45, 684-695.

Schurr, A., Payne, R.S., Miller, J.J., and Rigor, B.M. (1997a) Brain lactate, not glucose, fuels the recovery of synaptic function from hypoxia upon reoxygenation: an in vitro study. *Brain Res,* 744, 105-111.

Schurr, A., Payne, R.S., Miller, J.J., and Rigor, B.M. (1997b) Brain lactate is an obligatory aerobic energy substrate for functional recovery after hypoxia: Further in vitro validation. *J Neurochem,* 69, 423-426.

Schurr, A., Miller J.J., Payne R.S., and Rigor, B.M. (1999a) An increase in lactate output by brain tissue serves to meet the energy needs of glutamate-activated neurons. *J Neurosci,* 19, 34-39.

Schurr, A., Payne, R.S., Miller J.J., Rigor B.M. (1999b) Study of cerebral energy metabolism using the rat hippocampal slice preparation. *Methods: A Companion to Methods in Enzymology,* 18, 117-126.

Schurr, A., Payne, R.S., Miller, J.J., and Tseng, M.T. (2001) Preischemic hyperglycemia-aggrevated damage: evidence that lactate utilization is beneficial and glucose-induced corticosterone release is detrimental. *J Neurosci Res* 66, 782-789.

Schurr, A, and Payne, R.S. (2007) Lactate, not pyruvate, is neuronal arobic glycolysis end product: an *in vitro* electrophysiological study. *Neuroscience,* 147, 613-619.

Siesjö, B.K. (1981) Cell-damage in the brain - a speculative synthesis. *J Cereb Blood flow Metab,* 1, No. 2, 155-185.

Siesjö, B.K. (1988) Historical overview. Calcium, ischemia, and death of brain cells. *Ann NY Acad Sci,* 522,638-661.

Tsacopoulos, M., and Magistretti, P.J. (1996) Metabolic coupling between glia and neurons. *J Neurosci,* 16, 877-885

Volk, C., Kempski, B., and Kempski O.S. (1997) Inhibition of lactate export by quercetin acidifies rat glial cells *in vitro. Neurosci Lett,* 223, 121-124.

Yamamoto, C., & McIlwain, H. (1966) Electrical activities in thin sections from the mammalian brain maintained in chemically-defined media in vitro. *J Neurochem,* 13, 1333-1343.

Yodoya, E., Wada, M., Shimada, A., Katsukawa, H., Okada, N., Yamamoto, A., Ganaphaty, V., and Fujita, T. (2006) Functional and molecular identification of sodium-coupled dicarboxylate transporters in rat primary cultured cerebrocortical astrocytes and neurons. *J Neurochem*, 97, 162-173.

# 4

# Evoked Potentials

Ahmet Akay
*Ege University*
*Turkey*

## 1. Introduction

Evoked potentials are electrical activities that occur in the neural pathways and structures as a response to various external stimulations induced by light, sound, electric, smell, or taste. Evoked potentials are polyphasic waves that oftenly present with an amplitude between 0.1-20 μA which are formed within 2-500 ms. The source of these activities is probably the summation of the action potentials generated by the afferent tracts and the electrical fields or activities of the synaptic discharges or post-synaptic potentials on those tracts.

Understanding evoked potentials bears importance in terms of controlling the entire pathway from stimulation point to the cortical areas, in other words, to the primary cortex. By examining evoked potentials, we can find answers to many questions such as: Does the response against the stimulus reach intended destinations on time? Does the response show any loss of intensity? If there is a problem in the neural parthways, what is its exact location?

When a person receives a visual stimulus such as a flash light, the EEG (electroencephalogram) record concerning the occipital region (particularly at the O1-P3 and O2-P4 derivations) demonstrates waves that are called "photic driving response" which form within about 150 ms and can be observed after any kind of light stimulation. However, most of the responses elicited due to external stimulation are not observed very clearly because those tiny little responses that we call "evoked potentials" can not be seen in EEG signals which may have amplitudes reaching 100 μV.

Moreover, there are non-neural activities that suppress those signals such as EEG: ECG (electrocardiogram), EMG (electromyogram), and other biologic signals. In addition, when the noises of the electronic devices and the environment are also considered, the difficulty of isolating evoked potentials can be figured out more easily. Currently, there are two methods used for eliminating those external interferences and both of them should be used in combination: "filtration" and "averaging".

Today, novelties in the electronics and computerized devices present us these advantages: High-quality amplifiers, smaller devices, perfect averaging techniques, multichannel capability, quality filtration options (digital filter, adaptive filter, spectral analysis etc.), capability of recording in any kind of environment (eg. operating room, bedside, or noisy environments), routine use of evoked potential recording systems in clinics.

The three major types of evoked potentials used in clinical studies are visual evoked potentials (VEP), brainstem auditory evoked potentials (BAEP), and somatosensory evoked potentials (SSEP).

## 2. Recording sytem

### 2.1 Electrodes

In evoked potential recordings, Ag/AgCl or gold-plated surface electrodes with a hole are used. Needle electrodes should not be employed because they produce many artifacts and have high electrode-skin impedance (5000–7000 Ω). The electrode-skin impedance in surface electrodes is lower than 5000 Ω, within a range of 2000–3000 Ω (under intensive care settings or in comatose patients and during intraoperatif use, needle electrodes or disposable electrodes can be employed for following the evoked potentials).

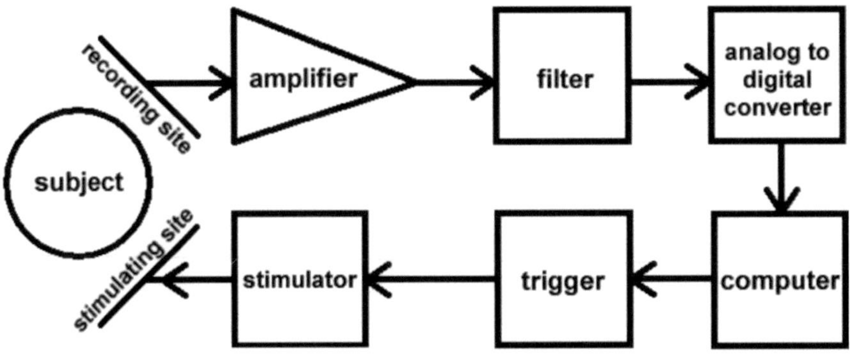


Fig. 1. Block diagram of the recording system.

Nonetheless, surface electrodes and needle electrodes do not have any difference with regard to recording quality of evoked potentials, both in terms of amplitude and waveform. In addition to the use of chloride gel in all electrodes, collodion is applied on hairy skin areas (for fixation purposes in long recordings).

Prior to the placement of the electrodes, the related skin surface should be cleaned with alcohol or acetone in order to adequately reduce the electrode-skin impedance. In case of need, abrasive gels can be applied for this purpose.

During recording, bipolar electrodes are preferred because lowest noise level can be achieved only by them. As the distance between the bipolar electrodes increase, signals grow more strong, however, the noise increases by the same rate, as well.

Stimulus electrodes are also bipolar and the distance between them should be 35 mm with the active electrode placed distally.

The electrode configuration and system of a classic 10/20 electrode EEG recording system, shown in the Figure 2, are used in evoked potential recordings, as well. However, if needed, the electrode configuration of a 32-electrode EEG recording system can also be employed. (F: Frontal region, C: Central region, T: Temporal region, P: Parietal region, O: Occipital region, A1 and A2: Ear lobes, Fz, Cz, Pz, Oz: Midline electrodes, The odd numbered electrodes are always placed on the left.)

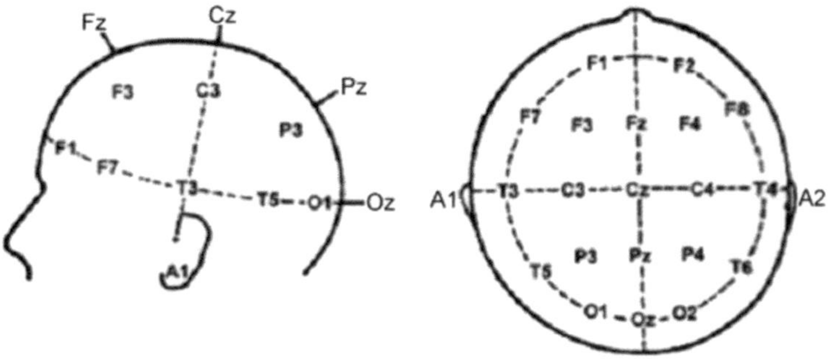


Fig. 2. International 10/20 EEG electrode positioning system.

## 2.2 Amplifier

In evoked potential recordings, differential amplifiers that can carry out 500,000x amplification which can be intensified stepwise, are used (an amplifier that amplifies the difference between voltages of the first and second inputs). One of the main characteristics of differential amplifiers is the capability of eliminating electrostatic and electromagnetic interferences from reaching the patient.

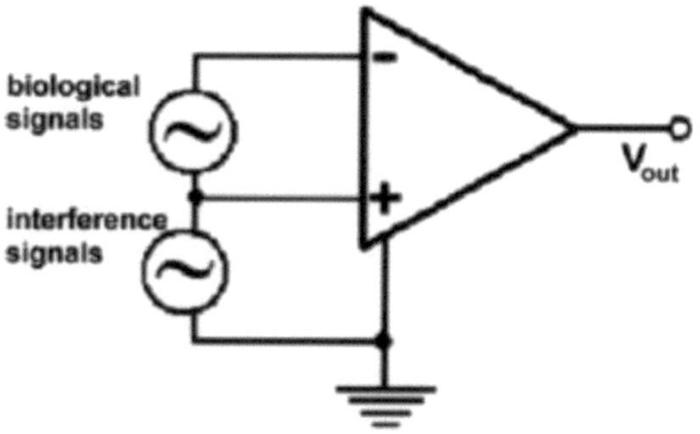


Fig. 3. Two main signals in the input of an amplifier.

The input of the amplifier has components of 6 different signals:

1. The biological signal that we aim to measure (evoked potential)
2. The biological signals that we do not want to measure (cortical, cardiac, muscular, and other biological activities)
3. 50 Hz interference signal and its harmonics
4. Interference signals arising from the electrode-tissue contact
5. Environmental interferences (electromagnetic, electrostatic, radio-frequency interferences)
6. Noise of the amplifier itself.

## 2.3 Filter circuit

It comprises serial connection of a low-cut filter (high-pass filter) and a high-cut filter (low-pass filter) including passive and active components, or a band-pass filter bearing the characteristics of those two filters.

| | Low-cut | High-cut |
|---|---|---|
| SSEP | 30 Hz | 3000 Hz |
| BAEP | 100 Hz | 3000 Hz |
| VEP | 0.2–1 Hz | 200–300 Hz |

Table 1. Filter values used in evoked potential recording systems.

Notch filters which is applied for eliminating 50/60 Hz mains electricity interference, is not used in any of the evoked potential recording procedures in order to not eliminate the 50/60 Hz components of the concerning evoked potential signals (Since low-cut frequency for BAEP is already 100 Hz, there is no need for 50/60 Hz notch filter) Instead of high-cut and low-cut filters, band-pass filters of 30-3000 Hz for SSEP, 100-3000 Hz for BAEP, and (0.2-1)-(200-300) Hz for VEP, can be used.

As shown in the Figure 1, filter circuit can be placed at the amplifier output or between the preamplifier stage and power amplifier stage. However, the best is to use a low-cut filter at the pre-amplifier output and a high-cut filter at the power amplifier output.

### 2.4 Analog-to-digital converter

Because computers can only work with numbers, the voltage changes at the filter output should be converted to digital data. Thus, analog-to-digital converter (ADC) performs this function. An analog-to-digital converter comprises "sampler" and "quantizer" circuits (Figure 4).

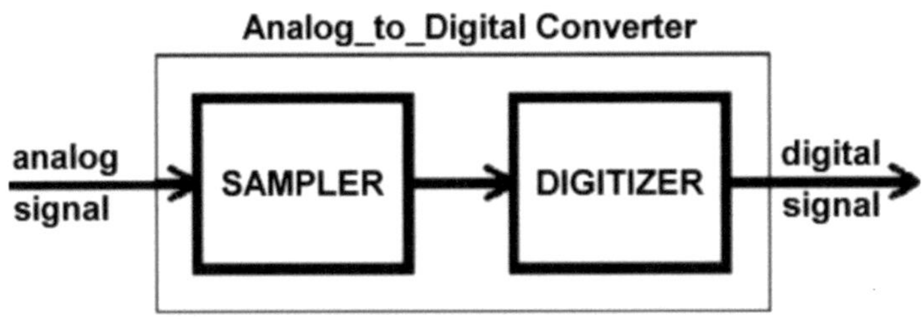


Fig. 4. Inside of the ADC circuit.

These two circuits should enable numerical ADC output, in other words "time series", to represent the original signal (the evoked potential we are trying to generate) in a complete way and thus carry the data included within the signal without a loss. In short, "sampling" and "quantization" ranges should be chosen sufficiently small (The vertical resolution of the ADC circuit, ie. "voltage resolution", should be lower than the least amplitude value of the signal; whereas its horizontal resolution, ie. temporal resolution, should be at least twice the highest frequency component) (Figure 5).

For example, lets say, the sampling sensitivity of our ADC circuit is 12-bit and the reference voltage is ± 5 V. In this case, the sampling range will be (5 + 5) volt / $2^{12}$ = 2 mV, which indicates that the circuit will detect the amplitude changes ≥ 2 mV. Since an amplitude value of 0.1 µV in an evoked potantial recording can reach a value of 10 mV after undergoing 100,000x amplification, an ADC circuit of 12-bit can easily be detected and converted to a digital value. However, if we use an 8-bit ADC circuit, because the sampling range of this

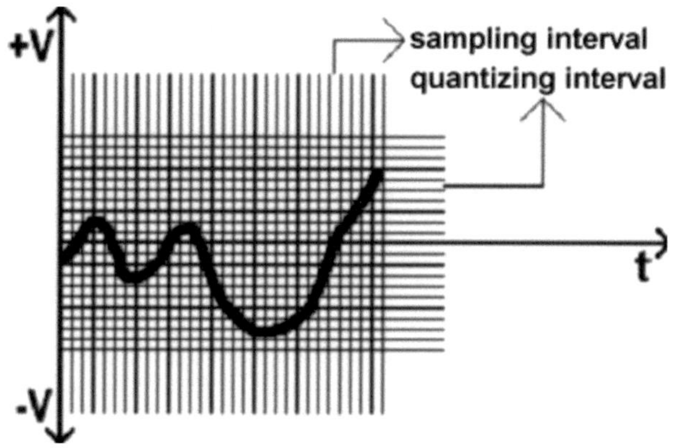


Fig. 5. Sampling & quantizing intervals of a signal.

would be (5 + 5) volt / $2^8$ = 39 mV, a 0.1 µV change in the evoked potential wave or amplitude will not be detected, and thus will be eliminated.

As you can see in our example, the sampling sensitivity of ADC circuits used in recording evoked potentials should be 12-bit. Therefore, 12-bit ADC circuits are the standard in this regard.

Lets give another example. If we have an ADC circuit with a sampling sensitivity of 1000 Hz, the subsequent quantization range will be 1/1000 = 1 ms, meaning that as a result of the Nyquest formula, our ADC circuit will not detect evoked potential changes faster than 2 x (1 ms) = 2 ms. Because a change of 2 ms corresponds to 1/0.002 = 500 Hz, in our target evoked potential, the changes faster than 500 Hz will not be converted into digital data and thus will subsequently vanish.

In short, if the high-cut frequency of our filter circuit is 600 Hz and the sampling frequency of our ADC circuit is 1000 Hz, it means that we will not be able to see the components of the evoked potential signal between 500-600 Hz. In conclusion, the quantization range used in the ADC circuit depends on the high-cut filter frequency in the filter circuit, and it should be at least twice the value of this frequency.

### 2.5 Computer

Triggers stimulation circuits at appropriate intervals; takes trigger-locked samples of same duration from digital signals elicited from the ADC circuit; after a certain amount of sampling, subjects them to "averaging" process; renders the obtained evoked potentials ready for visualization, evaluation, and storage.

#### 2.5.1 Triggering

It is a must that the stimulation circuits are triggered by a computer, in other words, stimulation times should be determined by a computer because the samples should be synchronous with those triggerings, which can be termed as being "trigger-locked". Otherwise, we can not determine the starting time of the samples, and thus fail to evaluate the signals. The samples (epoches) have 3 properties:

**1. Sample duration** SSEP: 40 ms for upper extremities, 60-80 ms for lower extremities, BAEP: 10 ms, VEP: 200-250 ms.

**2. Sample amount** SSEP: 500 samples, BAEP: 2000 samples and should be repeated twice, VEP: 200 samples and should be repeated thrice.

**3. Onset of sampling** After the the samples undergo *summation* and *averaging*, the obtained evoked potential signal should start at a certain time relative to the stimulus in order to be valid for evaluation (ie. it should be stimulation-locked). The starting time of the samples may be one of the following three:

**At the onset of stimulation** The computer starts sampling simultaneously with the triggering for stimulus. This is the most commonly preferred method.

**Before stimulation** The computer starts sampling prior to the stimulus. In this method, the aim is to see the isoelectric line (to predetermine it). It is applied when amplitudes of evoked potentials are wanted to be measured relative to the isoelectric line or when the events before stimulus are aimed to be determined.

**After the stimulation** The computer starts sampling after the stimulus. This is the less commonly used method. The aim here is to eliminate any interference of stimulus artifact over the evoked potential.

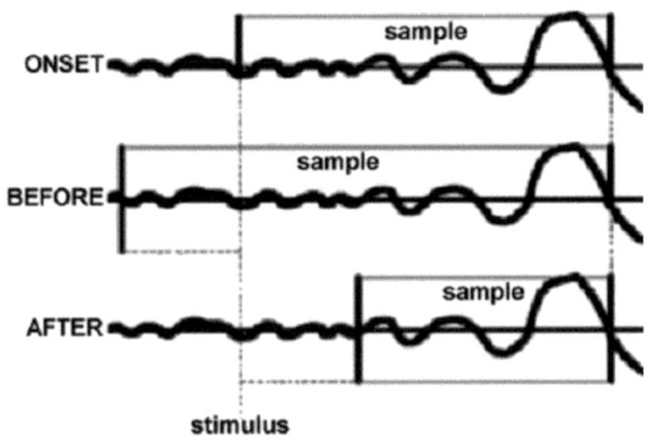


Fig. 6. Three different sampling methods.

### 2.5.2 Averaging

Despite the fact that all EEG signals are generated by the grey matter of the cerebral cortex (reflecting the cortical activity), both cortical and subcortical structures as well as the white matter creating the neural pathways contribute to the evoked potential signals. Since evoked potential signals which can also termed as EEEG (Evoked EEG), have markedly lower amplitude compared to the EEG signals with a normal background activity, they are embedded within the ECG traces and thus they can not be seen directly.

As known by many, EEG signals are spontaneous polyphasic waves whose amplitude-frequency-phase values constantly vary. However, evoked potential signals are changes that are non-spontaneous and have a specific waveform. Moreover, their occurrence times following the stimulus are known.

Therefore, when we superimpose numerous samples obtained from spontaneous "random" signals such as EEG, the resultant graphic will be an appearance that is entirely filled up to its lower and upper amplitude limits. The averaging of this graphic will produce only "nil", represented by a graphic consisted of an isoelectric line (the upper and lower areas will balance each other)! If we sum up the samples in sequence instead of applying superimposition, we acquire the same result (as shown in the figure below). Thus, first summing up "sample 1" and "sample 2", then "sample 1+2" and "sample 3", then "sample 1+2+3" + "sample 4", in short, by following the formula of (n-1) + sample n, and applying averaging, no signal will be observed in the end (n=infinite)!

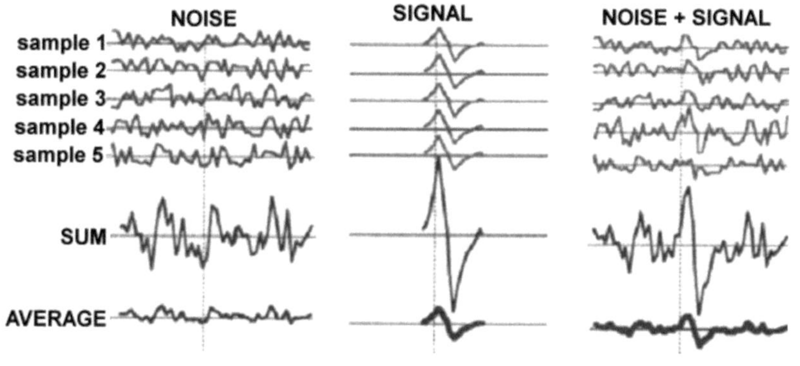


Fig. 7. Averaging of samples.

However, if we perform the same procedure for non-spontaneous and specific evoked potentials, the signal increases at the end of each summation, and finally, the averaging produces the same signal with its original waveform.

When the samples generated by the computers from the evoked potential recordings are subjected to the above mentioned processes, ie. averaging, spontaneous waves such as EEG vanish, whereas the evoked potential wave becomes more significant (as shown in the figure above).

Actually, averaging is a term used for increasing the signal-to-noise ratio (S/N ratio) that is markedly low such as 1/50 or even 1/100. At this point, some may ask the following question: Since it is a fact that infinite number of samples can not be acquired, how many samples should be used in this averaging process aiming to reveal the evoked potential signal?

We can calculate this practically as follows: for example, lets take the average amplitude for EEG waves with background noise as 50 μV and take the average amplitude of the related evoked potential as 5 μV (as in VEP). The "signal/noise ratio" of this system is 5 μV / 50 μV = 0.1, and we have to mulply it with at least 10 in order to elevate it to 1. This number that we multiply the result with is termed as "supression factor" and it is shown by $\sqrt{N}$. When $\sqrt{N}$ is 10, then N equals to 100, which represents the minimal "sample" amount that should be used for averaging.

Again, lets suppose that average amplitude of the EEG waves is 50 μV, whereas average amplitude of the evoked potential is 0.25μV (as in BAEP). In this case, signal/noise ratio is 0.25 μV / 50 μV = 0.005. We should multiply this value with 200 in order to elevate it to 1.

Therefore, suppression factor (√N) is 200 and N=4000. In other words, the minimum number of samples to be used in the BAEP recording should be 4000.

There is a shortcut formula to find the required minimal sample amount: "Amplitude of the background noise / Amplitude of the evoked potential = Suppression factor" The square root of the result provides us the minimal amount of samples.

### 2.6 Stimulation

First thing that should be reminded here is that the applied frequency should not conflict with the upper or lower harmonics of the mains electricity regardless of the type of the stimulus and the evoked potential test (this is the reason why stimulus frequency is applied as 4.71/s instead of 5/s for SSEP, 11/s instead of 10/s for BAEP, and 1.98/s instead of 2/s for VEP).

#### 2.6.1 Somatosensory stimulation

Square-wave stimulation of 10 μs – 2 ms duration is applied (oftenly, square waves with 100-200 μs are delivered). Stimulus frequency is at most 100/s (in practical cases, stimulus frequency is 1-5/s for upper extremities and 0.5-2/s for lower extremities).

The current intensity of the applied square wave does not exceed 20 mA and generally occurs between 10-15 mA. However, in medical disorders that increase the stimulation threshold required for generation of an action potential (ie. neural response), this current may need to be elevated (eg. it may be required to elevate it up to 50 mA in peripheral neuropathy).

Stimulus electrodes should be placed in a way to have a 35 mm distance to each other, while the active electrode should be placed distally.

#### 2.6.2 Auditory stimulation

Square waves of 100-200 μs are applied on a single ear through an ear phone (click sound). Simultaneously, the contralateral ear should receive white noise in a continuous fashion (a hissing sound covering all frequencies). Generally 10 stimuli are applied and it is enough that they are of 65-70 dB intensity.

#### 2.6.3 Visual stimulation

It is performed by a TV screen that is 70-100 cm distant to the patient and having a constant luminance along with checkerboard pattern where the white and black colors are displaced in an alternating fashion. If possible, the test room is preferred to be dark. The alternation rate of the colors is 1 or 2 colors a second (in faster alternations, evoked potential is delayed).

## 3. General principles

Before the test

1. The patient should wash his/her hair on the evening before the test or a couple of hours in advance.

2. Substances such as perfume, lotion, or cream should not be applied prior to the test.
3. Any accessories such as an auditory device, glasses, or lense should be brought to the clinic.
4. The patient should dress in a comfortable way and clothes with a turtle neck or bra should not be worn.
5. Drugs or foods containing caffeine should not be taken.
6. The people that will undergo visual evoked potential test, should not use sedatives.

During the test

1. In somatosensory, dermatomal, and auditory evoked potential tests, patient is told that the test could take a while and that he/she would take a nap during the test.
2. In somatosensory evoked potential test, the patient should be informed that a tingling can be felt in the stimulation points and flexion may be observed in the thumbs and toes.
3. The patient should be informed that there is no limitation of drug, food, or activity after the test.
4. Skin surfaces that will receive the electrodes should be rubbed with alcohol and acetone, and smoothened if required to.
5. In presence of muscular noise during the auditory evoked potential test and if the patient can not sleep, then sedation with chloride hydrate or diazepam should be performed.
6. Prior to the visual evoked potential test, the visual acuity and pupil width should be controlled in both eyes of the patient.

After the test

There is no limitation of drug, food, or acitivity.

## 4. Somatosensory evoked potentials

They are used for evaluating the synaptic terminals extending towards cortex, by stimulating the peripheral sensory pathways via delivery of an electric current. In short, it is aimed to acquire a response that can be recorded electrically in the central nervous system against a stimulation applied on vibration, position, or epicritic tactile senses.

As noted above, this method, applied for stimulating the central nervous system externally, is a short-term electrical shock that is applied on peripheral (sensory) nerves. Although Eps can be elicited by more natural stimulation methods such as mechanic, tactile, thermic, and pain, they have no practical value as of yet.

If we place the active electrode over the contralateral parietal region and reference electrode over the back of the hand in order to stimulate the median nerve via wrist, and acquire an evoked potential signal while obtaining samples with long duration, we can acquire a polyphasic complex with many ups and downs which starts 9-10 ms after the stimulus and continue until 500 ms.

In Figure 8, the "late components" are nonspesific waves which can vary even in the same individual, depend on the state of attention-consciousness of the individual, and are easily influenced by the used drugs. They occur not only from the primary cortex, ie. post-central region, but also as a result of the cortical association, activities of the components, and effects of ARAS (Ascending Reticular Activating System); they are associated with cortical integration.

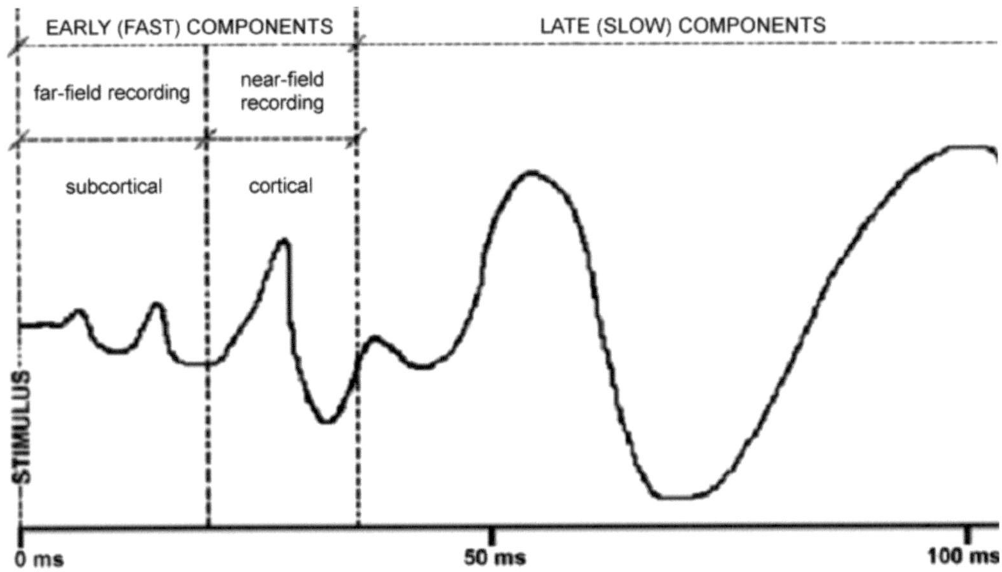


Fig. 8. Components of the SSEP.

Therefore, those late components of SSEP do not have the characteristics of a somatosensory-specific evoked potentials. In studies on evoked potentials, investigators do not focus on these waves, however, they become more important in psychologic, psychiatric, and pharmacologic studies.

When we take a look at the "early components" of the graphic, we see potentials with very small amplitude for 10-15 ms before the occurrence of components with a large amplitude that start nearly 20 ms after stimulus. Thus, those potentials with a large amplitude are cortical (post-rolandic) activities that are recorded both from under the active electrode and around it, and they are called as "near-field recordings".

On the other hand, small-amplitude waves that occur prior to the near-field potentials, are activities that arise from subcortical structures (brachial, plexus, spinal medulla, lemniscus medialis etc.); they are called as "far-field recordings". In other words, these are evoked potential activities that are located far from the active electrode and as per volume conductivity law, they are detected by and recorded by the active electrode. In short, we can call near-field records as "cortical components" and far-field records as "subcortical components".

Another point that needs explanation here is that there is a classification in the related terminology:

**Late components** Same as the late components we mentioned above.

**Middle components** The near-field portion of the above mentioned early components (cortical early component recording).

**Early components** The far-field portion of the above mentioned early components (subcortical early component recording).

Since the response generated after the stimulus first passes through the subcortical structures, subcortical components are observed earlier, and because they are located far from the active electrode, they do not have a high amplitude. Their polarity and amplitude may vary depending on the location of the reference electrode, and some components may not appear. For example, when the reference electrode is placed on the forehead, subcortical components become weak and polarities are reversed.

Is there a way to record subcortical components as "near-field" or in other words, can we obtain afferent components in detail? The only way for that is to place the active electrode close to the sources. As shown by Figure 10, if we place three active electrodes separately to the Erb point (ipsilateral), cervical region, and parietal region (contralateral), and carry out a synchronized recording, we can acquire evoked potentials from brachial plexus, spinal medulla, and cortical region separately.

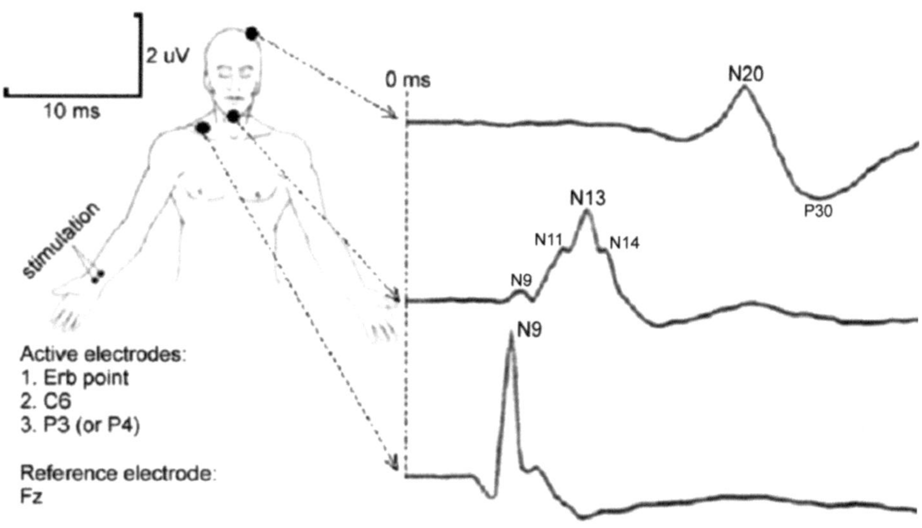


Fig. 9. Peripheral, subcortical, and cortical evoked potentials obtained from three different recording sites.

In clinical practice, active electrodes are P3–P4 or C3–C4 in the upper extremity test and C1–C2 or only Cz in the lower extremity test; whereas reference electrode is Fz or A1–A2. Again in clinical practice, the most commonly used upper extremity nerves are median and ulnar (at wrist level) nerves, whereas most commonly employed lower extremity nerves are tibial (at ankle level) and peroneal nerves (at knee level).

Spike potential observed in the record obtained from Erb point is named as N9 due to the fact that it is a negative wave occurring nearly 9 ms after the stimulus. Spike potential observed in the record obtained from cervical region is named as N13 due to the fact that it is a negative wave occurring nearly 13 ms after the stimulus. The spur on the ascending arm of the N13 is N11 and the spur on the descending arm of the N13 is N14. Moreover, N9 wave can be observed here, as a negative potential just before N11 (far-field record).

The first wave observed in the record obtained from the parietal region is N20, which is a negative wave that occurs 20 ms after the stimulus. Approximately 10 ms after this, a positive wave is seen which is named as P30. Moreover, N9 and N13 waves can also be observed as low-amplitude waves (far-field records), but as having a positive character this time (due to the location relative to the reference electrode).

In another designation, the first wave that is seen or should be seen is called as IP (initial positive) if it is positive, and as IN (initial negative) if it is negative. The subsequent wave is called PI if it is positive, and NI if negative. The following waves are named as NII, PII, NIII, NIV etc.

### 4.1 Possible sources of the waves

**Median nerve stimulation**

N9: Brachial plexus activity (action potential).
N11: Spinal medulla dorsal root activity (or dorsal root + cuneate fascicle activity).
N13: Dorsal funiculus activity (post-synaptic grey matter activity).
N14: Lemniscal tract and nucleus activity (lemniscal nucleus and prethalamic lemniscal medial tract activity).
N18: Thalamus posterolateral nucleus activity?
N20: Parietal cortex activity.
P30: Parietal cortex activity.

**Tibialis posterior stimulation**

N20: Spinal roots and spinal column activity.
P27: Nucleus gracilis activity.
N35: Parietal cortex activity.
N40: Parietal cortex activity.

Roughly speaking, the response enters spinal column 10 ms after the stimulus and reaches somesthetic cortex at 20 ms (it reaches primary cortex in 35-40 ms from the lower extremities).

### 4.2 Evaluation

First criterium to check, is the latency. Latency is the distance between the stimulus and peak of wave in milliseconds.

$$\text{Latency} = \frac{\text{Distance of the peak of wave from the stimulus (mm) x Sampling duration (s)}}{\text{Sampling length (mm)}}$$

This is an absolute latency and bilateral comparison is required. However, absolute latency values vary between individuals depending on the length of the extremity or height of a person. Therefore, in addition to absolute latency, "interpeak latency" or "central conduction time" values which are considered even more valuable, are measured.

For example; "N20 – N9", "N20 – N13", "N13 – N9" values obtained by median nerve stimulation are all interpeak latencies. By using this method, absolute latency differences

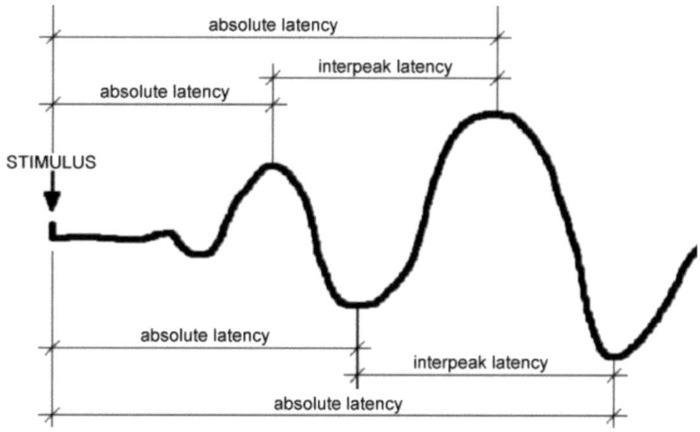


Fig. 11. Absolute & interpeak latencies.

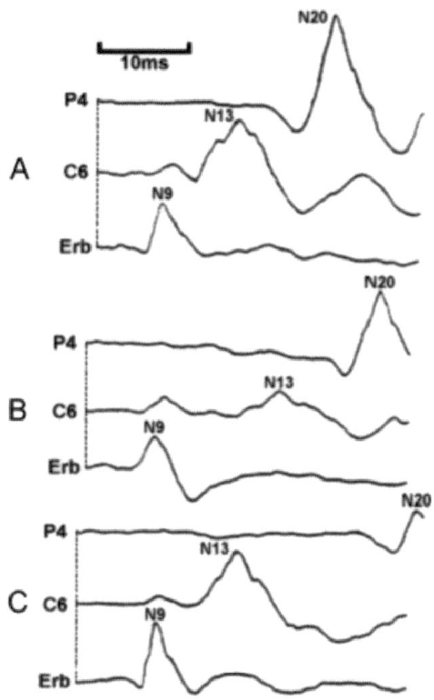


Fig. 12. Evaluation of SSEP recordings. **Evaluation of Figure 12A:** Amplitudes and waveforms, absolute latencies, and interpeak latencies are normal. Interpretation: Normal individual. **Evaluation of Figure 12B:** Erb record is normal; N13 absolute latency is prolonged; N13–N9 interpeak latency is prolonged; N13 amplitude is reduced leading to disrupted N11 and N14 notches; N20 absolute latency is prolonged, however, N20-N13 interpeak latency is normal. Interpretation: There is a lesion at cervical spinal cord level, located proximal to the brachial plexus and distal to the brainstem. **Evaluation of Figure 12C:** Erb and C6 records are normal; C6-Erb relationship is normal; N20 absolute latency is prolonged; N20-N13 interpeak latency is prolonged; N20 amplitude is reduced. Interpretation: There is a disruption in the contralateral tracts between the brainstem and the cortex.

arising from differences concerning height of individuals or length of extremities, is reduced, and the conduction variability of the peripheral nerve system is partially eliminated.

During evaluation, apart from the "absolute latency" and "central conduction time" values, morphologies and interpeak amplitudes of the waves are examined, as well. However, evaluating amplitudes does not bear much importance because even the same individual may exhibit different amplitude values at different times.

Lastly, the presence or absence of the components and morphologic intercomponent differences, which are also important findings, are evaluated (Figure 12).

In Figure 13, cervical and cortical SSEP recordings of a multiple sclerosis case are shown.

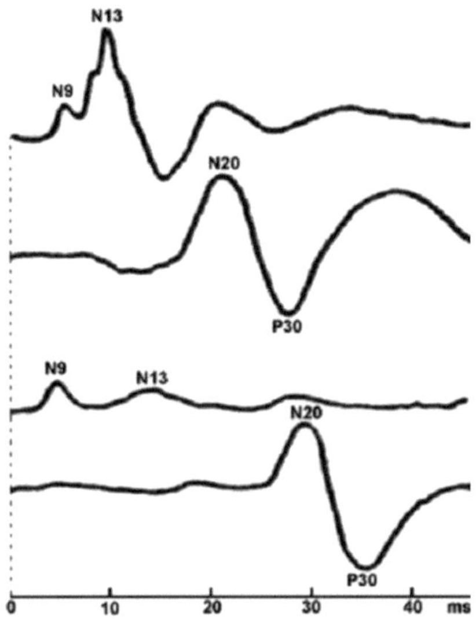


Fig. 13. SSEP changes in multiple sclerosis.

N11, N13, and N14 are weakened in the cervical recording and the interpeak latencies are prolonged. Cortical recording displays preserved N20 and P30 waveforms with prolonged absolute latencies.

Figure 14 is a SSEP recording of a cervical myelopathy case.

All components after N9, appear to be reduced, whereas all the absolute latencies starting from the N9 point are observed to be prolonged.

Evaluation criteria

1. Absolute latencies
2. Interpeak latencies
3. Interpeak amplitude values
4. Presence of components
5. Morphology of the components
6. Intercomponent morphologic differences
7. Bilateral evaluation

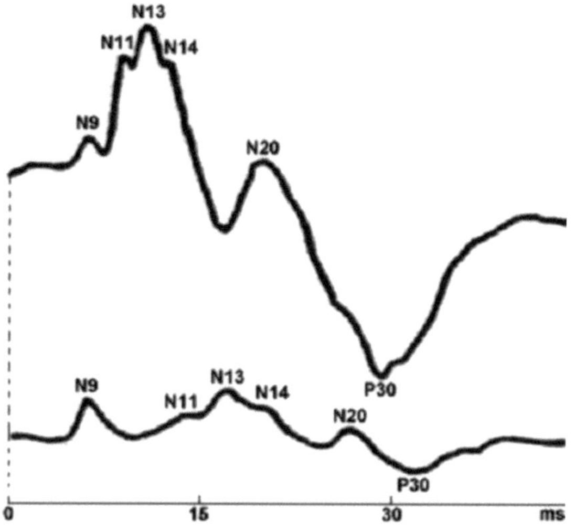


Fig. 14. SSEP changes in cervical myelopathy.

### 4.3 Clinical Indications

SSEP test is applied for checking the peripheral (thick ones) sensory fibers, spinal cord, and somesthetic cortex. It is useful in evaluating and supporting the already established diagnosis concerning the below mentioned cases.

Indications

- Plexus injuries
- Thoracic outlet syndrome
- Carpal tunnel syndrome
- Tarsal tunnel syndrome
- Evaluation of the peripheral nervous system
- Cervical and back pain
- Musculoskeletal injuries
- Brachial neuritis
- Spinal cord injuries
- Nerve root irritations and traumas
- Neuromuscular diseases
- Neuritis
- Radiculitis
- Motor/sensory deficits
- Vertebral subluxation complex
- Systemic neuropathies
- Lower back pain
- Plexus injuries and irritations

Complementary tests

- NCV
- USG
- BAEP and/or VEP

NCV (Nerve Conduction Velocity): It is used for measuring the conduction velocity through the peripheral motor and sensory nerve fibers.
USG (Ultrasonography): Musculoskeletal system ultrasonography of the related areas.

### 4.4 Other indications

1. Evoked potential tests are indispensable tools for diagnosis and following of multiple sclerosis, a demyelinating disease.
2. It is applied for monitoring purposes in operations involving spinal cord and vertebrae. The recordings in Figure 15 belong to a case of rheumatoid arthritis inducing compression on spinal cord.
3. Can be used in the early diagnosis of sensory problems in newborns.
4. Myelinization can be monitored (Figure 16).

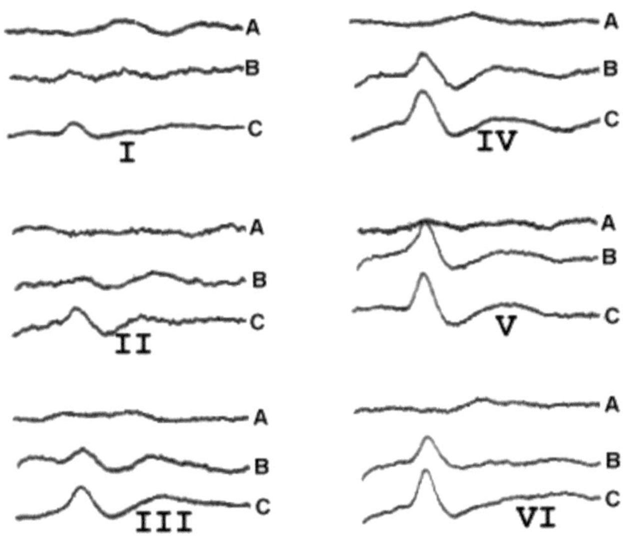


Fig. 15. SSEP changes during spinal cord operation.

A: Tibial nerve stimulation
B: Right ulnar nerve stimulation
C: Left ulnar nerve stimulation

I: Beginning of the operation
II: After left laminectomy
III: After right laminectomy
IV: End of the decompression procedure
V: Establishing stabilization
VI: End of the operation

The important point here is that patients under general anesthesia may be indifferent to stimuli applied at 3/s rate. Therefore, during application of SSEP technique for intraoperative monitoring, the stimulus rate should be 1 or 2 stimuli per second.

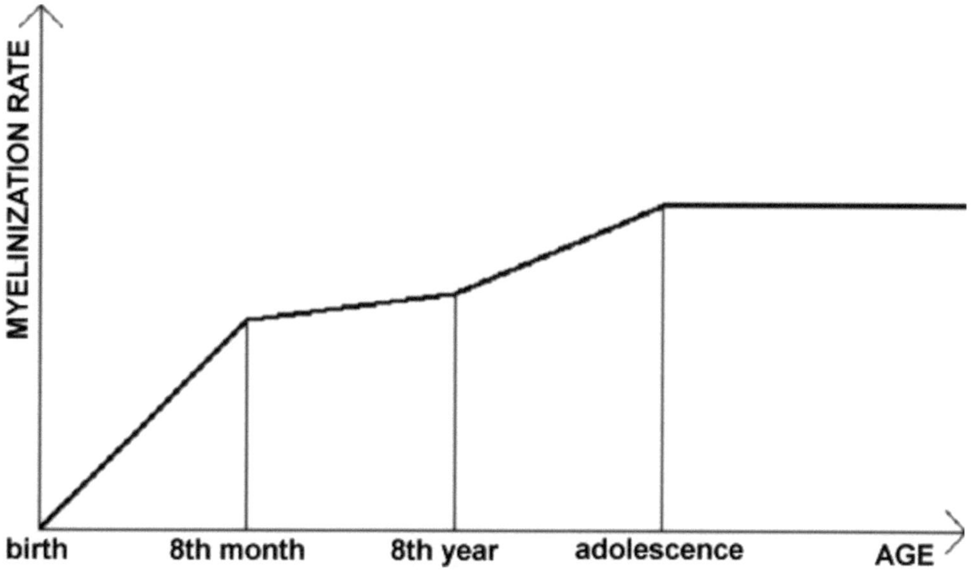


Fig. 16. Myelinization rate.

As shown in Figure 16 obtained from evoked potential recordings, myelinization is very fast during the interval from birth to 8th month, slowing down until the 8th year, and again fast from that point up to the adolescence period.

## 5. Auditory evoked potentials

This is an evoked potential test which is used for checking the auditory canals up to the primary cortex, ie. Heschl gyrus neighboring the temporal lobe, by applying auditory stimulus above hearing threshold to the external auditory canal.

The auditory stimulus is applied through a classic audiometric earphone by delivering a square wave of 100 - 200µs duration for 10 times a second. This is a "click" sound. Until finishing one ear, the other ear is subjected to white noise which is a "hissing" sound containing all frequencies at equal intensity.

The intensity of the sound applied for stimulus is generally above hearing threshold and range betwen 65-70 dB (in patients with a hearing loss, this value should be increased).

If the stimulus rate is higher than 10/s, absolute latencies and interpeak latencies are prolonged and amplitudes are reduced. When the intensity of the sound is decreased, the wave morphologies change and same events occur (practically, sound intensity is set based on the amplitude of the 5th wave).

For BAEP test, at least 2000 samples of 10 ms each, should be obtained for each ear, and the test should be repeated at least twice (In clinics, 1024 samples are obtained in normal cases and 4096 samples are obtained in pathologic cases. Sampling of both are repeated twice).

As mentioned before, a band-pass filter within range of 100-3000 Hz should be used. Again, as previously noted, the required amplification is a large one (500,000X), because the average amplitude of BAEP components are at 0.25 µV level.

Active electrode is the vertex electrode (Cz). Reference electrode is the one at the ipsilateral ear lobe or ipsilateral mastoid bone. It may be better if the mastoid electrodes are not used because they may lead to muscle artifacts. In this case, the electrodes used in BAEP recording will be as follows: Cz–A1–A2

The first thing to be done during recording is to monitor the first BAEP component (wave 1). If this wave can not be discerned, then the following steps can be taken:

1. Intensity of the sound is increased.
2. Poles of the earphone speaker are switched.
3. Stimulus rate (10/s) is reduced.
4. Reference electrode at the ear lobe is placed at the external ear canal.
5. In presence of unavoidable muscular noise, the patient is subjected to sedation.

Moreover, it should be born in mind that:

a. People above 60 years of age exhibit significantly prolonged latency.
b. Interpeak latencies are shorter in women than in men.
c. Last two of the BAEP components (there are 7 in total), which are named as "wave VI" and "wave VII", may never be seen.

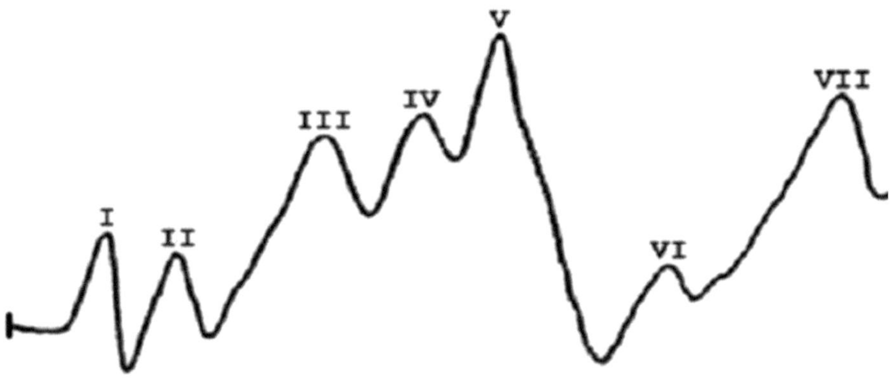


Fig. 17. Waveforms seen in BAEP recording.

Although the activated anatomic locations are completely certain, sources of the waves obtained by BAEP are not obvious. They may be as follows:

i. Distal action potential of the acoustic nerve (negative wave in the ipsilateral ear electrode).
Peripheral
1.3 ms latency
ii. Ipsilateral proximal acoustic nerve and/or cochlear nucleus activity.
Bulbar
2.4 ms latency
iii. Ipsilateral superior nucleus olivarius activity.
Pontine
3.3 ms latency
iv. Lateral lemniscal nuclear or axonal activity.
Pontine

4.4 ms latency
v. Inferior colliculus activity.
Mesencephalic
5.2 ms latency
vi. Medial geniculate body activity.
Thalamic
6.5 ms latency
vii. Thalamo-cortical projection activity.
Cortical
8.5 ms latency

In Figure 18, we see a normal BAEP recording with 5 components which has no pathology despite absence of two components.

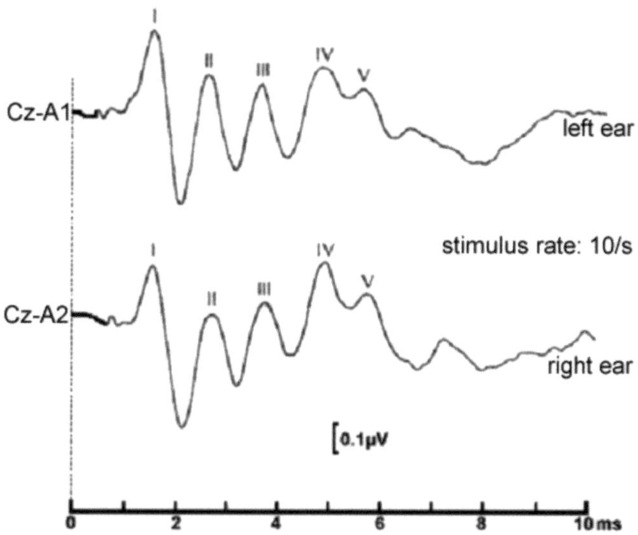


Fig. 18. Normal BAEP recording.

### 5.1 Indications

1. 1. Hearing loss, hearing imbalance
2. Balance disorders
3. Tinnitus
4. Assessment of type and level of hearing loss in children below 5 years of age
5. Metabolic, demyelinating, degenerative diseases and tumors of the brainstem
6. Ear canal lesions outside the brainstem
7. Monitorization during operations concerning brainstem
8. Control and follow-up after operations concerning brainstem
9. Headaches
10. Head traumas
11. Hyperflexion/hyperextension
12. Comas (with EEG). In Figure 19, you can see various coma levels reflected in BAEP recording.

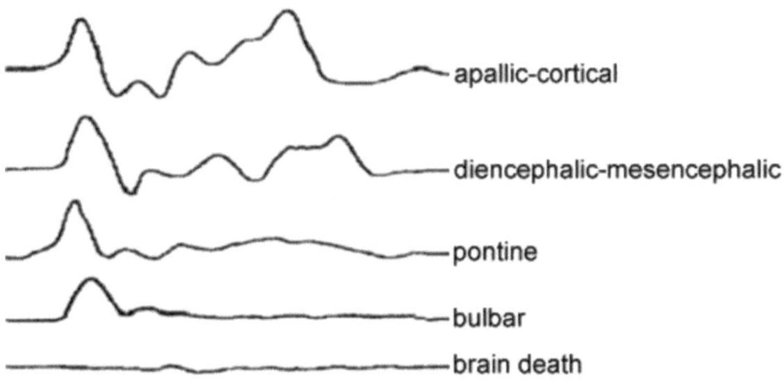


Fig. 19. Coma levels in BAEP recordings. It is noteworthy that as the coma deepens, BAEP components disappear from proximal to distal.

During the BAEP test, component amplitudes are not taken into consideration because amplitude values are of considerably variable nature. The most common pathology seen during the test is prolonged "I-III" or "I-V" intervals. In Figure 20, you can see a BAEP recording of an acoustic neurinoma case, causing a prolonged "I-V" interval.

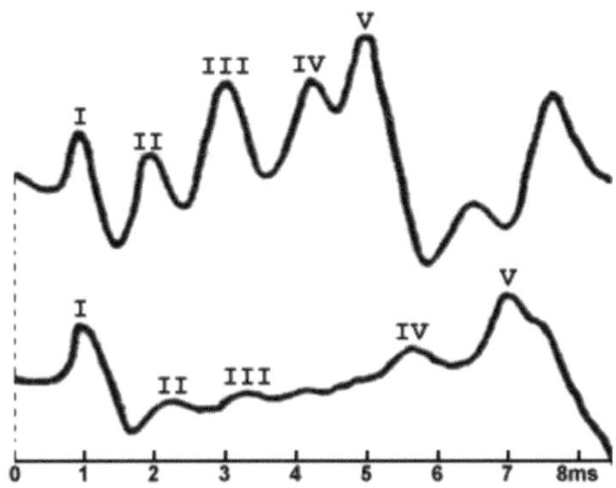


Fig. 20. BAEP changes in acoustic neurinoma.

We have to underscore once again that BAEP tests are not influenced by anesthetics, barbiturates, and attention-consciousness-sleep statuses.

## 6. Visual evoked potentials

Visual evoked potentials are obtained from the optic tract by recording the evoked potentials generated by retinal stimulation. The sources of the stimulus are as follows:

1. Stroboscopic flash light with regular flashing intervals: Applied on babies and uncooperative patients.
2. Flashing LED: Applied as an intraoperative stimulus source. However, it requires use of specially designed lenses.
3. Alternating checkerboard pattern stimulation: This is the stimulation method used most commonly and it is a more sensitive and stable technique. VEP test performed by applying this stimulation is also called as PSVEP (Pattern-Shift Visual Evoked Potential).

Testing environment should be dark, or at least dim. The patient sits in front of a 70-100 cm distant B/W monitor with a checkerboard pattern showing constant luminance and he/she continuously and carefully looks at this pattern. The checks alternate from black to white and from white to black at every 1 or 2 seconds. Each alternation acts as a stimulation and generates an evoked potential at the occipital lobe.

The size of the squares on the checkerboard pattern should be between 28' - 31' (practically, squares with a size of 30', ie. 0.5°, are commonly used). In patients with a reduced visual acuity, this size should be increased a little. It should be borne in mind that as the size changes, the latency and amplitude of the P100 wave changes, as well. As shown in Figure 21, as the squares get smaller, the latency is prolonged and amplitude is elevated.

Note: The polarities of the VEP curves shown in Figure 21 were placed in reverse order, meaning that P100 wave, which should have a lower position, was positioned upwards due to location of the positive potential.

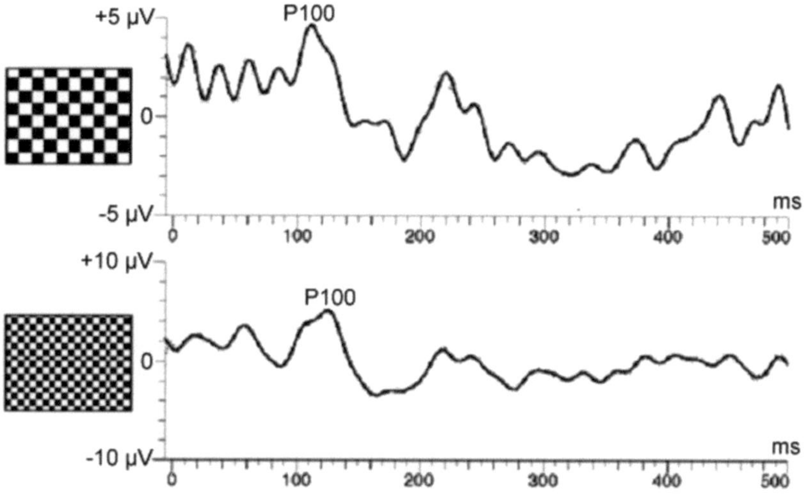


Fig. 21. The size of squares effects P100 quality.

One should also know that if the stimulus rate (normally 1 or 2 stimuli per second) is increased, then subsequently latency is prolonged. Moreover, latency and amplitude values are affected by factors such as brightness of the room, luminance of the screen, and visual fixation of the patient.

As mentioned before, average amplitude of VEPs is about 5-10 µV and it is enough for 10.000x amplification. In other words, this is the type of evoked potential that can be recorded most easily.

In VEP recording, active electrode is Oz, whereas reference electrode is oftenly Fz, and sometimes A1-A2. Routine test is always performed unilaterally (monocular). However, since this evaluation does not work in pathologies past the optic chiasm, binocular VEP test is carried out and the number of active electrodes over the occipital region is 5 in this test.

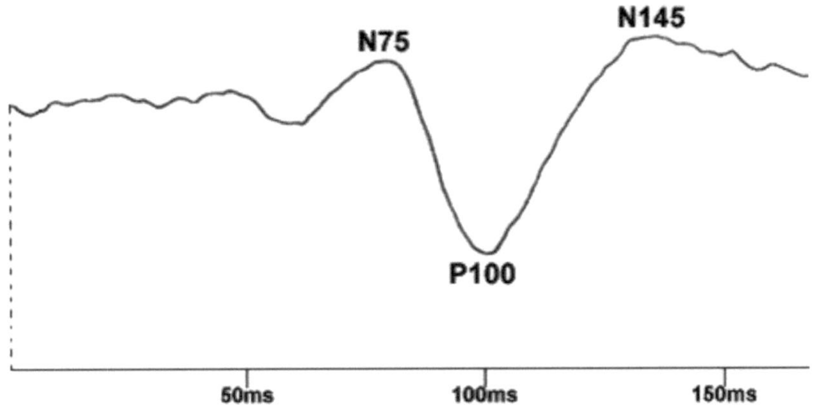


Fig. 22. Components of the VEP.

### 6.1 Evaluation

As seen in Figure 22, since N75 and N145 show high variability during 3-component VEP recording, only P100 wave, which is the essential component, is evaluated (VEP test is also called as "P100 test").

Bilateral comparison bears great importance in the evaluation. However, first, latency and amplitude values of the P100 wave should be identified.

It should be taken into consideration that women have a 5 ms shorter average P100 latency compared with the men, and that among people above 60 years of age, latency may reach high values such as 125 ms.

When there is an amplitude difference exceeding 2 μV between the VEP recordings of two eyes which can not be explained in terms of technical factors, it is a remarkable finding. However, one should always remember that abnormal amplitudes are almost always observed with abnormal latencies.

Main pathologies that may be seen in VEP are as follows.

1. Latency may be prolonged, but amplitude and form may remain normal. Multiple sclerosis, a demyelinating disease, is reflected on VEP in this fashion.

Figure 23 is the VEP recording of a patient with a prolonged P100 absolute latency in the left eye due to multiple sclerosis.

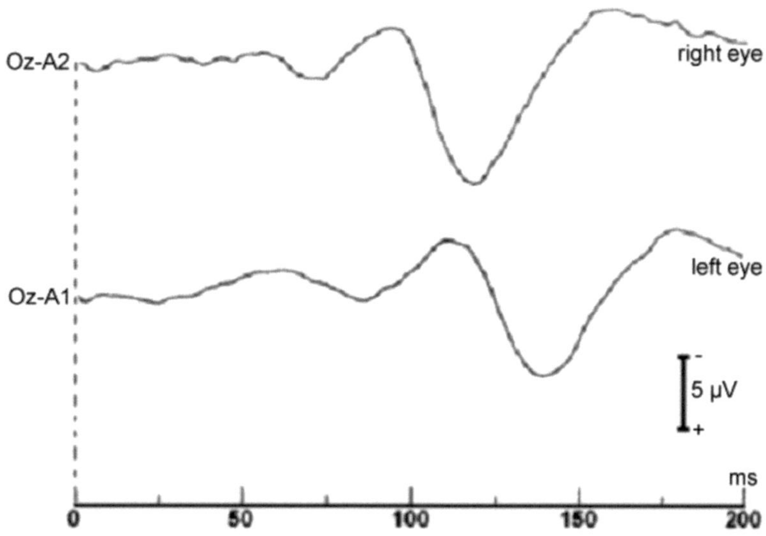


Fig. 23. Prolonged latency: Multiple sclerosis in left eye.

Even in the absence of visual complaints, 30% of multiple sclerosis patients display VEP pathology.

2. Amplitude may be reduced. Lesions compressing the optical nerve are reflected in the VEP recording in this fashion. However, amplitude may be reduced in refractive abnormalities, cataract, and retinopathy, as well. Moreover, even a decrease in the attention of the patient can lead to amplitude reduction.

You can see the prolonged latency and amplitude reduction in the VEP recording of a patient with right optic neuritis (Figure 24).

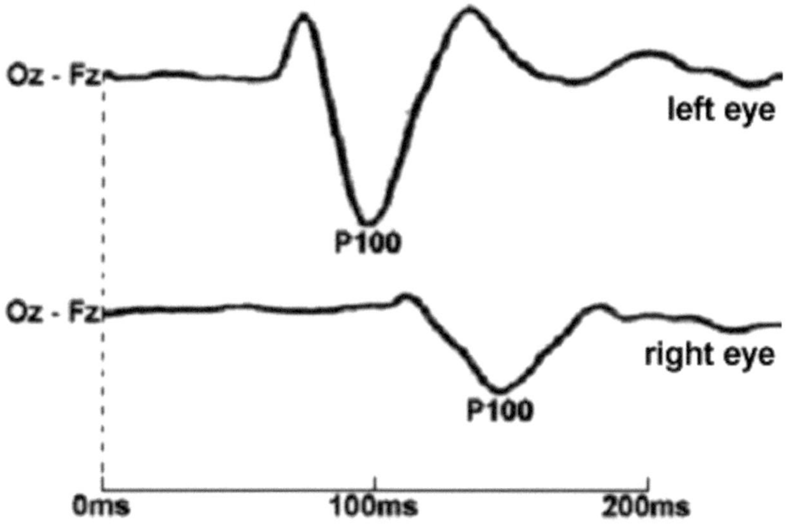


Fig. 24. Reduced amplitude & prolonged latency: Optic neuritis in right eye.

3. In cases involving compressive lesions, amplitude reduction may cause changes in the form, as well. Even in people with no complaints, tumors located at the optic tracts may lead to loss of N75 and prolonged P100.

### 6.2 Indications

1. Optic nerve damage
2. Optic neuritis
3. Headache
4. Head trauma
5. Brain aneurysm
6. Brain tumors
7. Blurred vision
8. Intraoperative monitoring

It may even be used in operations which do not involve optic tracts, but might influence them. However, as shown in Figure 25, the effect of general anesthesia over VEP is considerably high.

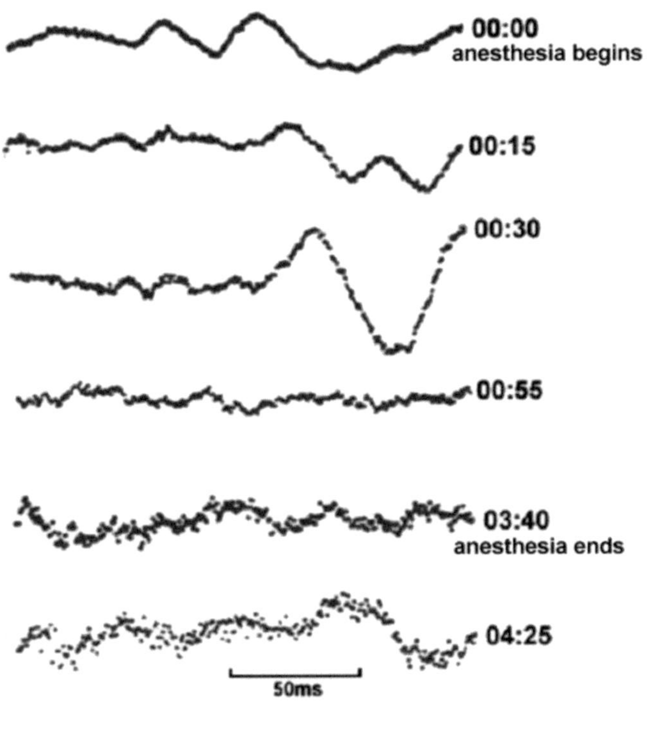


Fig. 25. Effect of general anesthesia on the VEP.

## 7. Conclusion

Which conditions indicate evoked potential tests?

1. Persistence of symptoms despite decided and ongoing treatment
2. Presence of subjective complaints without supportive objective findings
3. Negative X-ray, CT, MRI, or EMG results despite existing complaints
4. Presence of radicular complaints
5. Existing nerve irritation or damage requiring definition
6. Need for advanced diagnosis/treatment
7. Cases requiring confirmation of presence of pain

Advantages and disadvantages of the evoked potential tests

**Pros**

1. Although modern imaging methods other than PET can depict pathological localizations in detail, they can not provide data on functional/physiological structures (ie. metabolic cerebral diseases). Thus, evoked potential tests compensate for this shortcoming.
2. Non-invasive character
3. Objective measurement
4. Subcortical components of auditory and somatosensory evoked potentials are not influenced by general anesthesia, sleep, and states of consciousness.
5. Significantly low cost compared with the modern imaging modalities.

**Cons**

1. There is still no standard in technical regard. Even the fundamental terminological standards have not been completed yet, let alone being a "gold standard". However, currently; SSEP, BAEP, and VEP techniques have been almost standardized.
2. Tests are long and tedious for patients
3. The risk of technical error, therefore the likelihood of repeating the test, is high
4. While the characteristics of the acquired recordings are mostly known, their sources and mechanisms have not yet been completely or clearly understood (due to the complexity of the brain anatomy and nonlinear nature of the brain physiology).

## 8. References

Anbar, Michael. & Spangler Robert. A. & Scott Peter. (1985). *Clinical Biophysics*, Warren H. Green, ISBN 0-87527-316-5, Missouri, USA

Aston, Richard. (1991). *Principles of Biomedical Instrumentation and Measurement*, Macmillan Publishing Company, ISBN 0-02-946562-1, New York, USA

Carr, Joseph J. & Brown, John M. (2001). *Introduction to Biomedical Equipment Technology* (4th edition), Prentice Hall, ISBN 0-13-010492-2, New Jersey, USA

Chiappa, Keith H. (1997). *Evoked Potentials in Clinical Medicine* (3rd edition), Lippincott-Raven Publishers, ISBN 0-397-51659-2, Philadelphia, USA

Daube, Jasper R. (1996). *Clinical Neurophysiology*, F. A. Davis company, ISBN 0-8036-0073-9, Philadelphia, USA

Kimura, Jun. (2001). *Electrodiagnosis in Diseases of Nerve and Muscle: Principles and Practice* (3rd edition), Oxford University Press, ISBN 0-19-512977-6, New York, USA

Misulis, Karl E. & Fakhoury, Toufic. (2001). *Spehlmann's Evoked Potential Primer* (3rd edition), Butterworth-Heinemann, ISBN 0-7506-7333-8, Maryland, USA

Webster, John G. (2004). *Bioinstrumentation*, John Wiley & Sons, ISBN 0-471-45257-2, Maryland, USA

# 5

# Diagnostic Values of Electrophysiology in Ophthalmology

Morteza Movassat
*Tehran University of Medical Sciences, Farabi Hospital*
*Iran*

## 1. Introduction

The main function of the eye is converting received light energy to neuronal impulses by some chemical interactions in posterior segment; then, these impulses, after some processing, will be transferred to visual cortex by the visual pathways. Striate cortex located at posterior pole of brain is where which creates vision through a complicated physiological phenomena.

Electrodiagnosis in ophthalmology is a method that investigates this process functionally and can help in many complicated situations.

Two important characteristics make this paraclinic method different from others; to be both functional and objective. Many ocular tests as angiography, ultrasonography and OCT are objective but not functional, and some, as perimetry and contrast sensitivity test are functional but not objective. This is why electrodiagnostic tests are problem solving and conclusive in equivocal instances specially when encountered to forensic or legal cases with probability of simulation.

Electrodiagnosis in ophthalmology includes electroretinography (ERG), electro-oculography (EOG) and visual evoked potentials (VEP); ERG evaluates function of posterior segment of the eye specially sensory retina; EOG, also, evaluates function of the posterior segment of the eye with more focus on retinal pigment epithelium (RPE), and VEP evaluates function of visual pathways and striate cortex.

It should be reminded that aside from these advantages , these tests are not ones to be ordered without proper indications, and their results must be interpreted by someone familiar with pathogenesis of ocular diseases.

## 2. History

The history of recording of electroretinogram goes back to Einthoven and Jolly in 1908 and then, to Kahn and Lowenstein in 1924, with their works on modifying electrodes; but it was Granit's investigations during 1933-1947 that differentiated ERG's components in human. The work of Noell, Tomita, Brindly and Brown showed the origin of these components and paved the way for clinical use of ERG. In a separate research, Brown's group blocked central retinal artery of cat during ERG recording, and proved the relation between a-wave and photoreceptors (Brown & Wiesel, 1961 ). The relation between b-wave and Muller cells was shown by Miller and Dowling ( Miller & Dowling,1970 ); and Riggs introduced contact lens electrodes in 1941, and opened the perspective of practical use of ERG in ophthalmology; then Karpe emphasized on diagnostic value of ERG even in eyes with hazy media (Karpe,1982 ).

In electro-oculography, Kris's works helped to find the slow electrical changes of the eye in rest condition which cause a posterior-anterior electrical vector, and he showed that this potential changes differ in dark and light adapted eyes ( Kris, 1958) ; then Arden suggested comparing these potentials in light and dark adaptation and based a diagnostic index, which, today, we know it as Arden ratio ( Arden & Kelsey, 1962 ).

History of visual evoked potentials reaches to Adrian and Matthews in 1934, who explained responses of occipital lobes in electroencephalogram. Then Monnier, in 1952, by placing scalp electrodes on occiput, recorded waves with latencies of about 90-120 msec. Ciganek, later in 1961, described some components of VEP ( Ciganek, 1961 ) and Gastaut and Regis explained that the most invariable component of VEP is $P_2$ wave.Harding and colleagues designed a pattern/reversal stimulation for VEP and ruled out the hypothesis claiming that some components of VEP are ERG waves . Finally, Halliday brought experimental works of VEP to clinical use in 1972.(Halliday et al, 1972).

## 3. Biological and biochemical bases of tests

### 3.1 Electroretinography

Photoreceptors, rods and cones, containing photosensitive pigments, are responsible for converting light energy into neuronal impulses, and retinal pigment epithelium (RPE) has a fundamental role in this process. Extracellular matrix, filling subretinal space is medium for molecular interactions between choroid, RPE and sensory retina. RPE cells' membrane with Na+ and K+ ATPase affects inflow and outflow of ions in this matrix (Ostwald & Steinberg, 1980) and by this ionic transferring, initial conversion of light energy to neuronal impulses occurs. RPE also has an important role in absorption of scattered lights entering eyes which can interfere visual function. Opsin, a photosensitive protein derivative in outer segment of photoreceptors, is in close relation with ionic changes of extracellular matrix. By photo-chemical and then chemo-electrical interactions of these pigment components, resting potential of inner segment of photoreceptors changes to action potential. Inner segment-Muller cell's processes complex makes outer limiting membrane which separates molecularly interphotoreceptor space from neural retina (Lam,2005). Muller cells with long processes are present in many layers of retina, from outer to inner limiting membranes, and make glial structure of the sensory retina. By changing the potassium and carbohydrate level (Newman,1993), these cells share electrical response and thus affect ERG. Interphotoreceptor matrix, mentioned earlier, contains some soluble and insoluble compounds with a retinol-binding protein, showing the role of vitamin A metabolism in visual function. On the other hand, close anatomical and physiological relationship between choroid, RPE and sensory retina explains why pathology of each can affect others, and this is the cause of relative overlapping of results of ERG, EOG and VEP tests. In bright light or photopic vision, cones with three pigments, red, green, and blue sensitive are responsive; but in dim light or scotopic vision rods containing rhodopsin, are active.

Bipolars and ganglion cells, in association with horizontal, amacrine and Muller cells, receive impulses from photoreceptors and, after some processing, transfer them to visual pathways. These pathways begin from optic nerves and continue through chiasm, optic tracts, geniculate bodies and optic radiations, and terminate in visual cortex.

The role of horizontal cells, physiologically, is interesting. These cells connect neuronal cells together in a manner that makes possible for a large number of photoreceptors and bipolars to connect with a small groups of ganglion cells and higher centers neurons to produce "receptive field". Some parts in these fields work synergic and some parts antagonistic and this mechanism makes anatomical basis for center-surround antagonism and On/Off responses. In fact perception of movement, direction and form are complicated visual functions which need too many physiological interactions that are not completely understood.

### 3.2 Electro-oculography

Depolarization of the basal surface of RPE due to light stimulation causes a transepithelial negative charge with a posterior-anterior vector which can be measured as a positive charge in anterior pole of the eye. This slow changing potential is, in fact, resting potential of eye and if light adaptation occurs, this potential reaches to a maximum. Dividing maximum peak in light by minimum trough in dark gives Arden ratio which helps to differentiate normal from pathologic cases. Horizontal saccades of the eye during test help to eliminate other electrical charges affecting globes and cause electrodes, placed close to the canthi, receive only globes potentials. In contrast with ERG that shows action potentials in sensory retina, the EOG reflects resting potential of the eye as a dipole and shows RPE function.

### 3.3 Visual evoked potentials

Brain cortex with main intrinsic neuronal activity responds to external stimuli, and if stimulation has visual nature, the response will be visual evoked. By placing skin electrodes on occiput and stimulation of the eyes with light, the cortical responses to visual stimuli can be obtained. Any pathology in macular ganglion cells, optic nerves, chiasm, optic tracts, geniculate bodies, optic radiations and striate cortex can affect the VEP results. But this test specially helps when functional defects overcome anatomical changes and clinical examinations and neuro-imagings results are equivocal.Considering optic nerves fibers crossing in chiasm and also, combination of signals in cortex, VEP is a hemi-bilateral brain response to unilateral stimulation of the eye.

Occiput is an area of scull near to some parts of visual cortex which are responsive for foveal area and central 10°of visual field. Ganglion cells of retina and neurons of higher centers are in different kinds; magnocellular for perception of movement, parvocellular for visual acuity and color vision, and koniocellular for perception of form. This functional variety of ganglion cells in association with horizontal cells role, mentioned earlier, give us ability of not only seeing, but also distinction of the position of things in our environment. For evaluation of these complicated functions, the visual stimuli should have some characteristics other than simple light flashes. Formed stimuli with several patterns are designed for this mean. Pattern/reversal and pattern onset/offset checks, horizontal and vertical bars, full-field and quadrant-field patterns in black/white or colored, are several forms of stimulations used for pattern VEP.

## 4. Characteristics of normal electroretinogram

Full-field ERG is the most common used method of electroretinography. Stimulation of extensive area of fundus and obtaining whole response of retina gives full-field ERG.

### 4.1 ERG components

Three principal components and some less distinctive wavelets make standard ERG.

#### 4.1.1 a-wave

A prominent negative wave arising from inner segment of photoreceptors, also known as late receptor potential.This wave reflects the function of outer retina, RPE and choroid.

#### 4.1.2 b-wave

A more prominent but positive wave which originates from On bipolars and Muller cells. Ionic interactions between these cells, triggered by light stimulations, are main factor to produce this wave (Heckenlively&Arden ,2006). This component reflects the function of middle layers of retina which receive its vasculature from central retinal artery and vein.

#### 4.1.3 Oscillatory potentials

4-6 wavelets on ascending part of b-wave, representing inhibitory feedback circuit in inner plexiform layer due to bipolar-amacrine cells interactions. Initial wavelets originate from cones and subsequent ones originate from rods (Wachtmeister, 1998). These oscillations can be obtained by a separate protocol in both dark and light adaptations. Although mechanism of formation of these wavelets are not well understood, but their high sensitivity to hypoxia gives them a diagnostic value in retinal vascular disorders.

In addition to these major components of standard(full-field) ERG, there are some minor ones, usually exploited in research works. Of these, early receptor potentials originating in outer segment of photoreceptors, d-wave which is off-response in photopic ERG, d.c-component referring RPE function and e-wave or delayed off-response (Lam,2005) are noteworthy.

To separate responses of rods from cones, test is performed first in scotopic condition (with patching eyes for 20′in a dark room ), with blue, orange, red and white lights; then the eyes will be dazzled with bright light for about 4′ (light adaptation) for photopic ERG.

Both cone and rod photoreceptors respond to stimulations in both dark adapted (scotopic) and light adapted (photopic) eyes; but in scotopic vision rods' function is prevailed, while in photopic vision cones mostly are involved.

Two data of each component should be measured for interpretation of response:

- Implicit time (1.T.): time between the end of stimulation and wave peak, in m.sec.

- Amplitude: the height of wave in microvolts; in a-wave it is measured from iso-electric line and in b-wave from a-wave peak to b-wave peak. These data vary in different conditions of adaptation and, also due to several variables as age, race, refractive errors, pupil size and unit amplifier. For this reasons, it is recommended to evaluate normal range in each electrodiagnostic center; but international society for clinical electrophysiology of vision (ISCEV) declares normal data every 3 years which can be referred to.

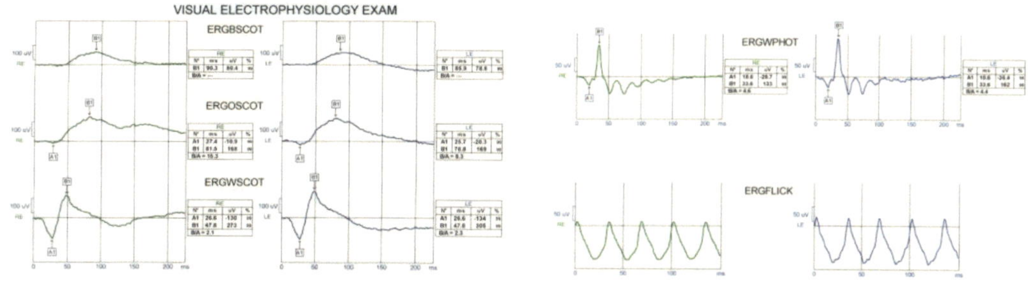


Fig. 1. Normal standard ERG.Right, scotopic with blue, orange ,and white lights.Left, photopic(up) and flicker(down).

| | Implicit time a- wave(ms) | Amplitude a- wave(micro V) | Implicit time b-wave(ms) | Amplitude b-wave(b-a) (micro V) |
|---|---|---|---|---|
| ERG-25dB (rod response) | | | | Average=232±60 |
| ERG-0dB (mixed response) | Average=25.2±1 | Average=197±25 | Average=46.9±3 | Average=365±80 |
| | Implicit time a- wave(ms) | Amplitude a- wave(micro V) | Implicit time b-wave(ms) | Amplitude b-wave(b-a) (micro V) |
| Photopic ERG | Average=19.1±2 | Average=-25.0±5 | Average=31.6±1 | Average=90±15 |
| Flicker ERG | | | Average=34.2±1 | Average=118±17 |

Table 1. Normal values of ERG in ISCEV protocol.

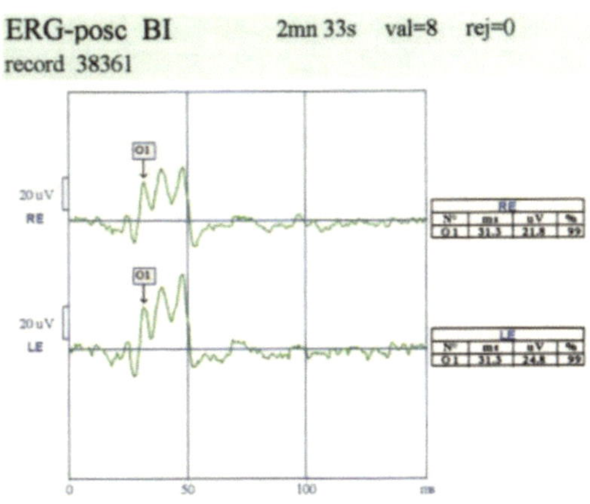


Fig. 2. Normal oscillatory potentials.

### 4.2 Specialized techniques of ERG

#### 4.2.1 Flicker (focal) ERG

Some differences in physiology of cones and rods can help to separate their responses in ERG. Retractory period of rods is about 100 msec., which means rods can not respond to stimulations with frequency higher than 10 Hz, but cones with much shorter retractory period can respond to stimulations with frequency up to 30 Hz(flicker ERG). By using different frequencies of stimulation, these two systems can be differentiated physiologically but not anatomically; of course, because of high concentration of cones in macula, flicker ERG practically shows macular function.

#### 4.2.2 Bright flash ERG

Severe haziness of ocular media as seen in corneal leukoma, pathologic cataract, condensed vitreous opacities and deformed ocular tissues due to trauma may be candidates for surgical procedures to gain better vision. The main question will be visual potential or outcome in these eyes. Also in recent globe lacerations, the catastrophe of sympathetic ophthalmia of the other eye, although very rare, should be kept in mind. ERG and VEP, by using bright or intensified flashes, which can pass ocular haziness, are helpful for making decision.

#### 4.2.3 Chromatic ERG

In suspected cases of color blindness, ERG with different wavelengths can show color vision abnormalities objectively; this method helps in vocational and legal cases.

#### 4.2.4 Pattern ERG

Representing ganglion cells function, which are more concentrated in macula, pattern ERG is a test to evaluate inner retina and optic nerve disorders. Visual acuity measurement in preverbal children, evaluation of nerve fibers loss in glaucoma, and diseases involving inner retina, as seen in longstanding retinal detachments are special clinical indications of this test. Stimuli with frequency of 3 Hz, give transient response with three components of $N_{35}$ , $P_{50}$ and $N_{95}$ waves; the numbers show wave's implicit time. Stimuli with frequency of 5 Hz or higher give steady-state sinusoidal response. In ganglion cells disorders, amplitude of $P_{50}$ component is reduced, while in optic nerve lesions $N_{95}$ wave shows pathology.Steady-state response changes are comparable with $N_{95}$ component in transient response.

Stimuli are pattern/reversal checker-board with 48'size checks and 100% contrast which covers 10-16 degrees of central visual field.Pupil dilation is not necessary (Lam,2005).

#### 4.2.5 Multifocal ERG (m.f.ERG)

Using physics and mathematics, m.f.ERG is a method designed to evaluate small local lesions in fundus, specially cone involvements. 61 to 241 white/black scaled hexagons stimulate posterior pole of the eye conforming central 50 degrees of visual field in a pseudorandom, m-sequence program.Simulating random, but known by system's software, it works in a manner that in each time of stimulation each hexagon has 50% chance to be on or off. After amplifying responses, they will be matched together for finding the area of retina related to each hexagon. In fact m.f.ERG waveforms are not true recorded responses, but mathematical data in which, response of each hexagon is measured by adding all recordings following a white frame and then subtracting all recordings following a black frame (Lam,2005). For this type of analysis, the number of hexagons in each frame should be odd and equal to number of stimulations in each test. After matching responses (adding and subtracting) the sum response of all hexagons but one, will be zero and only one response remains which correlates with its related location in fundus. Stimulation with frequencies up to 75 Hz give first order kernels (k1) which represent function of outer retina, and stimulation with higher frequencies give second order kernels ($k_2$) showing function of ganglion cells.Test with more hexagons in each frame gives more precise localization of lesion, but noise-to-signal ratio will be higher.

Pupil dilation and maintained central fixation are critical to obtain accurate topographical responses. Although binocular test is possible, monocular results are more assured.

Each $k_1$ response includes $N_1$, $P_1$ and $N_2$ components in which $N_1$ and $P_1$ accord roughly to a-wave and b-wave in standard ERG.

Print-outs may be designed as concentric rings showing 2, 5, 10, and 15 degrees of central visual fields which are more used for small lesions in fovea and perifovea; or it may be designed in four quadrants, used in more peripheral involvement in posterior pole.

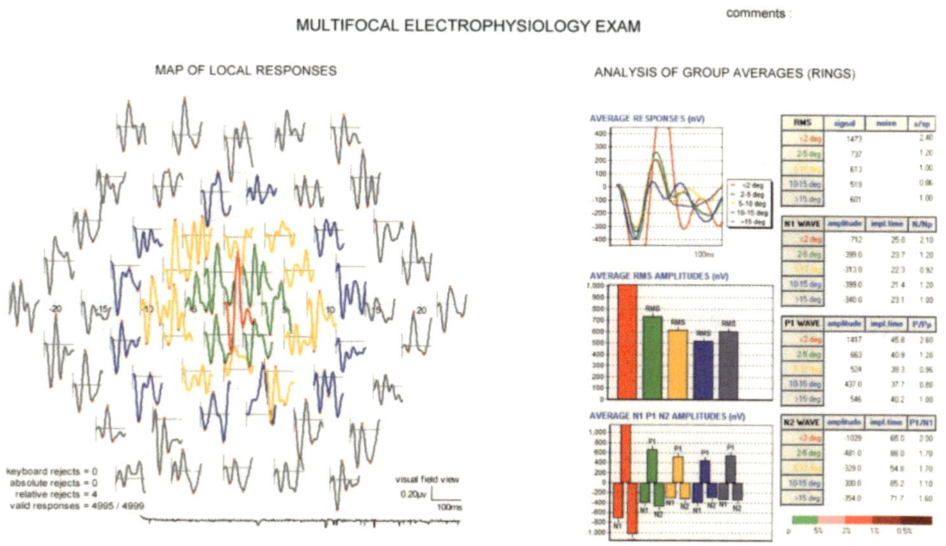


Fig. 3. Normal m.f.ERG.Concentric rings show the locations of the responses.

#### 4.3 Recording of electroretinogram

Electroretinography unit consists of stimulator, electrodes, connectors, amplifier, computer and printer.

#### 4.3.1 Stimulator

Usually a standing monitor with a chin-rest 33 away from the screen.Flash or pattern stimulations are given to the eyes in different colors and forms. Of course flash stimulations in a Ganzfeld bowl are preferred in full-field ERG for better stimulation of center-directed elements in retina.For kids and patients not able to sit in front of monitor, stimulations can be given by a portable flasher.

### 4.3.2 Electrodes

Several kinds of electrodes are available. For active or positive electrodes, Burian-Allen and Dawson-Trick-Litzkow (DTL) are more known.These are solid contact lenses which touch the cornea via a conductive gel.

In case of pattern ERG gold foil or fibers are used for active electrodes, mounting inferior lid border which makes possible better receiving of pattern stimuli by patient. Reference or negative electrodes are skin plaques and are placed on lateral wall of orbits posterior to globes. Ground or earth electrode is to reduce the noise and may be placed on auricle.

Cornea should be anesthetized with topical anesthetics and pupils should be in full dilation in all methods of ERG except pattern ERG. The sites of electrodes on skin should be cleaned carefully and conducting gel should be used for electrode-skin attachment.

### 4.3.3 Connectors

Made of fine wire which connect electrodes with amplifier.

### 4.3.4 Amplifier

Amplifier is to empower and making recordable the responses which are weak and not obtainable if not amplified. The characteristics of amplifier are important in any unit and its range of amplifying affects the range of normal data in each system.

### 4.3.5 Computer

Computer may be as a desktop or laptop, containing several softwares for several kinds of programs including type of stimulation, receiving responses, averaging data, analyzing components, and finally, saving results in files.

### 4.3.6 Printer

Printer is last part of unit and gives print-outs of results, showing responses and data of components.

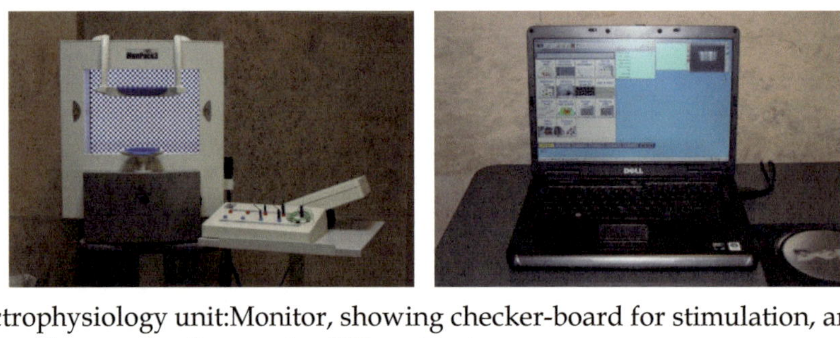

Fig. 4. Electrophysiology unit:Monitor, showing checker-board for stimulation, amplifier and laptop with several softwares for different tests.

## 5. Characteristics of normal electro-oculogram

EOG is sum up of many square-shaped waveforms due to horizontal back and forth saccades of the eyes fixing 2 red diodes located 15 degrees to the right and left of the primary gaze on monitor or in a bowl (Lam,2005).

### 5.1 EOG Component

After some saccades for orientation of patient, test starts in darkness for about 10′ in which, potential gains its minimum (dark trough); then continues in light for about 10′ in which, maximum potential (light peak) is reached. The light peak potential divided by dark trough potential gives Arden ratio. The time length of each saccade is about 1.5 sec. and patient has a while for rest between some of them.

Normal range of Arden ratio is about 1.8-2.2 in ISCEV protocol; ratios between 1.8 and 1.6 are considered borderline and ratios less than 1.6 are abnormal.

### 5.2 EOG recording

#### 5.2.1 EOG electrodes

Four silver-silver chloride skin electrodes are attached to skin via a conductive gel, close to four canthi. One ground electrode is placed on forehead or auricle to decrease noise. In each horizontal saccade, the electrode close to cornea becomes active and the opposite one becomes reference electrode.The electrode close to medial canthus of one side is matched with electrode close to lateral canthus of the other side in connecting to amplifier, causing homonymous electrical polarization in each saccade.

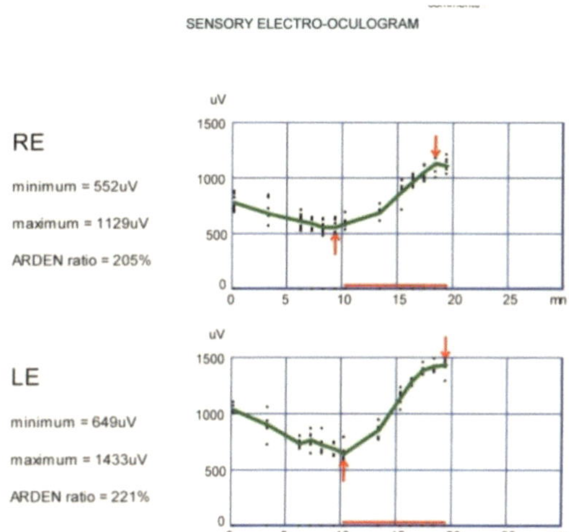


Fig. 5. Normal EOG, showing dark trough and light rise.

#### 5.2.2 Monitor or a bowl

A monitor or a bowl with a chin-rest 33 away of screen, with fixation lights, and ability to be dark or light. Patient should sit in front of monitor to follow the fixation light. In background luminance of about 50-100 cd/sqm, pupils should be dilated; but in higher luminance, about 400-600 cd/sqm, dilation is not needed.

**5.2.3 Other parts**, including connectors, amplifier, computer and printer are same as ERG test.

Considering duration of the test and its method, EOG can not be performed in poor physical conditions, severe strabismus, severe nystagmus, preverbal children and under general anesthesia.

## 6. Characteristics of normal visual evoked potentials

Visual, formed or unformed, stimulations of the eye, usually mono-ocularly, and then, obtaining electrical responses from striate cortex, is known as VEP test. Standard VEP is performed with flash or pattern stimuli with their special indications and limitations; also, there are some special new methods finding their clinical utilities in recent years.

### 6.1 Recording of visual evoked potentials

#### 6.1.1 Electrodes

Usually intra-dermic disposable needles. Active electrodes are placed one centimeter away of inion on either side, and referring electrodes are placed on mid-point of a hypothetical line between inion and nose base. Ground electrode, reducing noise, is placed on auricle.

**6.1.2** Connectors connect the electrodes with amplifier which empowers responses up to recordable level.

**6.1.3** Stimulation unit, a monitor with ability to give flash or pattern stimulations; in cases not able to sit in front of monitor, stimulations can be given by a portable stimulator.

In pattern VEP, patient sits one meter away of monitor, wearing his or her correction, and fixes with one eye the fixation spot at the center of monitor; the other eye is patched. In flash method, patient puts his or her chin on chin-rest 33 away of monitor and looks with one eye to the flashing screen.

Stimulation with frequencies of 5 Hz or less give transient VEP, but higher frequencies give steady-state VEP which has special indications.

Neurologists prefer positive downward peak, but positive upward peaks are recommended in ophthalmology.

If performed binocularly, amplitude of waves increases some.

**6.1.4** Laptop with several softwares to choose the kind of test and analyzing the responses.

**6.1.5** Printer gives printed results and data of components.

### 6.2 Methods and components of VEP

Because of high noise-to-signal ratio, averaging of responses to multiple stimulations, usually 64, is recommended. Due to the same reason variability of responses specially in amplitude, between two eyes and also, between different subjects is expected.

Dilation of pupils is not recommended unless in severe miosis, which can cause delayed responses.

### 6.2.1 Flash VEP

Indicated in cases with poor vision or poor fixation ability and nystagmus, this method gives an overall information about visual pathways. The response includes $N_1$, $P_1$, $N_2$, $P_2$, and $N_3$ components; most prominent and diagnostic one is $P_2$ wave.

### 6.2.2 Pattern onset/offset VEP

With fixed black/white checks stimulations, interrupted by iso-luminant blank screen, this method of pattern VEP is indicated in visual acuity evaluation in uncooperative cases. The response consists first positive, second negative, and third positive components with implicit time about 75 msec., 125 msec. and 150 msec.

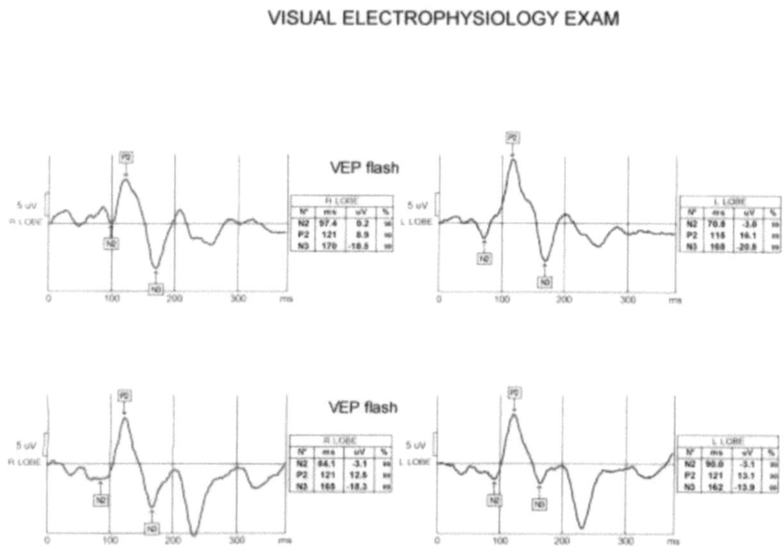


Fig. 6. Normal flash VEP; right eye(up )and left eye(down) responses.

### 6.2.3 Pattern/ reversal VEP(P/R VEP)

Most preferred and most commonly used method of VEP is P/R VEP. Comparing with other methods, responses of P/R VEP are more consistent, and by using several forms of patterns, even the precise location of lesion can be guessed. Check sizes can vary, but usually 15′ , 30′, and 60′ checks are used; about 64 stimulations with reversing sites of black and white squares are projected to the eye and after averaging, responses will be obtained which consist of $N_{75}$, $P_{100}$ and $N_{135}$ components. $P_{100}$ wave is the most prominent and the most diagnostic component of P/R VEP.

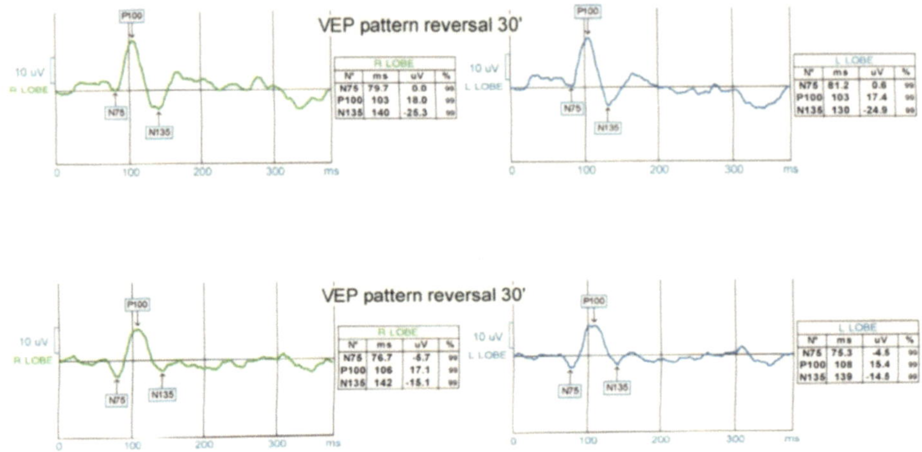


Fig. 7. Normal P/R VEP; right eye(up) and left eye( down) responses.

#### 6.2.4 Multifocal VEP

Similar to m.f.ERG, alternating black/white checks, in a special design of pseudorandom and m-sequence, is used for stimulation, and software of computer cross-correlates the responses with sectors in fundus and visual pathways. In fact m.f.VEP is an objective evaluation of visual field, which is helpful in cases with poor cooperation for perimetry.

#### 6.2.5 Sweep VEP

Stimulation of eyes with high-frequency, temporal reversing patterns gives steady-state VEP response.

By using two methods of spatial and contrast frequency (Lam,2005), this test can measure visual acuity in preverbal children. In spatial frequency method, rate of temporal frequency is fixed but the width of black/white bars decreases gradually; in contrast frequency method, spatial and temporal frequencies are fixed while contrast of bars decreases. Recording responses during spatial or contrast changes, gives information about visual functions of the case, which are roughly comparable with Snellen chart and contrast sensitivity test.

| | Implicit time $P_2$(ms) | Amplitude $P_2$(microV) |
|---|---|---|
| Flash VEP | Average=112±11 | Average=9±5 |
| | Implicit time $P_{100}$(ms) | amplitude$P_{100}$(microV) |
| Pattern 60' | Average=103±7 | Average=12±6 |
| Pattern 30' | Average=106±3 | Average=16±7 |
| Pattern 15' | Average=110±5 | Average=13±7 |
| Pattern 7' | Average=125±10 | Average=10±6 |

Table 2. Normal values of flash and P/R VEP in ISCEV protocol.

## 7. Clinical applications and indications of tests

As mentioned earlier, because of close anatomical and functional relationships between choroid, RPE, sensory retina, and visual pathways which originate from ganglion cells in retina, electrodiagnostic , ERG, EOG and VEP, results are overlapping in many disorders. But, considering pathogenesis of diseases, the most indicated test should be performed. Therefore, physicians who order tests should be familiar with chorioretinal and visual pathways disorders and clinical examinations are recommended strongly.

### 7.1 Disorders affecting ERG

#### 7.1.1 Rod-cone degeneration or R.P. disease

A hereditary retinal dystrophy, mostly autosomal recessive, less autosomal dominant and least sex-linked, which starts with night blindness and continues with visual field constriction, reduced visual acuity, and fundus changes of pigment spicules and arterial narrowing. R.P disease may be seen in many systemic metabolic and neurologic disorders. Of these, Usher syndrome, Refsum's disease, Bassen-kornzweig syndrome, Hurler and Sanfilippo mucopolysaccharidosis, Laurence-Moon and Bardet-Biedl neurologic syndromes should be mentioned (Spaide, 1999).

ERG changes: delayed and reduced waves, first in scotopic and then in photopic responses.

In autosomal dominant form which has better prognosis, ERG may be some detectable, even up to middle-age, but in other forms, flat or non-detectable ERG is common finding when the disease passed initial stages.

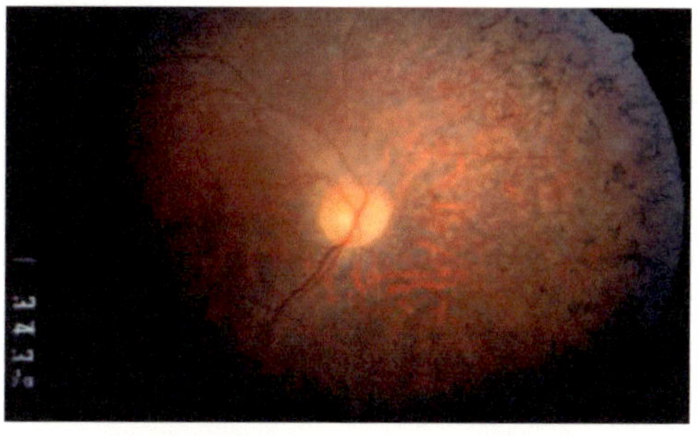

Fig. 8. RP disease or rod-cone degeneration.

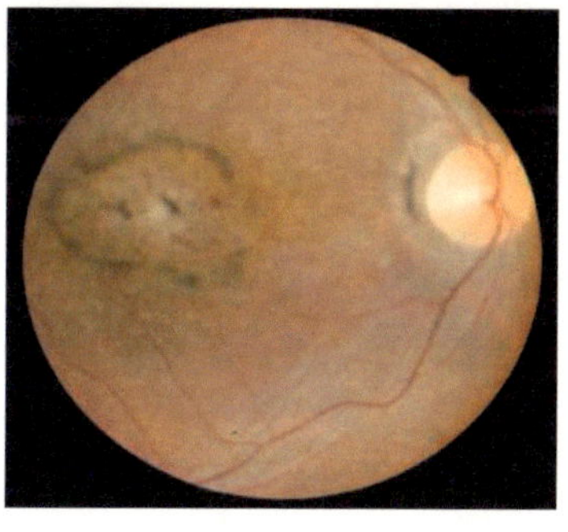

Fig. 9. Inverse RP disease.

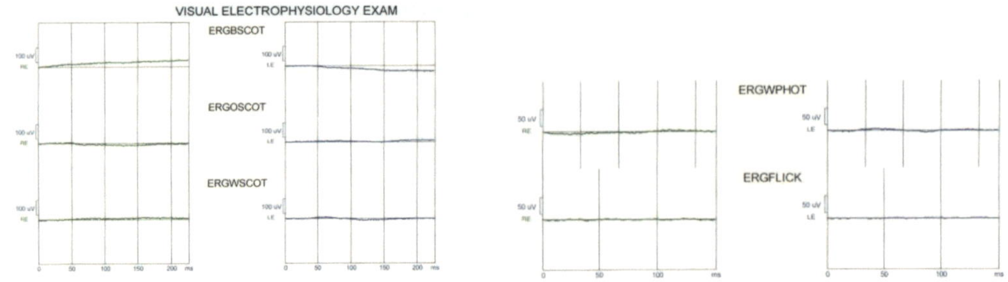


Fig. 10. Flat or non-detectable ERG in RP disease(right, scotopic ; left up, photopic; down, flicker).

### 7.1.2 Cone-rod degeneration

Also known as inverse R.P., starts with photophobia and reduced visual acuity that show cone involvement before rod degeneration. A rare form of disease involves cone system only.

ERG changes: Here, delay and amplitude reduction is more severe in flicker ERG, but finally, flat ERG in both scotopic and photopic responses is usual; m.f.ERG can help in primary stages without gross fundus changes, differentiating this disease from other disorders.

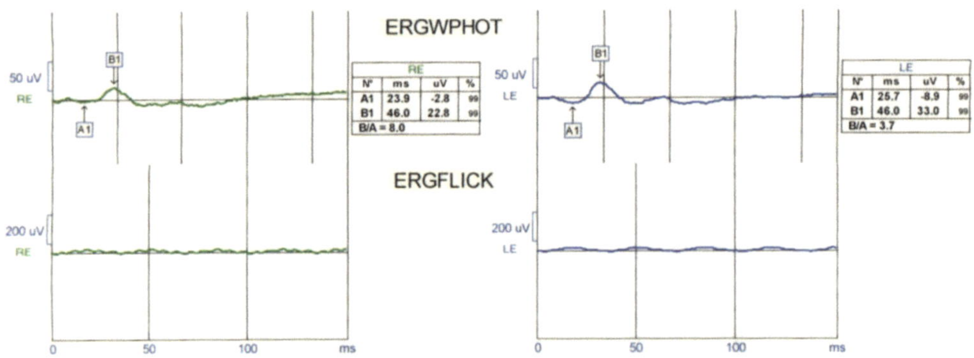


Fig. 11. Photopic and flicker ERG in cone-rod degeneration; flicker response(down) is severely reduced.

### 7.1.3 Avitaminosis A

Avitaminosis A with clinical symptoms and signs and ERG changes similar to R.P. disease; rarely seen today, but may occur in malabsorption. If treated timely, it is reversible.

### 7.1.4 Leber's Congenital Amaurosis (LCA)

LCA is ,in fact, congenital form of R.P disease. Patients suffer from low vision, manifesting with wandering eye movements or nystagmus and poor reactions to visual stimulations in neonatal life. Vast majority of cases are inherited in autosomal recessive trait (Ryan, 2006); and most of them have a high degree of hyperopia. Fundus changes, if observed, are mild but may progress in older ages.

ERG changes: Nearly flat or completely non-detectable ERG is routine response, differentiating it from delayed visual maturity (Movassat et al,2008 ).

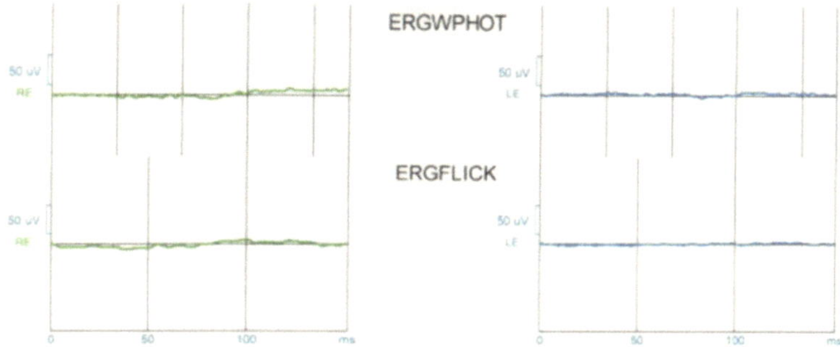


Fig. 12. Flat ERG, photopic and flicker, in LCA.

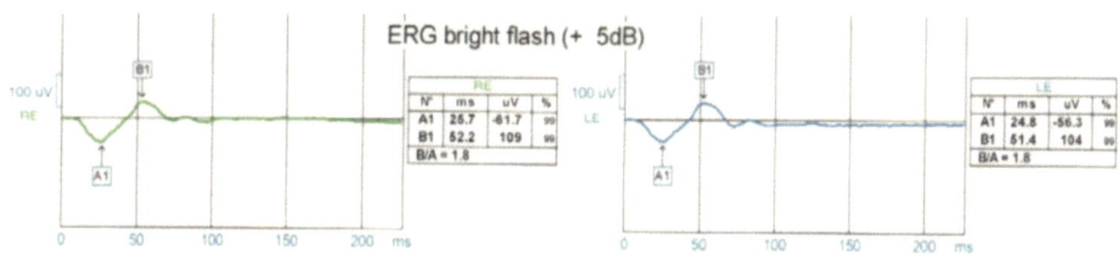


Fig. 13. Normal photopic ERG in delayed maturity.

### 7.1.5 Congenital Stationary Night Blindness (CSNB)

A group of hereditary diseases, with congenital non-progressing night blindness, and usually good visual acuity. Normal fundus is common finding, but in some types, white pigmentary changes without arterial narrowing (fundus albipunctatus) may be seen.

ERG changes: Abnormal scotopic, but normal photopic and flicker responses . Type 1 CSNB has totally flat scotopic ERG with all wavelengths, but type 2 has flat response with blue light, but negative ERG(a-wave only) with white light in scotopic ERG (Ryan, 2006).

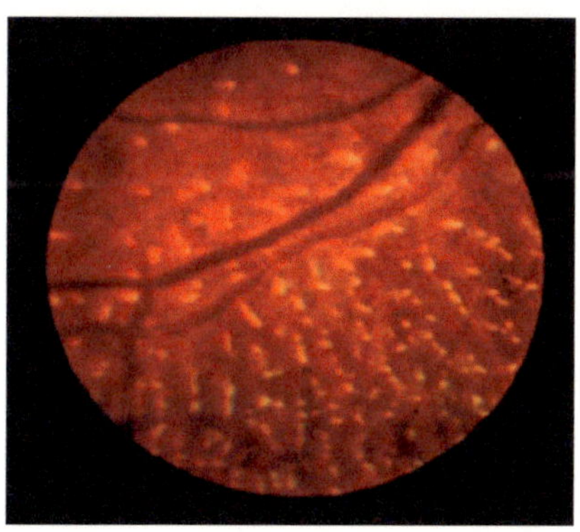

Fig. 14. Fundus albipunctatus.

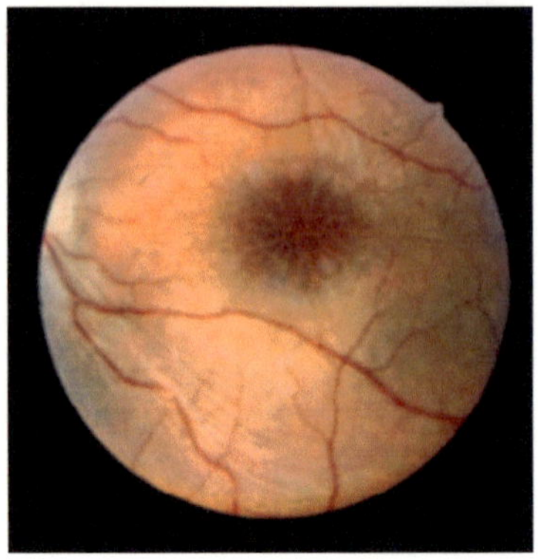

Fig. 15. X-linked retinoschisis.

X-linked retinoschisis with foveal cystic change is a subgroup of CSNB, with negative ERG that is characteristic when confronted with fundus changes.

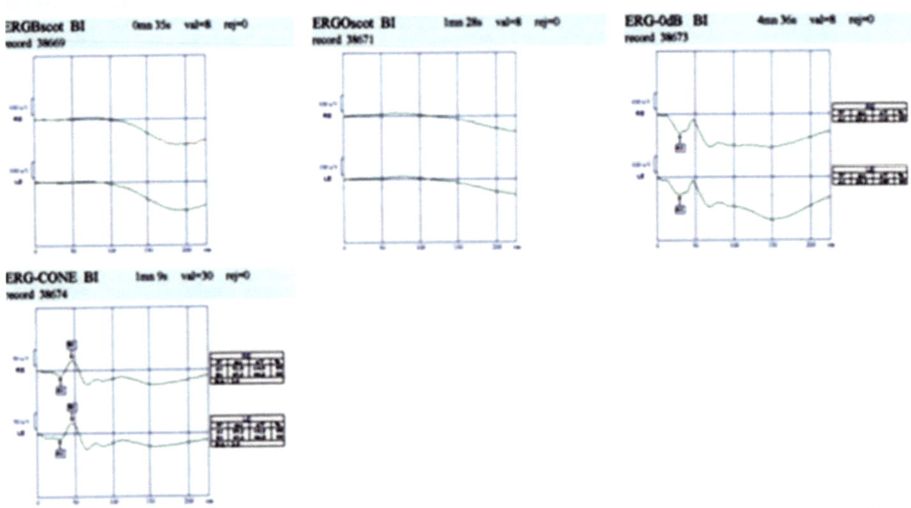


Fig. 16. Scotopic(up) and photopic(down) ERG in CSNB, showing negative ERG with white light in scotopic condition.

### 7.1.6 Achromatism

This group of anomalies is due to physiologically abnormal cone system, which causes color blindness. In complete, or typical rod monochromatism, all three types of cones have dysfunction. Although rare, this autosomal recessive monochromatism causes total color blindness associated with reduced visual acuity. In cone monochromatism, color blindness is incomplete, and cones not involved, work normally and patient has some color vision ability.

ERG changes: Normal scotopic, subnormal photopic , but non-detectable flicker responses are characteristic for rod monochromatism. In cone monochromatism flicker responses are reduced but not totally non-detectable.

### 7.1.7 Chorio-retinal vascular disorders

Central retinal artery (CRA), supplying blood of inner retina , if occluded causes painless total visual loss due to retinal ischemia. Branch retinal artery occlusion causes field defects due to ischemic changes in involved area. Central or branch venous occlusions causing severe blood circulation defects, although not so emergent as arterial occlusions, may result in serious late-onset complications which need close follow up. High blood pressure, diabetes and hyperlipidemia are predisposing factors for vascular disorders of retina.

ERG changes:Non-detectable b-wave, but normal a-wave(negative ERG) is ERG response in central retinal artery occlusion. In ophthalmic artery occlusion, affecting both choroid and retina, ERG is totally non-detectable.

Delayed and then reduced b-wave, initially in scotopic, and then in all conditions, is ERG response in branch or central retinal venous occlusions. Severe reduction of b-wave amplitude is a poor prognostic index, and b/a amplitude ratios less than 1 predicts neovascular complications, recommending prophylactic laser therapy (Lam, 2005). In stasis or incomplete occlusions, delayed b-wave in full-field and flicker ERG reflects the severity of ischemia.

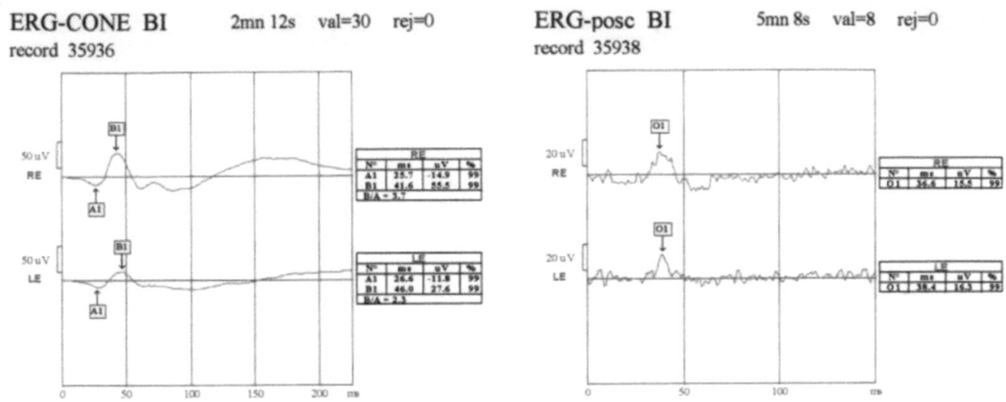


Fig. 17. Photopic(left) and oscillatory(right) potentials in a hypertensive case with branch retinal vein occlusion in left eye(down).

ERG helps in diabetes at two whiles. In patients with no diabetic retinopathy, normal or reduced oscillatory potentials indicate the ischemic condition of the retina and help for follow up planning (Lam, 2005 ;Movassat et al.,2008 ). In patients with non-proliferative retinopathy, changes of b-wave help to evaluate the degree of retinal ischemia and forecast occurrence of proliferative retinopathy, which help for timely laser therapy; m.f.ERG, also, can evaluate macular dysfunction objectively, and in association with angiography and OCT, is useful in proper treatment of diabetic macular edema.

### 7.1.8 Choroidal dystrophies

Of this group, autosomal recessive gyrate atrophy, helicoid peripapillary degeneration, X-linked recessive choroideremia, and central areolar choroidal atrophy, are diseases which can affect RPE and outer retina.

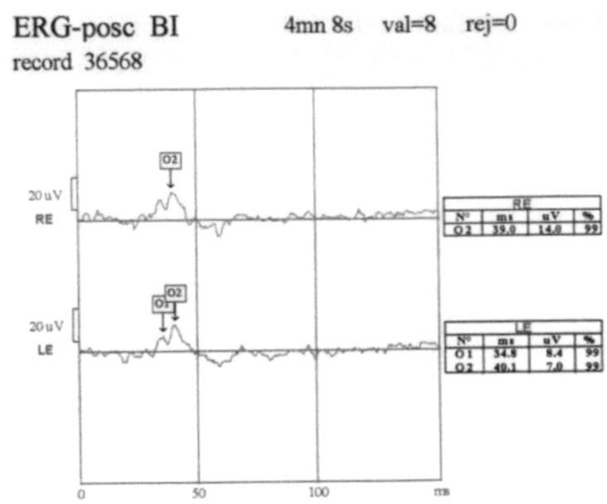


Fig. 18. Abnormal oscillatory potentials in a diabetic case without retinopathy.

ERG changes: Delayed and reduced waves, first in scotopic and then in photopic responses are usual. Ocurring later with less severity than seen in retinal dystrophies, ERG responses reflect the stage of disease.EOG results parallels with ERG, showing RPE involvement too.

### 7.1.9 Chorioretinal inflammations

Congenital or acquired, disseminated or localized, chorioretinal inflammations and infections destruct the choroid, RPE, and retina and, if scar formation be extensive, the visual outcomes will be poor.

ERG changes: In localized macular involvements, m.f.ERG can evaluate the tissue destruction, and has both diagnostic and prognostic values.

In disseminated forms, full-field ERG can help for differential diagnosis and, also, can be used for follow up in cases receiving treatment.

### 7.1.10 Intra-ocular foreign bodies and drug-induced retinal toxicity

Intra-ocular metallic foreign bodies can cause metallosis which is more severe in case of copper (chalcosis), but more encountered in case of iron (siderosis).

Involving epithelial cells of the eye, they cause inflammation, and finally may terminate to severe permanent visual loss.

ERG changes: Following a short period of supernormal responses, delayed and reduced amplitude of components, specially in b-wave and first in scotopic condition, indicate starting of metallosis. It should be reminded that ocular traumas itself, can reduce ERG responses, and in risky removal of foreign bodies, it is recommended to wait for a few weeks and repeat the test for better evaluation. Non-detectable responses indicate poor results of surgery, but do not mean hopeless eye.

Of systemic drugs with retinal toxicity, chloroquine and hydroxychloroquine, indicated in rheumatoid arthritis and systemic lupus erythematosus, are ones to be mentioned. These drugs which bind with melanin may cause severe permanent visual loss before fundus changes. Diminished foveal reflex, bull's eye and peripheral pigmentary changes appear when permanent paracentral scotomas are produced. Periodic ocular examinations, perimetry and ERG test are recommended in these cases.

ERG changes: Full-field ERG in progressed retinal toxicity, and flicker ERG in earlier stages can show the pathology.

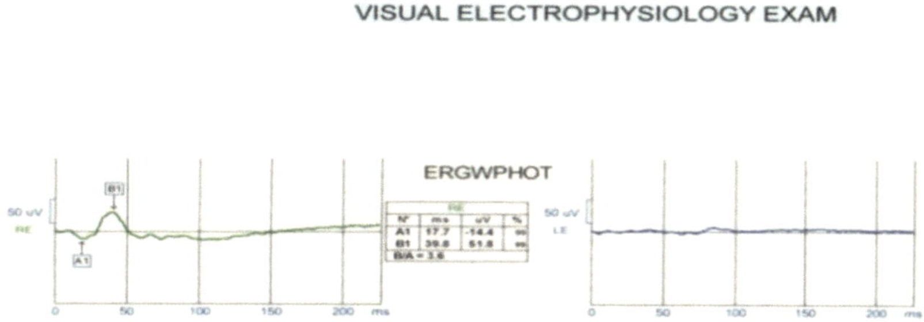


Fig. 19. Flat ERG in left eye due to siderosis bulbi.

In asymptomatic patients with normal visual acuity, m.f.ERG is a choice test in preclinical toxicity, showing reduced responses in rings pertained to fovea and perifovea (Lam, 2005).

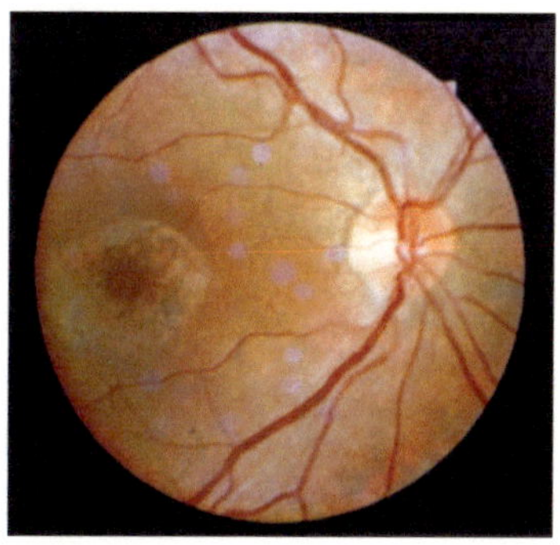

Fig. 20. Bull's eye due to chloroquine toxicity.

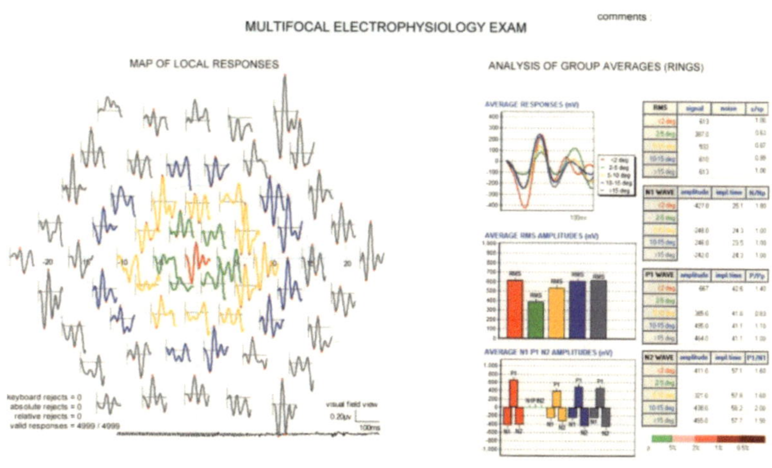


Fig. 21. Reduced response of m.f.ERG in chloroquine toxicity in perifovea.

### 7.1.11 Hazy ocular media

Deformed ocular tissues and hazy media in cases which need additional ocular surgery are dilemma in ophthalmology. In one side is a, probably, hopeless globe with risk of sympathetic ophthalmia with legal or forensic point of view, and in other side is an injured eye which may be treatable, although with very poor outcome. Other situations similar with these , are eyes with pathologic cataract, non-absorbing vitreous hemorrhagia, probably associated with fundus lesions, and longstanding corneal opacities with potential retinal lesions or amblyopia. In all these cases taking a proper decision is very difficult and is not only a clinical matter. In these situations functional and objective tests as, ERG and VEP, can help.

ERG changes:Any positive response of bright flash full-field ERG and VEP recommends to preserve the traumatized globe. In other causes of hazy media mentioned, comparing electrodiagnostic results with clinical conditions gives clue to prognose the outcome of procedure if indicated.

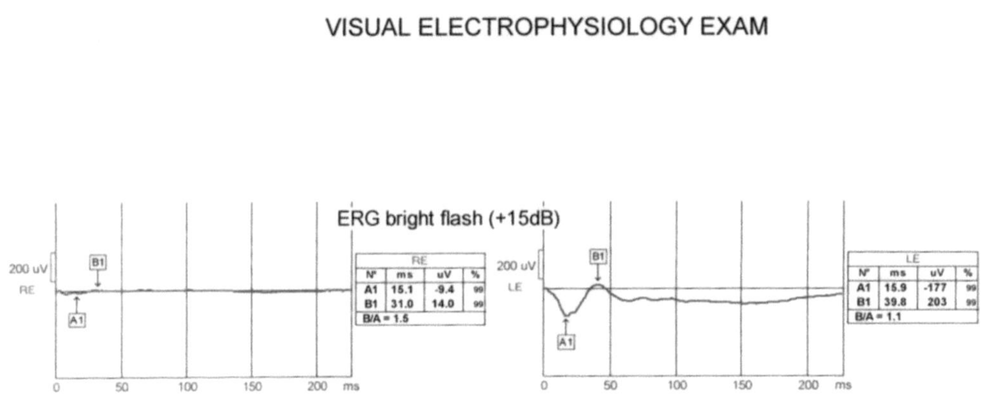


Fig. 22. Bright flash ERG in globe laceration of the right eye.

## 7.2 Disorders affecting EOG

In addition to outer retina disorders affecting EOG as ERG, there are some diseases, specially macular dystrophies and degenerations, in which EOG is a valuable diagnostic test.

### 7.2.1 Best vitelliform disease

An autosomal dominant dystrophy due to lipofuscin accumulation in RPE , which causes an egg-yolk-like appearance in macula. Several progressing stages from vitelliform to pseudohypopion and then to vitelliruptive and finally choroidal neovascularization and scar formation make the course of disease. In spite of characteristic macular changes, patients may have nearly good vision. With more tissue destruction, visual acuity reduces and macular hemorrhagia, edema and scar formation cause serious visual complications.

EOG changes: Severely decreased light rise of EOG, causing reduced Arden ratio, with normal full-field ERG is a characteristic dichotomy in Best disease (Spaide, 1999; Lam, 2005).

When RPE changes cause macular photoreceptors' dysfunction, flicker ERG and m.f.ERG show some reduced amplitude.

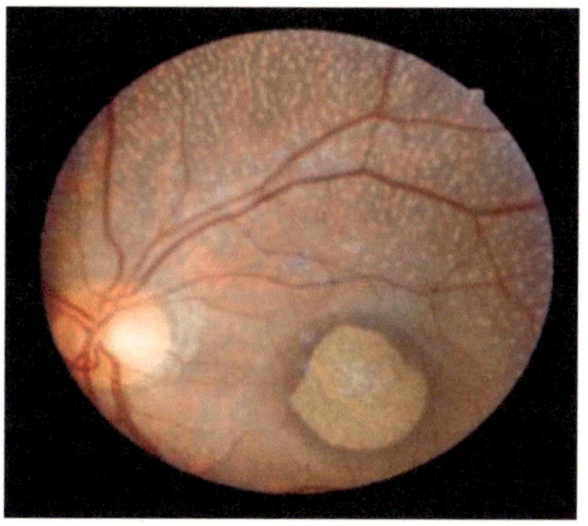

Fig. 23. Stargardt disease.

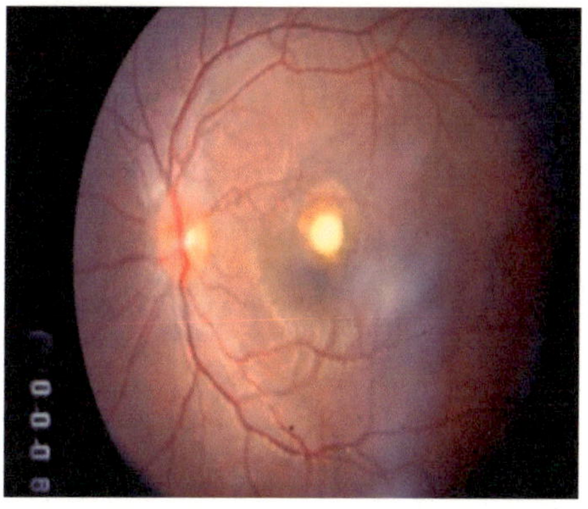

Fig. 24. Best vitelliform disease.

### 7.2.2 Stargardt and fundus flavimaculatus

This autosomal recessive macular dystrophy differs clinically with Best in early-onset decreased vision, even in pre-clinical stage. With characteristic beaten-metal macular appearance, usually surrounded with fishtail-like flecks, this disease is the most prevalent macular dystrophy.

EOG changes: Low Arden ratio, but not so severe as seen in Best disease.Flicker ERG, m.f.ERG and pattern ERG are abnormal, indicating involvement of macular sensory retina in Stargardt disease.

### 7.2.3 Pattern macular dystrophies

This group includes several diseases, with some similarity to Best disease in inheritance and clinical course. Of these, granular, reticular and specially, butterfly pattern dystrophies have characteristic macular appearance which, with almost good visual acuity, are easily diagnosed.

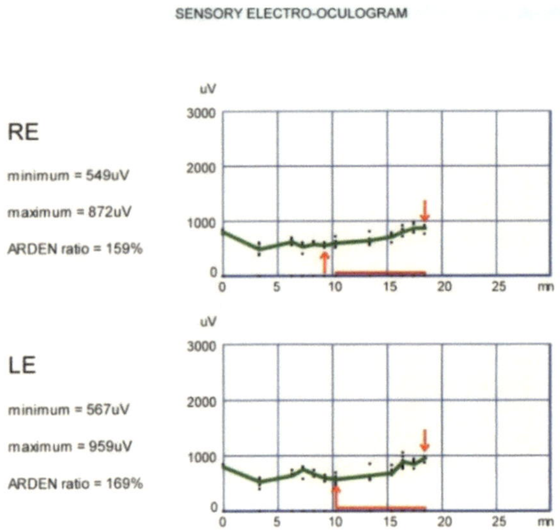


Fig. 25. EOG response in Stargardt disease.

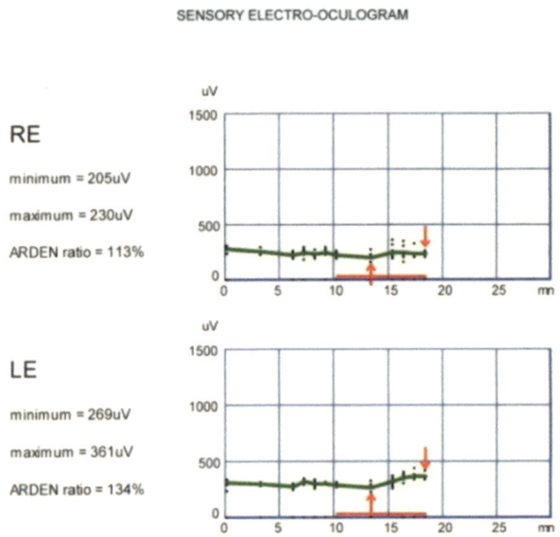


Fig. 26. EOG response in Best disease.

EOG changes: Nearly normal or subnormal EOG response is usual.In severely abnormal response of EOG, close follow up is recommended to foresee serious complications.There are some other RPE dystrophies and degenerations in which EOG can help for differential diagnosis.

### 7.3 Disorders affecting VEP

Involvement of visual pathways is probable in all cases of unexplained visual loss. VEP test can help for diagnosis in disorders affecting retinal ganglion cells, optic nerves, chiasm, optic tracts, geniculate bodies, optic radiations and striate cortex.

### 7.3.1 Optic neuritis

Optic neuritis, isolated or in systemic nervous system (CNS) disorders as multiple sclerosis (MS), HIV infection, neuromyelitis optica and so on, may occur as papillitis or retrobulbar neuritis. Visual loss varies from mild to severe, even no light perception. Pain during eye movement and afferent pupillary defect are positive clinical ocular findings. M.S disease is the most common cause of optic neuritis. MRI is a valuable paraclinic test in these patients, but its results may be equivocal and not conclusive in mild involvements.

VEP changes: Changes of $P_{100}$ component of pattern/reversal VEP can be a valuable diagnostic index in optic neuritis. In mild retro-bulbar neuritis without severe visual loss, delayed $P_{100}$ wave helps to diagnose the problem. In recurrent optic neuritis, delay and reduced amplitude of $P_{100}$-or-$P_2$ wave have prognostic value (Lam, 2005).

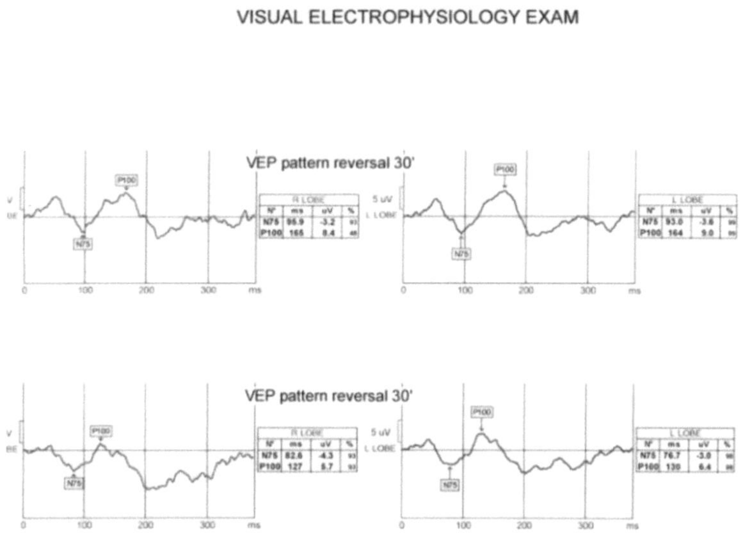


Fig. 27. P/R VEP in M.S. disease; delayed $P_{100}$ wave specially in right eye(up).

In MS cases without any ocular complaint, delayed $P_{100}$ component may be seen which confirms visual pathways involvement (Gronseth& Ashman, 2000; Movassat et al,2009). In suspected new attack of disease, also changes of VEP is helpful for diagnosis.

### 7.3.2 Optic neuropathies

This group of diseases with vast etiologic factors, causes suddenly or gradually visual loss; optic disc swelling or pallor may be seen in some cases.Of those with more clinical interest are ischemic optic neuropathy (ION), traumatic optic neuropathy (TON), toxic optic neuropathy (due to methanol ,lead, and nutritional or $B_{12}$ vitamin deficiency), hereditary optic neuropathy, and compressive optic neuropathy.

VEP changes: Delayed and reduced $P_{100}$-or-$P_2$ component show abnormalities, specially in challenging situations. In ischemic and toxic neuropathies, VEP can help to evaluate the recovery or deterioration; in traumatic neuropathy, it helps to evaluate the visual function and also, in follow up of cases; and in hereditary optic neuropathy like the Leber neuropathy it helps for differential diagnosis. In Leber hereditary optic neuropathy which involves both eyes with an interval of weeks to months (Lam, 2005), in addition to VEP changes, $N_{95}$ component of pattern ERG is also reduced, showing pathology of ganglion cells of retina too.

Optic neuropathy in glaucoma, although related to high intra-ocular pressure, is another disease in which VEP, specially m.f.VEP, can help to decide when to shift to other drugs or to surgery or when therapy should be started in ocular hypertension.

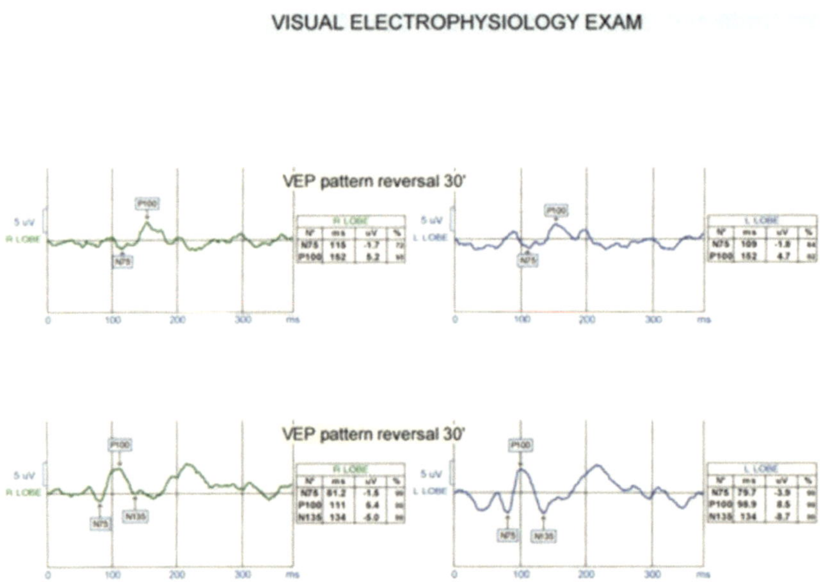


Fig. 28. P/R VEP in ischemic optic neuropathy in right eye(up); reduced and delayed $P_{100}$ wave is diagnostic.

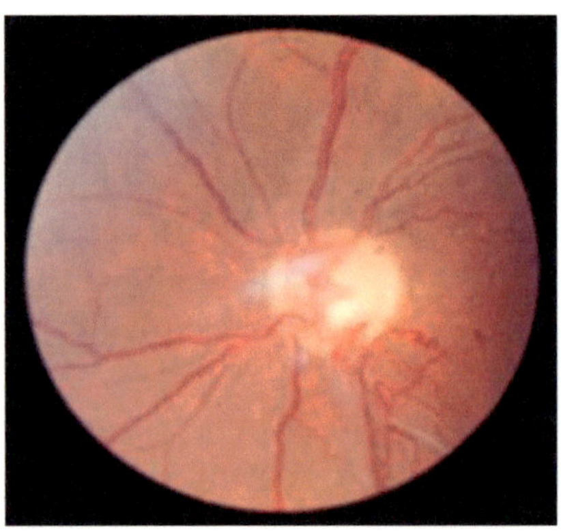

Fig. 29. Leber's optic neuropathy.

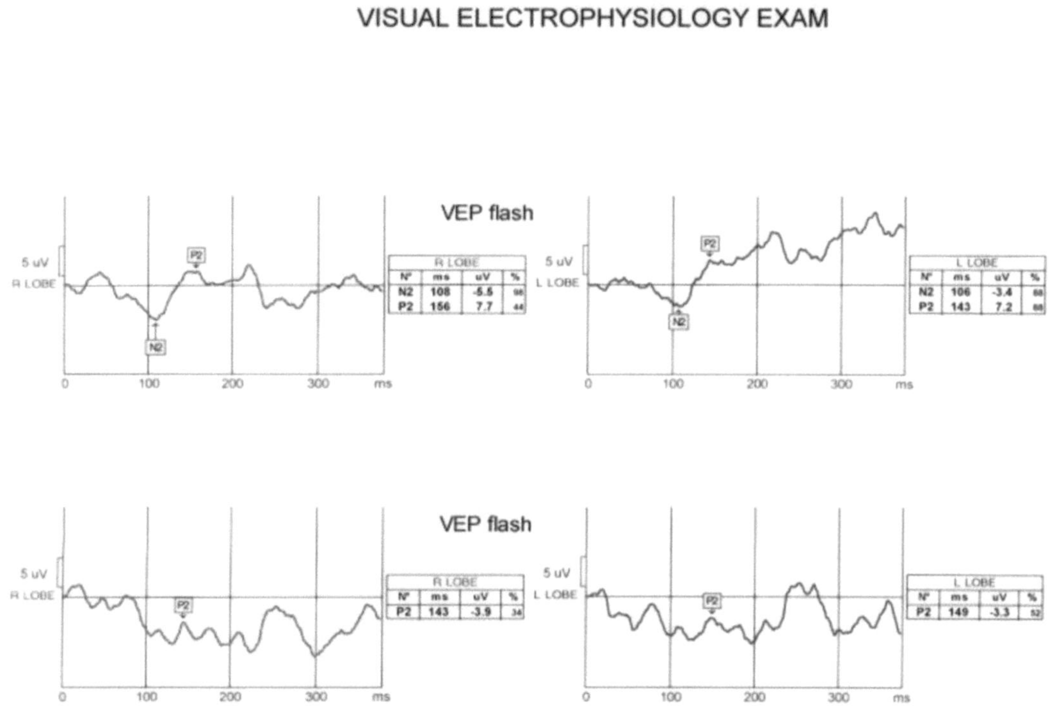


Fig. 30. Flash VEP in Leber's optic neuropathy.

### 7.3.3 Central Nervous System (CNS) disorders

Several diseases in this group can affect visual pathways and striate cortex, but visual complications are not initial and predominant manifestations in many of them. In cortical blindness due to CNS lesions and in Alzheimer disease, affecting visual memory, visual symptoms may draw attention before other manifestations. Neuro-degeneration in Alzheimer (Prisi et al,2001) may cause agnosia which may be first symptom of disease. Also in patients suffering from stroke, encephalitis and head trauma the geniculate bodies, optic radiations and visual cortex may be involved.

VEP changes: VEP, specially m.f.VEP helps to document the visual problems. Also pattern ERG can show retinal ganglion cells degeneration.

## 8. References

Arden GB, Kelsey JH (1962). Changes produced by light in the standing potential of the human eye *JPhysiol*, 1962 May; 161(2):189-204, ISSN: 0022-3751

Brown KT, Wiesel T N(1961). Analysis of the intraretinal electroretinogram in the intact cat eye. *J Physiol*, 1961 Sep; 158(2):257-280, ISSN: 0022-3751

Ciganek ML (1961). The EEG response (evoked potential) to light stimulus in man. *Electroencephalogr Clin Neurophysiol*, 1961 Apr; 13:165-72 , ISSN: 0013-4694

Halliday AM, McDonald WI, Mushin J (1972). Delayed visual evoked response in optic neuritis. *Lancet*, 1972 May 6; 1 (7758): 982-985, ISSN: 0140-6736

Heckenlively John R. and Arden Geoffrey B. (2006).*Principles and practice of clinical electrophysiology of vision*, the MIT Press, ISBN: 0-262-08346-9, England

Karpe G. (1982). Basis of clinical electroretinography. *Acta Ophthalmol* 1982: 60:123-132, ISSN:1755-3768

Kris C (1958). Corneo-fundal potential variations during light and dark adaptation.*Nature*, 1958 Oct 11, 182: 1027-1028, ISSN: 0028-0836

Lam Byron L. (2005). *Electrophysiology of vision; clinical testing and applications*, Taylor and Francis, ISBN: 0-8247-4068-8, USA.

Miller RF, Dowling JE (1970). Intracellular responses of the Muller (glial) cells of mudpuppy retina: Their relation to b-wave of the electroretinogram. *J Neurophysiol*, 1970 May; 33 (3): 323-41 ISSN: 0022-3077

Movassat Morteza, Roohipour Ramak, Nili-Ahmadabadi Mehdi (2008). A case series study of Leber's congenital amaurosis, clinical description and ERG. *Iranian journal of ophthalmology*, 2008; 20(3):33-38 ISSN: 1735-4153

Movassat Morteza, Modarresi Mohsen, Mansouri Mohammad-Reza, Nili-Ahmadabadi Mehdi, Rajabi Mohammad-Taher (2008).Oscillatory potentials in diabetic retina without retinopathy. *Iranian Journal of Ophthalmology*, 2008;20 (1): 20-24 ISSN: 1735-4153

Movassat Morteza, Piri Niloufar, Nili-Ahmadabadi Mehdi (2009).Visual evoked potential study in multiple sclerosis disease, *Iranian Journal of Ophthalmology* 2009; 21(4): 37-44, ISSN: 1735-4153

Newman EA (1993). Membrane physiology of retinal glial (Muller) cells. *J Neurosci,* 1993 Aug; 13(8): 3333-45, ISSN: 0270-6474

Ostwald TJ, Steinberg RH (1980). Localization of frog retinal pigment epithelium Na+ K+ ATPase.*Exp Eye Res*, 1980; 31: 351-360, ISSN: 0014-4835

Pinckers A, Broekhuyse R.M. (1983). The EOG in rheumatoid arthritis.*Acta Ophthalmol*, 1983 Oct; 61(5): 831-7, ISSN: 1755-3768

Ryan, Stephen J. , Hinton David R. (2006). *Basic science and inherited retinal diseases*, Elsevier Mosby. ISBN-13: 978-0-323-02598-0;-10: 0-323-02598-6 USA

Spaide Richard F. (1999). *Diseases of the retina and vitreous.* W.B Saunders Company. ISBN: 0-7216-8005-4

Wachtmeister L. (1998). Oscillatory potentials in the retina: what do they reveal. *Prog Retinal Eye Res* 1998; 17: 485-521 ISSN: 1350-9462

# 6

# Right Ventricular Pacing and Mechanical Dyssynchrony

Kevin V. Burns, Ryan M. Gage and Alan J. Bank
*United Heart and Vascular Clinic, St. Paul, MN, USA*

## 1. Introduction

Since the development of the first wearable cardiac pacemaker in 1957, electrical pacemaker devices have become common treatment options for a number of cardiac conditions. Dual chamber pacemakers are routinely used to treat patients with atrioventricular (AV) node dysfunction or bundle branch block by electrically stimulating the right ventricle (RV). In the United States, 180,000 patients per year receive RV pacemakers (Birnie et al. 2006). On average, pacing reduces symptoms, and improves quality of life, exercise capacity, and survival (Gammage et al. 1991; Lamas et al. 1995; Sweeney et al. 2007). However, chronic RV pacing may be detrimental to cardiac function and lead to heart failure (HF) in some patients.

The mechanisms responsible for RV pacing-induced HF are not fully understood. However, since RV pacing induces a slower myocyte-to-myocyte propogation of the electrical activation wavefront throughout both the RV and left ventricle (LV), rather than rapid propagation through the His-Purkinje network, surface electrogardiograms exhibit a wide QRS complex and bundle branch block pattern, characteristic of electrical dyssynchrony. Locations nearest to the pacing lead are activated significantly earlier than more distant areas of the LV, compromising efficient pumping function of the heart. This pattern of dyssynchronous electrical and mechanical activation of LV may lead to the reduced LV function and increased incidence of HF.

## 2. Cardiac structure and function

The pumping action of the heart is normally initiated by the spontaneous depolarization of myocardial cells in the sinoatrial (SA) node. After transduction through the AV node, depolarization is rapidly spread throughout the LV via the bundle of His, the left and right bundle branches, and the Purkinje network. Electrical activation is nearly simultaneous within the LV, with the apex activated just a few milliseconds before the base (Sengupta et al. 2005), and the endocardium activated just a few milliseconds before the epicardium (Ashikaga et al. 2007; Sengupta et al. 2005). Repolarization, occurs in the reverse fashion, with the base repolarizing first, followed rapidly by the apex (Sengupta et al. 2005).

The LV is comprised of layered myocardial fibers arranged in a double helical pattern, with counter-directional fiber layers meeting at the apex. When viewed from the apex, fibers are arranged in a counter clockwise direction in the epicardium and a clockwise direction in the endocardium (Ashikaga et al. 2004; Buckberg 2002; Torrent-Guasp et al. 2004). The orientation of the myocardial fibers results in intricate three-dimensional motion during contraction and relaxation. This motion can be described as the summation of motion in three planes: 1) longitudinal shortening or lengthening in the long-axis plane extending from apex to base, 2) radial thickening or thinning in the short axis plane, and 3) rotation about the long axis, as viewed from short-axis projections of motion. Similar to electrical activation, longitudinal systolic shortening begins in the apex and rapidly progresses to the base (Sengupta et al. 2005). The rapid electrical transmission throughout the ventricle results in synchronous radial motion at any cross-sectional level of the long axis of the LV (Tops et al. 2007).

Rotational motion is controlled not only by the fiber orientation, but also by the relative strength of the forces generated by the contracting epicardium and endocardium. At the apex of the LV, the epicardium produces greater force during contraction than the endocardium because it contains a greater mass, and also has the mechanical advantage of being located farther from the center of rotation (i.e., it has a longer lever arm). This creates a counter clockwise rotation at the apex. Conversely, the endocardium exhibits greater strain than the epicardium at the base of the LV, and generate a clockwise rotation during systole. The difference in rotation at the base and apex creates a twisting motion, defined as torsion. As epicardial fibers relax, twisted fibers recoil rapidly with continued active contraction of the endocardial layers. This creates suction during the isovolumic relaxation period, and enhances early diastolic filling (Buckberg et al. 2006). Thus, rotational motion is an important link between systolic and diastolic function.

The 3-dimensional motion created by the contraction of the helically structured myocardium generates efficient pumping action with minimal fiber shortening. It is estimated that, as a result of these mechanics, the heart can generate an ejection fraction (EF) of 50% or more with a fiber shortening of only 15% (Buckberg 2002; Torrent-Guasp et al. 2004). Maintaining this efficient pumping mechanism may be critical to ensuring proper cardiac function.

## 3. Methods of quantifying LV function

The motion of the heart can be quantified in a number of ways. Invasive methods such as placing sonomicrometer crystals in the myocardium enable accurate tracking of motion during the cardiac cycle. Not only does the invasive nature of this type of test limit its utility, but also the procedure of implanting crystals may alter subsequent cardiac motion. Magnetic resonance imaging (MRI) is a common non-invasive alternative to measure cardiac structure and motion. While spatial resolution is excellent, temporal resolution of the beating heart is more limited. (Marwick and Schwaiger 2008) The procedure is relatively costly, restricting clinical and research use. In addition, the electromagnetic field used in this procedure can interfere with the electronics of the pacing device, and generate heat within the leads, potentially damaging the myocardium. (Kolb et al. 2001) Echocardiography is a relatively inexpensive and commonly used imaging technique that can be safely used in patients with cardiac devices. This chapter will focus on echocardiographic techniques used to measure many aspects of cardiac function which are affected by RV pacing.

### 3.1 Tissue Doppler imaging

Projections of the three-dimensional motion onto the longitudinal plane of the LV, parallel to the long axis, have been studied extensively using tissue Doppler imaging (TDI) (Sogaard et al. 2002b; Yu et al. 2004). This technology measures the velocity of myocardial motion along the path of incidence of the ultrasound beam. The motion of the heart during a full cardiac cycle is commonly displayed as either the velocity (tissue velocity imaging; TVI) or displacement (tissue tracking; TT) of the region of interest with respect to the transducer. In normal hearts, velocity or displacement curves from different regions of interest throughout the LV have the same general shape, so that peaks and troughs occur nearly simultaneously. Because of this, TDI is commonly used to assess dyssynchrony within the LV. Examples of TVI and TT curves for a normal and dyssynchronous heart are shown in Figures 1 and 2.

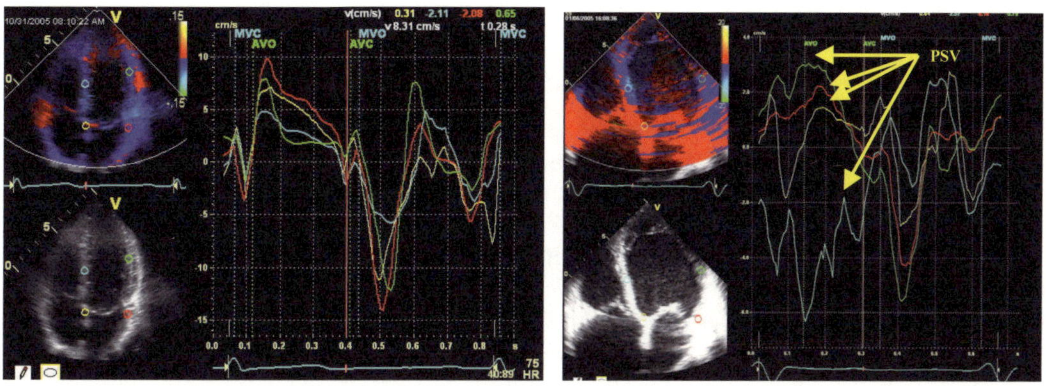


Fig. 1. Apical 4-chamber TVI images of a normal heart (left panel), and a dyssynchronous heart (right panel.) In the normal heart, the systolic velocity curves of each wall segment overlap and reach peak systolic velocity (PSV) at the same time. In the dyssynchronous heart, peak velocity occurs at different times (marked with arrows in the right panel) for each wall segment.

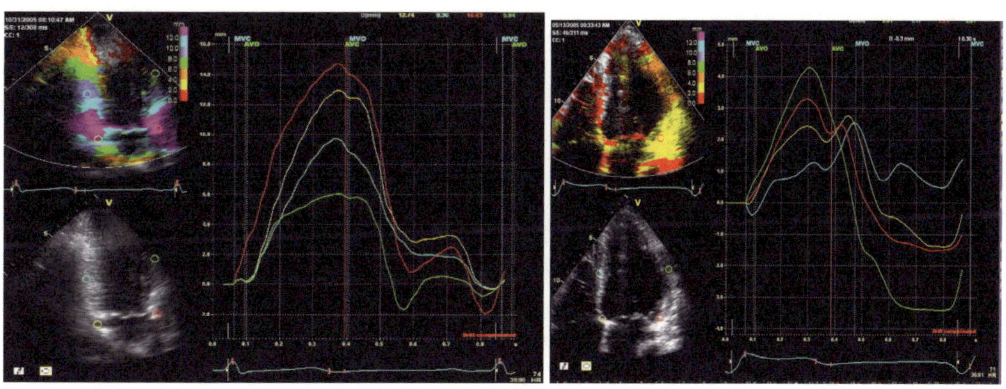

Fig. 2. Apical 4-chamber TT curves of a normal (left panel) and dyssynchronous (right panel) heart. In the normal heart, all wall segments reach peak displacement at the same time, at aortic valve closure. In the dyssynchronous heart, wall segments do not reach peak displacement at the same time, and may reach a peak after aortic valve closure.

The use of TVI for assessing the synchrony of the contracting myocardium is widely supported in the literature (Bax et al. 2004; Gorcsan et al. 2004; Suffoletto et al. 2006; Yu et al. 2005). However, it is sometimes difficult to identify which systolic velocity is the peak velocity, due to multiple or jagged peaks in the velocity curves. Displacement curves can be derived from TVI data by integration of the velocity profiles over time to produce TT curves. The displacement curves generated in this manner are often smoother, with less noise, than velocity curves. The identification of times to peak wall displacement may be less variable with this technique (Bank and Kelly 2006; Bogunovic et al. 2009).

In both TVI and TT modes, active contraction cannot be differentiated from passive motion (such as that due to tethering with the adjacent myocardium or translational movement of the heart). Measurements are also limited to one dimension, along the line of incidence of the ultrasonic beam, which, in some images, may not coincide with the long axis of the heart. In spite of these limitations, TDI techniques are commonly used to assess dyssynchrony, particularly in patients with HF, who may benefit from cardiac resynchronization therapy (CRT).

### 3.2 Speckle tracking echocardiography

Speckle tracking echocardiography (STE) has more recently been applied to analyze heart function (Helle-Valle et al. 2005; Suffoletto et al. 2006). STE is based on the identification and tracking of stable speckle patterns in the two-dimensional ultrasound image, which are assumed to correspond to fixed points within the myocardial tissue. The relative motion of these speckles represents the strain of the myocardium, which is fairly independent of ultrasound angle of incidence. To perform the analysis, the endocardial border is manually traced at a single time point during the cardiac cycle, and the thickness of the region of interest is set to encompass the entire myocardium. Speckles within the region of interest are then tracked throughout the cardiac cycle. The region of interest is divided into segments, and the average motion of the speckles within each segment is displayed. Motion is most commonly displayed as strain, but strain rate, displacement, velocity and rotation can also be derived from STE data. Examples of normal and dyssynchronous radial strain patterns are presented in Figure 3.

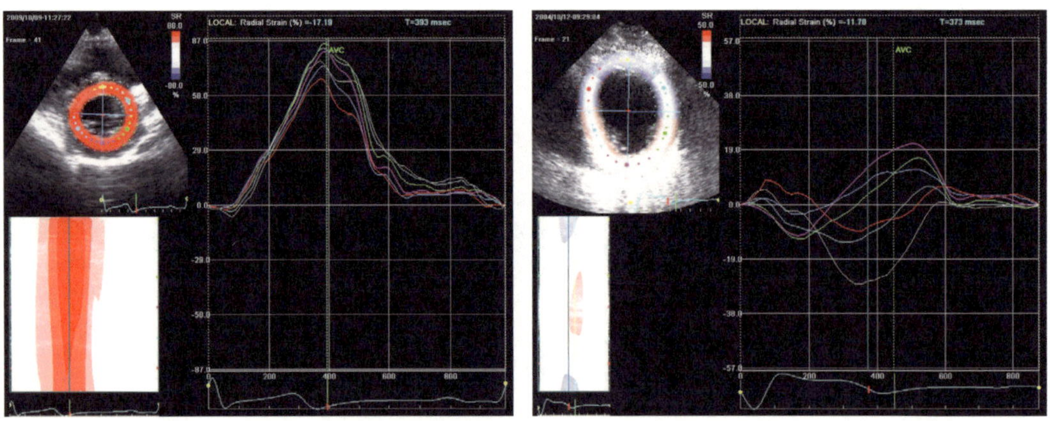

Fig. 3. STE images of radial strain in a normal (left panel) and dyssynchronous (right panel) heart. In the normal heart, strain curves overlap, while in the dyssyncronous heart strain patterns are very different for different wall segments.

STE has been frequently used to assess radial function using short axis images of the LV. The magnitude of radial systolic function can be expressed as the average strain of all wall segments in an image, and dyssynchrony in the radial plane can be expressed by describing the heterogeneity of the curves from multiple segments. Using the same short axis images, rotational motion around a central point in the LV can be measured with STE. Both radial and rotational motion measurements, derived from STE, have recently been used in a variety of settings to assess cardiac function (Borg et al. 2008; Chung et al. 2006; Delhaas et al. 2004; Dohi et al. 2008; Kanzaki et al. 2006; Suffoletto et al. 2006; Tops et al. 2007).

## 4. Normal LV mechanics

As the helically arranged myocardial fibers contract, the walls of the LV shorten longitudinally, thicken radially, and rotate about the long axis. Although this coordinated motion is complicated, it can be simplified using two-dimensional echocardiographic projections. The magnitude of motion and timing between different wall segments can be measured with TDI and STE so that longitudinal, radial and rotational motion can be assessed.

### 4.1 Longitudinal motion

Motion of the LV parallel to the long axis of the LV is referred to as longitudinal motion. When the ultrasound transducer is placed at the LV apex, the longitudinal motion of the LV can be approximated as the motion either towards or away from the transducer. For this reason, TDI is well-suited to measure longitudinal motion. A 12-segment model of the LV is commonly used, in which regions of interest are placed in the basal and mid-ventricle areas of the lateral, anterior, anteroseptal, septal, inferior and posterior walls. Global LV systolic function in the longitudinal plane can be assessed using TT. The average displacement of all 12 segments (global systolic contraction score; GSCS) that occurs between the closing of the mitral valve (the end of the previous beat) and the closing of the aortic valve (the end of systole) can be used to assess the magnitude of useful systolic longitudinal shortening (Sogaard et al. 2002a). A normal adult LV will shorten by 8-10 mm during systole, while the LV of HF patients may shorten 4-5 mm or less (Bank et al. 2009).

Longitudinal dyssynchony is typically measured with TDI, using the same 12-segment model. In either TVI or TT mode, the curves describing the motion of the regions of interest move in unison in the normal heart. Several methods of quantifying deviations from synchronous movement have been proposed. The most common method was proposed by Yu, et al. and involves calculating the standard deviation of the times to peak systolic velocity among the 12 regions of interest (SD-TVI) (Yu et al. 2005; Yu et al. 2006). A cut-off of 32 ms has been used to indicate clinically significant dyssynchrony (Yu et al. 2005).

Dyssynchrony can be also be measured with TT in a method analogous to the Yu method (SD-TT), which may result in a more reproducible measurement (Bank et al. 2009; Kaufman et al. 2010). SD-TT may range from less than 50 ms in a normal heart to over 80 ms for a CHF patient's heart (Bank et al. 2009). Tissue displacement curves tend to be smoother than velocity curves, with fewer jagged peaks, and thus less difficulty occurs in differentiating isovolumic peaks from systolic peaks (Kaufman et al. 2010).

Recently, TT has also been used to investigate the coordinated motion within a particular wall of the LV, rather than the more typical method of assessing motion between several different walls (Bank et al. 2010b; Burns et al. 2011). A pattern of paradoxical motion within a wall has been termed intramural dyssynchrony, and is depicted in Figure 4. This particular measurement of dyssynchrony appears to be a good indicator of pacing-induced LV dysfunction (Burns et al. 2011).

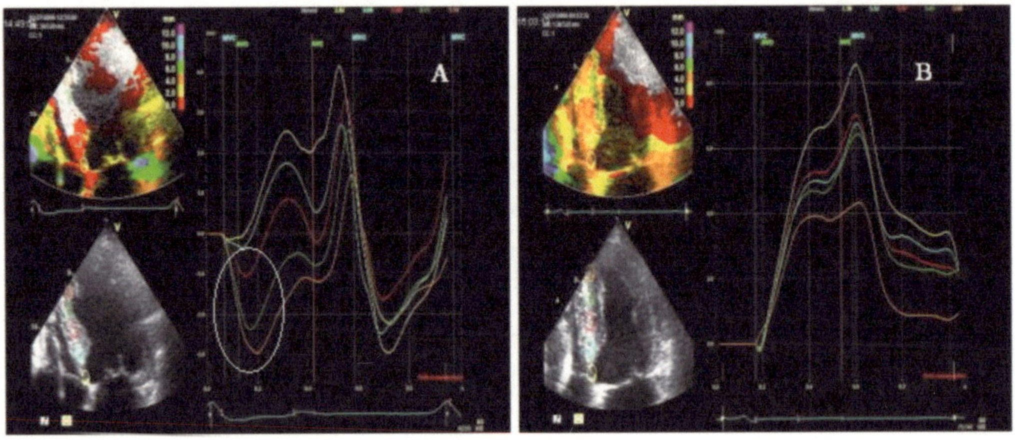

Fig. 4. Intramural dyssynchrony within the septum of a chronically RV-paced patient before (panel A; paradoxical motion is circled), and after (panel B) upgrade to CRT.

### 4.2 Radial motion

Not only does the LV shorten and lengthen longitudinally, but it also moves in a perpendicular direction; either towards or away from an imaginary line representing the central long axis. Most of this radial motion is not parallel to the angle of incidence of the ultrasound beam, so cannot be accurately assessed with TDI. Instead, STE can be used to measure the relative position of speckles within the myocardium during the cardiac cycle. When nearby speckles move closer to one another, the wall thickness is reduced, and negative radial strain is measured. Positive radial strain corresponds to speckles moving farther apart as the myocardial wall thickens.

Global LV function has been assessed using STE by computing the mean radial strain in six myocardial segments comprising the short axis image of the LV at the papillary muscle level (Bank et al. 2009; Kaufman et al. 2010). Mean radial strain is approximately 50% in normal, healthy subjects and 15% in CHF patients (Kaufman et al. 2010; Ng et al. 2009). The standard deviation of the time to peak radial strain among the six myocardial segments (SD-RS) can also be used as a measure of LV radial dyssynchrony (Bank et al. 2009; Donal et al. 2008; Kaufman et al. 2010; Suffoletto et al. 2006). In healthy hearts, SD-RS is typically under 20 ms, while it can be over 80 ms in CHF patients (Donal et al. 2008; Kaufman et al. 2010).

### 4.3 Rotational motion

During contraction, the LV also rotates about its long axis as the myocardial fibers longitudinally shorten and radially thicken. The helical structure of the fibers, and the twisting motion generated by the contraction of these fibers was described as early as the 1600's by Leonardo DaVinci (Geleijnse and van Dalen 2009). The more recent work of Torrent-Guasp and others has led to renewed appreciation for the relationship between cardiac structure and function, and the importance of LV rotational motion on systolic and diastolic performance (Torrent-Guasp et al. 2004).

When viewed from the apex in the short axis plane, the base of the normal heart rotates primarily counter-clockwise during systole, while the apex rotates primarily in a clockwise direction. Peak rotation in both planes occurs at, or just before aortic valve closure. Peak rotation at the base has been reported to range from -2.0° to -4.6°. Peak rotation at the apex may range from 5.7° to 11.2°. Maximum systolic torsion in normal hearts has then been found to range from 6.1° to 14.5° (Helle-Valle et al. 2005; Kanzaki et al. 2006; Nakai et al. 2006; Notomi et al. 2005; Notomi et al. 2005; Notomi et al. 2006; Takeuchi et al. 2006). An example of the rotational motion of a normal, healthy heart is presented in Figure 5 below.

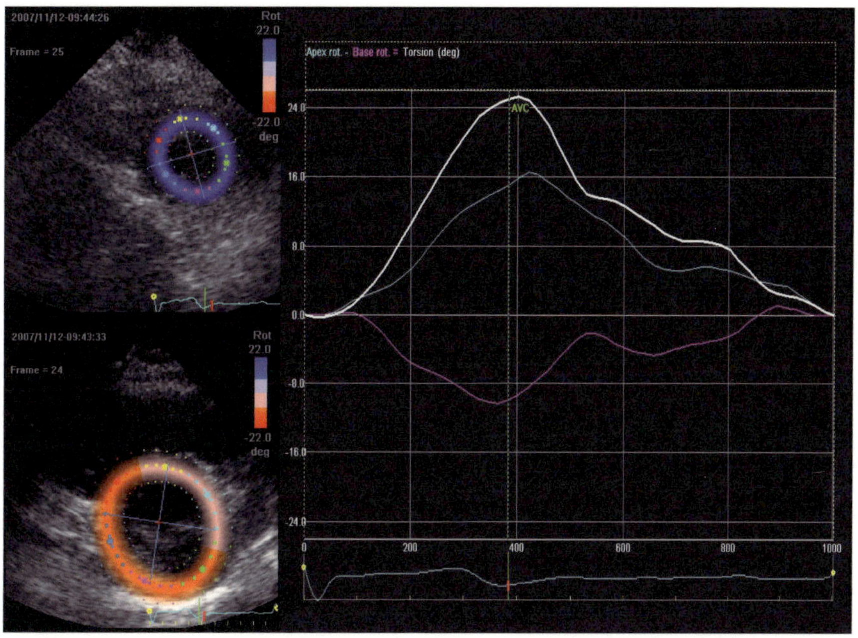


Fig. 5. Rotational motion in a normal heart. The base of the LV (pink line) rotates in a counter-clockwise direction during systole, while the apex (blue line) rotates in the opposite direction. The net difference between the rotation of the base and apex is torsion (while line).

An important consequence of systolic torsion may the subsequent recoil of the LV during early diastole (Notomi et al. 2008; Shaw et al. 2008). Notomi et al. demonstrated in canines that untwisting coincided with relaxation of the LV, and preceded suction-aided filling (Notomi et al. 2008). The magnitude of untwisting rate also correlated with systolic torsion, relaxation time constant, and intraventricular pressure gradient. A reduced and delayed peak untwisting rate was found to occur with increasing age (Notomi et al. 2006) and in patients with dilated cardiomyopathy (Saito et al. 2009). However, in patients with isolated diastolic dysfunction, peak untwisting increased in mild cases, but was depressed in severe cases (Park et al. 2008). Diastolic dysfunction in these patients did not effect the time at which peak untwist rate occurs within the cardiac cycle. In patients with chronic mitral regurgitation, however, peak untwisting was both reduced in magnitude and delayed (Borg et al. 2008). Thus the timing and magnitude of peak diastolic untwisting rate may provide useful information about LV diastolic function.

## 5. Effects of RV pacing

In the United States, approximately 180,000 RV pacemakers are implanted each year (Birnie et al. 2006). Cases of sinus node dysfunction account for 58% of these procedures, while 31% are due to high grade AV block (due to ablation procedures, or other causes) (Birnie et al. 2006). RV pacing has been shown to improve symptoms, exercise capacity, quality of life and survival in these patients (Gammage et al. 1991; Lamas et al. 1995; Sweeney et al. 2007). However, permanent RV pacing has been associated with an increased risk of LV dysfunction, hospitalization, HF, and death (Hayes et al. 2006; Lieberman et al. 2006; O'Keefe et al. 2005; Sweeney et al. 2003; Tse and Lau 1997; Wilkoff et al. 2002). In 2002, the results of the DAVID trial revealed that RV paced patients with LV dysfunction, requiring a defibrillator, who were actively paced in DDDR-70 mode had a 60% greater risk for hospitalization or death than patients who received minimal back-up pacing in VVI-40 mode (Wilkoff et al. 2002). The percentage of patients who develop pacing-induced LV dysfunction is not clear. However estimates range from 25-50% (O'Keefe et al. 2005; Thackray et al. 2003; Tops et al. 2006; Tse and Lau 1997). Zhang and colleagues reported that, of 79 patients who were paced from the RV more than 90% of the time, 25% developed systolic HF within the 8-year follow-up period (Zhang et al. 2008b). It has also been noted that although chronically paced subjects can exhibit reduced systolic function, similar to HF patients, their ventricles do not appear to dilate as much (Bank et al. 2010a; Burns et al. 2011). Thus RV pacing may induce a unique HF phenotype.

### 5.1 Effects of RV pacing on systolic function

Since RV pacing artificially stimulates the ventricles at a location other than the His-Purkinje system, the action potential is propagated more slowly through myocytes rather than through the specialized conduction system. Electrical activation then becomes heterogeneous, with early activation near the pacing site, and delayed activation at distant locations. The resultant LV mechanical contraction becomes dyssynchronous. Studies by Prinzen and Wyman in acutely paced dogs, demonstrated that pacing results in heterogeneous electrical activation, strain and perfusion of the LV (Prinzen et al. 1990; Prinzen et al. 1999; Wyman et al. 1999). Specifically, pacing results in low systolic strain near the pacing site, and pre-stretch and increased systolic strain in the LV wall farthest from the pacing site. Dyssynchronous mechanical activation, along with reduced systolic function, has also been reported in chronically paced humans, as discussed in more detail later in this chapter.

### 5.2 Effects of RV pacing on longitudinal systolic function

Studies of the effects of RV pacing on longitudinal mechanics have focused on measuring mechanical dyssynchrony. In a study of 26 patients with normal LV function who were acutely paced from multiple locations within the heart, our lab found that RV apical pacing reduced LV systolic function and increased dyssynchrony (Bank et al. 2010b). As described in the animal studies above, we also found that abnormalities were most prominent near the pacing site, as demonstrated in Figure 6. Pacing from the LV free wall best preserved LV function and synchrony, while simultaneous pacing from both the RV apex and LV free wall yielded intermediate results.

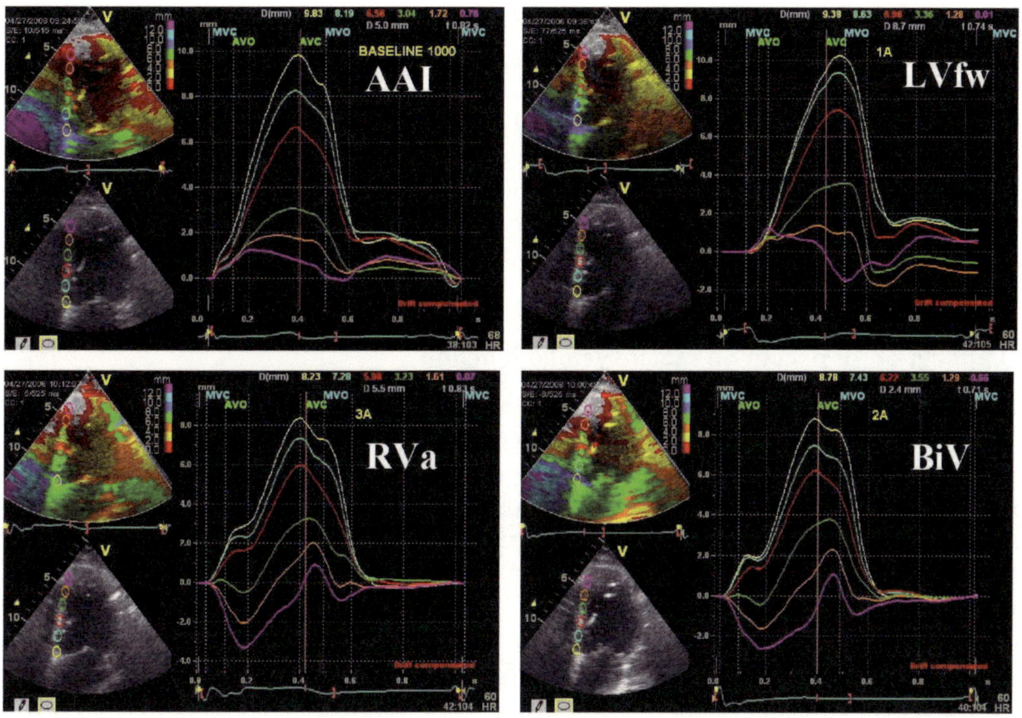


Fig. 6. Intramural TT of the septal wall from a patient with normal LV function paced from the right atrium (AAI), LV free wall (LVfw), RV apex (RVa), and both the LVfw and RVa simultaneously (BiV). Note that the apical regions on the septum are most impaired in cases where the RVa is actively paced (RVa and BiV).

Other studies have also found that paced subjects have greater systolic dyssynchrony, as quantified by SD-TVI, while paced from the RV, even when paced subjects had normal EF (Kawanishi et al. 2008; Zhang et al. 2008b). The degree of longitudinal systolic dyssynchrony was similar to that of a group of HF patients with EF of less than 35% (Zhang et al. 2008a). Thus, chronic pacing-induced dyssynchrony may put an unusual and excessive stress on the left ventricle, leading to remodeling and eventual heart failure.

In a study of 34 high degree AV block patients, paced for an average of 7 years, longitudinal dyssynchrony was increased as compared to non-paced control subjects. Plasma levels of B-type natriuretic peptide (BNP; a marker of abnormal ventricular wall stretch) were also increased, and EF was reduced (Kawanishi et al. 2008). Mechanical dyssynchrony was modestly correlated with BNP, but no correlations between dyssynchrony and EF were presented. In contrast, Ng and colleagues recently reported no difference in SD-TVI between non-paced controls and RV-paced subjects, however other measurements of dyssynchrony were not reported (Ng et al. 2009). In our lab we compared patients with high degree AV block, but otherwise normal LV function prior to the initiation of RV pacing to 25 non-paced, age and gender matched controls (Burns et al. 2011). Paced subjects had been paced for at least 1 year prior to the study, and detailed echocardiographic analysis was performed. Chronically paced subjects had significantly lower EF, and greater longitudinal dyssynchrony than non-paced controls.

Acute RV pacing has been shown to increase intramural dyssynchrony in normal hearts, without an increase in between-wall dyssynchrony (Bank et al. 2010b). After chronic pacing, intramural dyssnchrony has been shown to persist, while intraventricular dyssynchrony may also become apparent (Burns et al. 2011). Thus, intramural dyssynchrony may be an important mechanism in pacing-induced LV dysfunction. However, it remains unclear if mechanical dyssynchrony is the primary cause of LV dysfunction in RV paced patients, what percentage of RV paced patients with mechanical dyssynchrony will develop LV dysfunction, and which patients might be at greatest risk for developing pacing-induced LV dysfunction.

### 5.3 Effects of RV pacing on radial systolic function

Radial function and dyssynchrony have also been investigated in RV paced patients. Tops, et al. observed that peak radial strain, and the time to reach peak radial strain in 6 short-axis segments became heterogeneous after long-term RV pacing (Tops et al. 2007). These investigators found that radial strain was most reduced and peaked earliest in septal and anteroseptal regions, and increased in magnitude and delayed in lateral and posterior regions. In our lab, we have found that patients with chronic RV pacemakers have reduced EF and mean peak systolic radial strain. The radial dysfunction is similar between RV paced patients, and HF patients having the same ejection fraction (Burns et al. 2011). In both our study, and that of Ng (Ng et al. 2009) radial dyssynchrony was not different between non-paced controls and RV paced subjects. It appears that radial dysfunction in this case may be reflective of the global reduction in systolic function, and may not be unique to RV pacing.

### 5.4 Effects of RV pacing on rotational systolic function

The effects of various pacing modalities on LV torsion have been evaluated in animal models. Sorger et al. compared acute right atrial pacing to RV pacing and biventricular pacing using MRI in 5 canine hearts (Sorger et al. 2003). These authors concluded that torsion was highly sensitive to the site of excitation. Torsion has also been assessed qualitatively using sonomicrometric images in porcine hearts (Liakopoulos et al. 2006; Tomioka et al. 2006). Torsion was normal in right atrial and high septal RV pacing, however this motion was disrupted by pacing from other RV sites. These studies suggest that torsion is a sensitive indicator of alterations in the normal LV activation sequence due to non-physiologic pacing.

In chronically paced humans, it has been found that both basal and apical peak rotation, and peak systolic torsion were lower than in age-matched non-paced controls (Burns et al. 2011). In addition, apical rotation was found to be in the reverse direction from normal in about 1/3 of paced patients. By comparison, HF patients who had similar EF to the chronically paced subjects, did not exhibit reversed rotational direction, and had higher peak systolic torsion than paced subjects (Figure 7). This study suggests that pacing alters rotational function, and the alteration is not simply due to reduced systolic function.

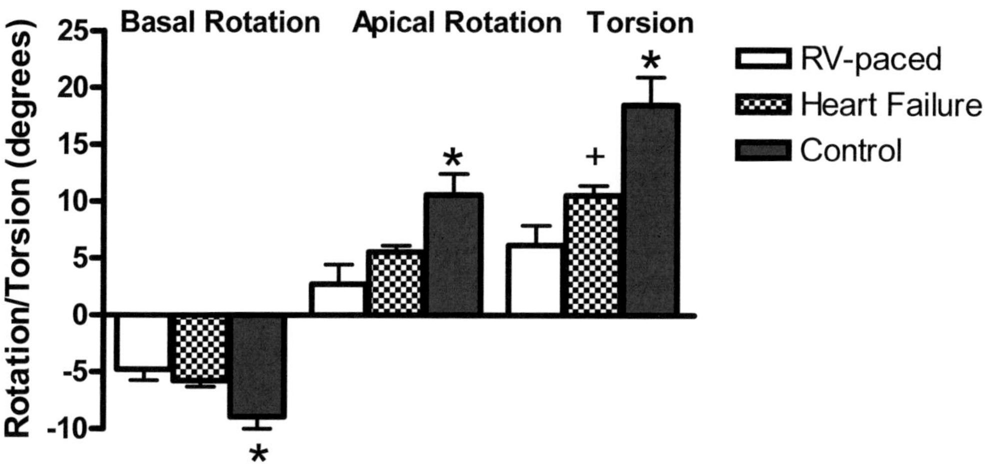


Fig. 7. Rotational function in chronically RV paced patients, heart failure patients with EF matched to the paced group, and healthy controls. * Indicates $p<0.05$ when compared to RV paced and heart failure groups. + Indicates $p<0.05$ when compared to RV paced group.

## 6. Minimizing the risk of pacing-induced dyssfunction

The long-term risks associated with RV pacing have been well documented, and several treatment alternatives have been explored, including minimizing pacing frequency, alternate RV lead location, and biventricular pacing.

### 6.1 Reducing pacing frequency

One method of minimizing the negative affects of chronic RV pacing is to reduce the number of heart beats that are artificially paced. A sub-study from the DAVID trial revealed that outcomes in that trial were explained primarily by pacing frequency (Sharma et al. 2005). Patients paced more than 40% of the time were more likely to die or be hospitalized for HF than those paced less frequently, regardless of the pacing mode. Similarly, the primary objective of the MOST trial was to compare single chamber RV pacing to dual chamber pacing. However, in a sub-study which included 707 dual chamber patients with narrow pre-pacing QRS durations, both HF hospitalizations and incidence of atrial fibrillation increased significantly with increasing pacing frequency (Sweeney et al. 2003). Again, those paced more than 40% of the time had worse outcomes than those paced less. Finally, the SAVE PACe trial tested an algorithm specifically designed to minimize the frequency of ventricular pacing (Sweeney et al. 2007). Minimal RV pacing significantly reduced the development of atrial fibrillation. However this study included a follow-up period of only 1.7 years, so mortality and HF rates were low, and no difference was noted between the minimally-paced, and frequently-paced groups. In total, these studies demonstrate that reducing the frequency of RV pacing is beneficial. However, in patients with high grade AV block, for example, ventricular pacing is required, and the frequency cannot be reduced. In these cases, other methods of attenuating the negative effects of RV pacing can be explored.

### 6.2 Alternate lead location

The RV apex is a readily accessible location to implant pacing leads, and has been the standard pacing site. However mounting evidence has indicated that this results in a dyssynchronous contraction pattern in the LV, and increases the risk of developing HF. As a result, many investigators have explored alternate lead locations within the RV, which may create a more physiological activation pattern and reduce the risks associated with apical RV pacing. The RV outflow tract (RVOT), the RV septum, and the His bundle have been the most commonly studied alternate pacing sites.

The most common alternate pacing site has been the RVOT. Several studies have demonstrated acute improvements in LV function and dyssynchrony, as compared to apical pacing. In a cross-over study of the acute effects of RVOT pacing, compared to apical pacing in 20 patients, Yamano and colleagues found RVOT pacing resulted in superior radial synchrony using STE, as well as better coronary blood flow dynamics (Yamano et al. 2010). Leong, et al. also showed that longitudinal LV function was better in RVOT pacing that in apical pacing in a randomized trial of 58 patients who were followed for an average of 29 months (Leong et al. 2010). Tse, et al., measured regional wall motion abnormalities in a long-term study of 24 patients with complete atrioventricular block paced from either the RV apex or RVOT for a period of 18 months (Tse et al. 2002). Changes in perfusion and dyssynchrony were not different between pacing sites after 6 months, but RVOT pacing resulted in significant reductions in perfusion defects and dyssyncrony after 18 months.

However, several studies have also failed to find any benefit from RVOT pacing. An early study of 16 patients by Victor and colleagues, in 1999, showed that pacing from the RVOT resulted in no difference in QRS duration, ejection fraction, New York Heart Association (NYHA) functional class, or exercise capacity after three months of pacing (Victor et al. 1999). Similarly, Stamber et al. performed a multi-center, randomized trial of apical RV pacing compared to RVOT pacing (Stambler et al. 2003). Patients in this trial were randomly assigned to three months of pacing from one site, followed by three months of pacing from the other site. No significant differences were found in NYHA functional class, ejection fraction or exercise capacity between the two pacing sites. Importantly, 2 recent studies have failed to demonstrate any survival (Dabrowska-Kugacka et al. 2009) or LV remodeling (Gong et al. 2009) benefit of RVOT pacing over RV apical pacing.

Pacing from the RV septum has also been investigated as a potentially superior pacing site, as compared to the RV apex. Schwaab, et al., showed in 1999 that QRS complex duration and EF were both improved acutely with pacing from the RV septum as compared to the RV apex (Schwaab et al. 1999). Only 14 patients were included in this cross-over study. In a recent pair of studies, Inoue and colleagues have used STE to demonstrate that septal pacing resulted in better longitudinal function, less longitudinal dyssynchrony, and better rotational function than apical pacing (Inoue et al. 2010; Inoue et al. 2011). Similarly, Cano, et al. showed that LV dyssynchrony was lower in a 32 patients randomly assigned to septal pacing, as compared to 28 apically paced patients (Cano et al. 2010). However, after a 1-year follow-up, no differences were detected in quality of life scores, NYHA classification, or exercise capacity. In another study by Cho and colleagues, however, TDI measures of longitudinal dyssynchrony were not different between apically and septally paced patients (n=45 and 34, respectively) (Cho et al. 2011).

A few smaller studies have suggested that pacing at or near the His bundle may also produce less dyssynchrony and better LV function than RV apical pacing. A recent study indicated that His bundle pacing is practical, and can be achieved in approximately 85% of patients, and results in nearly normal LV activation patterns (Kronborg et al. 2011). In an acute study of LV mechanics, His bundle pacing resulted in less dyssynchrony and better LV function, as compared to acute RV apical pacing in 23 patients (Catanzariti et al. 2006). Similarly, His bundle pacing was found to reduce LV dyssychrony using TDI, as well as preserve coronary circulation and reduce mitral regurgitation, as compared to RV apical pacing in a cross-over study of 12 patients who were paced for 3 months from each site (Zanon et al. 2008).

In summary, many studies have demonstrated benefits of pacing from sites other than the RV apex, but several studies have also contradicted these results. Alternate site pacing studies have been fairly small, with limited follow-up time. Large scale, randomized, prospective trials comparing RV pacing sites are needed to clarify the potential benefits.

### 6.3 Biventricular pacing

Another method of inducing a more synchronous contraction of the LV is to utilize biventricular pacing, or CRT. As is common in HF patients with dyssynchronous contraction, pacing both the LV and RV in a coordinated fashion may retain synchrony in patients requiring permanent pacing, and prevent LV dysfunction.

The benefits of CRT over standard dual chamber RV pacing were investigated in the HOBIPACE trial, a randomized, cross-over study of 30 patients with AV block and existing LV dysfunction (Kindermann et al. 2006). In these patients, after 3 months of treatment, CRT was found to be superior in terms of LV volumes, EF, quality of life scores, and exercise capacity. Yu and colleagues extended these findings to also include patients without LV dysfunction prior to pacing (Yu et al. 2009). Their study included 177 patients randomly assigned to either CRT of RV apical pacing. Patients receiving CRT had significantly better preserved LV volumes and EF after one year of pacing.

Long-term clinical effects of CRT, as compared to RV apical pacing, were recently examined by Brignole and coworkers (Brignole et al. 2011). In this study, 186 patients undergoing AV node ablation were randomly assigned to CRT or RV apical pacing, and followed for 20 months. Significantly more of the RV paced patients met the clinical composite endpoint of death due to HF, hospitalization due to HF, or worsening HF. This was true both in subgroups of patients meeting standard criteria for CRT (EF≤35%, QRS≥120ms, and NYHA class≥III), and in those not meeting those guidelines.

Although most studies have concluded that CRT reduces LV dysfunction in patients requiring permanent pacing, as compared to pacing from the RV apex, these studies have been relatively small and a number of unanswered questions remain. Many patients paced from the RV apex do not experience any adverse effects, but currently there is no method of determining which patients will develop HF from RV pacing, and benefit from CRT. Thus the added expense of CRT may not be justified in many patients. Also, studies comparing CRT to dual chamber pacing from alternate lead positions have not been carried out. Further, since CRT utilizes more energy in order to pace both ventricles, battery life is shorter, so more frequent change-out procedures will be required. Similarly, the extra lead required in CRT may increase the incidence of lead-related complications, as compared to dual chamber pacing. The cost-benefit analysis for routinely implanting CRT devices rather than RV pacermakers has not been performed.

## 7. Treatment of pacing-induced heart failure patients

Several studies have indicated that patients who are paced less frequently have better-preserved LV function than those paced more frequently (Sharma et al. 2005; Sweeney et al. 2003; Sweeney et al. 2007). However, the effect of reducing the frequency of pacing in patients who have already developed LV dysfunction remains uncertain. In addition, in cases of high degree AV block, nearly 100% ventricular pacing is required. To date, the best treatment for HF that is associated with chronic RV pacing is CRT. An LV lead can be added, and the patient can be paced from both the RV and LV, thus improving the synchrony of contraction.

In most large, multi-center randomized trials of CRT, patients chronically paced from the RV have been excluded. However, a number of smaller studies have suggested that these patients may experience similar benefits to CRT. Foley et al., reported that survival and hospitalizations rates were similar between a group of 58 RV paced patients upgraded to CRT, and 336 de novo CRT patients (Foley et al. 2009). In addition, significant improvements in a composite clinical score, EF, and LV volumes were reported in both groups, and were similar between groups. Improvements in dyssynchrony have also been reported in previously RV paced CRT patients (Eldadah et al. 2006; Vatankulu et al. 2009).

Improvements in rotational function may also be important mechanisms in functional improvement following upgrade from RV pacing to CRT. As previously discussed, rotational motion is significantly impaired following chronic RV pacing, and apical rotation is reversed in about 30% of patients (Burns et al. 2011). However, it has also been shown, in de novo CRT patients, that CRT improves rotation, and corrects rotational direction (Russel et al. 2009). Although it has not been demonstrated in clinical trials, it is logical that improvements in rotational function are important to the CRT response of previously-paced RV pacing.

We studied 31 previously RV paced HF patients upgraded to CRT and compared them to 49 patients receiving CRT for HF without previous pacing (Bank et al. 2010a). Previously RV paced patients had smaller ventricles despite similar EFs prior to CRT. Following CRT, previously RV paced patients improved their EF to a significantly greater extent than non-paced patients (12.8 ± 9.2% vs 7.4 ± 7.6%). RV paced patients had much more intramural dyssynchrony within the septum before CRT, and as shown previously in this chapter in Figure 4, a much greater reduction following about 1 year of CRT (Bank et al. 2010a). In addition, improvements in intramural dyssynchrony within the septum correlated to improved EF in previously paced patients, while other measures of dyssynchrony did not. This suggests that this pattern of intramural dyssynchrony may result in reduced LV function in chronic RV pacing, and may be readily corrected with CRT in affected patients. These patients likely developed iatrogenic HF from pacing, which was more readily corrected by improving electrical and mechanical dyssynchrony.

## 8. Summary

The increased risk of LV dysfunction associated with RV pacing has been well established. Similarly, both impaired LV systolic function and mechanical dyssynchrony have been shown to exist in groups of RV paced patients. Intramural dyssynchrony within the septum appears to be a common finding in chronically paced individuals, and may be an important mechanism in pacing-induced LV dysfunction. Similarly, rotational function appears to be more affected by RV pacing, than by other causes of heart failure. The correction of both intramural dyssynchrony and rotational dysfunction may be significant factors in the successful treatment of pacing-induced dysfunction using CRT.

## 9. References

Ashikaga, H., B. A. Coppola, B. Hopenfeld, E. S. Leifer, E. R. McVeigh and J. H. Omens. 2007. "Transmural dispersion of myofiber mechanics: implications for electrical heterogeneity in vivo." *Journal of the American College of Cardiology* 49(8):909-916.

Ashikaga, H., J. C. Criscione, J. H. Omens, J. W. Covell and N. B. Ingels Jr. 2004. "Transmural left ventricular mechanics underlying torsional recoil during relaxation." *American Journal of Physiology.Heart and Circulatory Physiology* 286(2):H640-7.

Bank, A. J. and A. S. Kelly. 2006. "Tissue Doppler imaging and left ventricular dyssynchrony in heart failure." *Journal of Cardiac Failure* 12(2):154-162.

Bank, A. J., Kaufman, C.L., Kelly, A.S., Burns, K.V., Adler, S.W., Rector, T.S., Goldsmith, S.R., Olivari, M,P., Tang, C., Nelson, L. and Metzig, A. 2009. "Results of the PROspective MInnesota Study of ECHO/TDI in Cardiac Resynchronization Therapy (PROMISE-CRT) Study." *Journal of Cardiac Failure* 15(5):401.

Bank, A.J., Kaufman, C.L., Burns, K.V., Parah, J., Johnson, L., Kelly, A.S., Shroff, S. and Kaiser, D. 2010a. "Intramural dyssynchrony and response to cardiac resynchronization therapy in patients with and without previous right ventricular pacing." *European Journal of Heart Failure* 12(12):1317.

Bank, Alan, Schwartzman D., Burns, K.V., Kaufman, C.L., Adler, S.W., Kelly, A.S., Johnson, L. and Kaiser, D. 2010b. "Intramural dyssynchrony from acute right ventricular apical pacing in human subjects with normal left ventricular function." *Journal of Cardiovascular Translational Research* 3(4):321-329.

Bax, J. J., G. B. Bleeker, T. H. Marwick, S. G. Molhoek, E. Boersma, P. Steendijk, E. E. van der Wall and M. J. Schalij. 2004. "Left ventricular dyssynchrony predicts response and prognosis after cardiac resynchronization therapy." *Journal of the American College of Cardiology; Journal of the American College of Cardiology* 44(9):1834-1840.

Birnie, D., K. Williams, A. Guo, L. Mielniczuk, D. Davis, R. Lemery, M. Green, M. Gollob and A. Tang. 2006. "Reasons for escalating pacemaker implants." *The American Journal of Cardiology* 98(1):93-97.

Bogunovic, N., D. Hering, F. van Buuren, D. Welge, B. Lamp, D. Horstkotte and L. Faber. 2009. "New aspects on the assessment of left ventricular dyssynchrony by tissue Doppler echocardiography: comparison of myocardial velocity vs. displacement curves." *The International Journal of Cardiovascular Imaging* 25(7):699-704.

Borg, A. N., J. L. Harrison, R. A. Argyle and S. G. Ray. 2008. "Left ventricular torsion in primary chronic mitral regurgitation." *Heart (British Cardiac Society)* 94(5):597-603.

Brignole, M., G. Botto, L. Mont, S. Iacopino, G. De Marchi, D. Oddone, M. Luzi, J. M. Tolosana, A. Navazio and C. Menozzi. 2011. "Cardiac resynchronization therapy in patients undergoing atrioventricular junction ablation for permanent atrial fibrillation: a randomized trial." *European Heart Journal.*

Buckberg, G. D. 2002. "Basic science review: the helix and the heart." *The Journal of Thoracic and Cardiovascular Surgery* 124(5):863-883.

Buckberg, G. D., M. Castella, M. Gharib and S. Saleh. 2006. "Active myocyte shortening during the 'isovolumetric relaxation' phase of diastole is responsible for ventricular suction; 'systolic ventricular filling'." *European Journal of Cardio-Thoracic Surgery : Official Journal of the European Association for Cardio-Thoracic Surgery* 29 Suppl 1:S98-106.

Burns, K. V., C. L. Kaufman, A. S. Kelly, J. S. Parah, D. R. Dengel and A. J. Bank. 2011. "Torsion and dyssynchrony differences between chronically paced and non-paced heart failure patients." *Journal of Cardiac Failure* 17(6):495-502.

Cano, O., J. Osca, M. J. Sancho-Tello, J. M. Sanchez, V. Ortiz, J. E. Castro, A. Salvador and J. Olague. 2010. "Comparison of effectiveness of right ventricular septal pacing versus right ventricular apical pacing." *The American Journal of Cardiology* 105(10):1426-1432.

Catanzariti, D., M. Maines, C. Cemin, G. Broso, T. Marotta and G. Vergara. 2006. "Permanent direct his bundle pacing does not induce ventricular dyssynchrony unlike conventional right ventricular apical pacing. An intrapatient acute comparison study." *Journal of Interventional Cardiac Electrophysiology : An International Journal of Arrhythmias and Pacing* 16(2):81-92.

Cho, G. Y., M. J. Kim, J. H. Park, H. S. Kim, H. J. Youn, K. H. Kim and J. K. Song. 2011. "Comparison of ventricular dyssynchrony according to the position of right ventricular pacing electrode: a multi-center prospective echocardiographic study." *Journal of Cardiovascular Ultrasound* 19(1):15-20.

Chung, J., P. Abraszewski, X. Yu, W. Liu, A. J. Krainik, M. Ashford, S. D. Caruthers, J. B. McGill and S. A. Wickline. 2006. "Paradoxical increase in ventricular torsion and systolic torsion rate in type I diabetic patients under tight glycemic control." *Journal of the American College of Cardiology* 47(2):384-390.

Dabrowska-Kugacka, A., E. Lewicka-Nowak, S. Tybura, R. Wilczek, J. Staniewicz, P. Zagozdzon, A. Faran, D. Kozlowski, G. Raczak and G. Swiatecka. 2009. "Survival analysis in patients with preserved left ventricular function and standard indications for permanent cardiac pacing randomized to right ventricular apical or septal outflow tract pacing." *Circulation Journal : Official Journal of the Japanese Circulation Society* 73(10):1812-1819.

Delhaas, T., J. Kotte, A. van der Toorn, G. Snoep, F. W. Prinzen and T. Arts. 2004. "Increase in left ventricular torsion-to-shortening ratio in children with valvular aortic stenosis." *Magnetic Resonance in Medicine : Official Journal of the Society of Magnetic Resonance in Medicine / Society of Magnetic Resonance in Medicine* 51(1):135-139.

Dohi, K., K. Onishi, J. Gorcsan 3rd, A. Lopez-Candales, T. Takamura, S. Ota, N. Yamada and M. Ito. 2008. "Role of radial strain and displacement imaging to quantify wall motion dyssynchrony in patients with left ventricular mechanical dyssynchrony and chronic right ventricular pressure overload." *The American Journal of Cardiology* 101(8):1206-1212.

Donal, E., F. Tournoux, C. Leclercq, C. De Place, A. Solnon, G. Derumeaux, P. Mabo, A. Cohen-Solal and J. C. Daubert. 2008. "Assessment of longitudinal and radial ventricular dyssynchrony in ischemic and nonischemic chronic systolic heart failure: a two-dimensional echocardiographic speckle-tracking strain study." *Journal of the American Society of Echocardiography : Official Publication of the American Society of Echocardiography* 21(1):58-65.

Eldadah, Z. A., B. Rosen, I. Hay, T. Edvardsen, V. Jayam, T. Dickfeld, G. R. Meininger, D. P. Judge, J. Hare, J. B. Lima, H. Calkins and R. D. Berger. 2006. "The benefit of upgrading chronically right ventricle-paced heart failure patients to resynchronization therapy demonstrated by strain rate imaging." *Heart Rhythm : The Official Journal of the Heart Rhythm Society* 3(4):435-442.

Foley, P. W., S. A. Muhyaldeen, S. Chalil, R. E. Smith, J. E. Sanderson and F. Leyva. 2009. "Long-term effects of upgrading from right ventricular pacing to cardiac resynchronization therapy in patients with heart failure." *Europace : European Pacing, Arrhythmias, and Cardiac Electrophysiology : Journal of the Working Groups on Cardiac Pacing, Arrhythmias, and Cardiac Cellular Electrophysiology of the European Society of Cardiology* 11(4):495-501.

Gammage, M., S. Schofield, I. Rankin, M. Bennett, P. Coles and B. Pentecost. 1991. "Benefit of single setting rate responsive ventricular pacing compared with fixed rate demand pacing in elderly patients." *Pacing and Clinical Electrophysiology : PACE* 14(2 Pt 1):174-180.

Geleijnse, M. L. and B. M. van Dalen. 2009. "Let's twist." *European Journal of Echocardiography : The Journal of the Working Group on Echocardiography of the European Society of Cardiology* 10(1):46-47.

Gong, X., Y. Su, W. Pan, J. Cui, S. Liu and X. Shu. 2009. "Is right ventricular outflow tract pacing superior to right ventricular apex pacing in patients with normal cardiac function?" *Clinical Cardiology* 32(12):695-699.

Gorcsan, J.,3rd, H. Kanzaki, R. Bazaz, K. Dohi and D. Schwartzman. 2004. "Usefulness of echocardiographic tissue synchronization imaging to predict acute response to cardiac resynchronization therapy." *The American Journal of Cardiology; the American Journal of Cardiology* 93(9):1178-1181.

Hayes, J. J., A. D. Sharma, J. C. Love, J. M. Herre, A. O. Leonen, P. J. Kudenchuk and DAVID Investigators. 2006. "Abnormal conduction increases risk of adverse outcomes from right ventricular pacing." *Journal of the American College of Cardiology* 48(8):1628-1633.

Helle-Valle, T., J. Crosby, T. Edvardsen, E. Lyseggen, B. H. Amundsen, H. J. Smith, B. D. Rosen, J. A. Lima, H. Torp, H. Ihlen and O. A. Smiseth. 2005. "New noninvasive method for assessment of left ventricular rotation: speckle tracking echocardiography." *Circulation; Circulation* 112(20):3149-3156.

Inoue, K., H. Okayama, K. Nishimura, A. Ogimoto, T. Ohtsuka, M. Saito, G. Hiasa, T. Yoshii, T. Sumimoto, J. Funada and J. Higaki. 2010. "Right ventricular pacing from the septum avoids the acute exacerbation in left ventricular dyssynchrony and torsional behavior seen with pacing from the apex." *Journal of the American Society of Echocardiography : Official Publication of the American Society of Echocardiography* 23(2):195-200.

Inoue, K., H. Okayama, K. Nishimura, M. Saito, T. Yoshii, G. Hiasa, T. Sumimoto, S. Inaba, J. Suzuki, A. Ogimoto, J. Funada and J. Higaki. 2011. "Right ventricular septal pacing preserves global left ventricular longitudinal function in comparison with apical pacing." *Circulation Journal : Official Journal of the Japanese Circulation Society* 75(7):1609-1615.

Kanzaki, H., S. Nakatani, N. Yamada, S. Urayama, K. Miyatake and M. Kitakaze. 2006. "Impaired Systolic torsion in dilated cardiomyopathy: Reversal of apical rotation at mid-systole characterized with magnetic resonance tagging method." *Basic Research in Cardiology* 101(6):465-470.

Kaufman, C. L., D. R. Kaiser, K. V. Burns, A. S. Kelly and A. J. Bank. 2010. "Multi-plane mechanical dyssynchrony in cardiac resynchronization therapy." *Clinical Cardiology* 33(2):E31-8.

Kawanishi, Y., T. Ito, M. Suwa, F. Terasaki, R. Futai and Y. Kitaura. 2008. "Effect of left ventricular dyssynchrony on plasma B-type natriuretic peptide levels in patients with long-term right ventricular apical pacing." *International Heart Journal* 49(2):165-173.

Kindermann, M., B. Hennen, J. Jung, J. Geisel, M. Bohm and G. Frohlig. 2006. "Biventricular versus conventional right ventricular stimulation for patients with standard pacing indication and left ventricular dysfunction: the Homburg Biventricular Pacing Evaluation (HOBIPACE)." *Journal of the American College of Cardiology* 47(10):1927-1937.

Kolb, C., B. Zrenner and C. Schmitt. 2001. "Incidence of electromagnetic interference in implantable cardioverter defibrillators." *Pacing and Clinical Electrophysiology : PACE* 24(4 Pt 1):465-468.

Kronborg, M. B., P. T. Mortensen, J. C. Gerdes, H. K. Jensen and J. C. Nielsen. 2011. "His and para-His pacing in AV block: feasibility and electrocardiographic findings." *Journal of Interventional Cardiac Electrophysiology : An International Journal of Arrhythmias and Pacing.*

Lamas, G. A., C. L. Pashos, S. L. Normand and B. McNeil. 1995. "Permanent pacemaker selection and subsequent survival in elderly Medicare pacemaker recipients." *Circulation* 91(4):1063-1069.

Leong, D. P., A. M. Mitchell, I. Salna, A. G. Brooks, G. Sharma, H. S. Lim, M. Alasady, M. Barlow, J. Leitch, P. Sanders and G. D. Young. 2010. "Long-term mechanical consequences of permanent right ventricular pacing: effect of pacing site." *Journal of Cardiovascular Electrophysiology* 21(10):1120-1126.

Liakopoulos, O. J., H. Tomioka, G. D. Buckberg, Z. Tan, N. Hristov and G. Trummer. 2006. "Sequential deformation and physiological considerations in unipolar right or left ventricular pacing." *European Journal of Cardio-Thoracic Surgery : Official Journal of the European Association for Cardio-Thoracic Surgery* 29 Suppl 1:S188-97.

Lieberman, R., L. Padeletti, J. Schreuder, K. Jackson, A. Michelucci, A. Colella, W. Eastman, S. Valsecchi and D. A. Hettrick. 2006. "Ventricular pacing lead location alters systemic hemodynamics and left ventricular function in patients with and without reduced ejection fraction." *Journal of the American College of Cardiology* 48(8):1634-1641.

Marwick, T. H. and M. Schwaiger. 2008. "The future of cardiovascular imaging in the diagnosis and management of heart failure, part 1: tasks and tools." *Circulation.Cardiovascular Imaging* 1(1):58-69.

Nakai, H., M. Takeuchi, T. Nishikage, M. Kokumai, S. Otani and R. M. Lang. 2006. "Effect of aging on twist-displacement loop by 2-dimensional speckle tracking imaging." *Journal of the American Society of Echocardiography : Official Publication of the American Society of Echocardiography* 19(7):880-885.

Ng, A. C., C. Allman, J. Vidaic, H. Tie, A. P. Hopkins and D. Y. Leung. 2009. "Long-term impact of right ventricular septal versus apical pacing on left ventricular synchrony and function in patients with second- or third-degree heart block." *The American Journal of Cardiology* 103(8):1096-1101.

Notomi, Y., P. Lysyansky, R. M. Setser, T. Shiota, Z. B. Popovic, M. G. Martin-Miklovic, J. A. Weaver, S. J. Oryszak, N. L. Greenberg, R. D. White and J. D. Thomas. 2005. "Measurement of ventricular torsion by two-dimensional ultrasound speckle tracking imaging." *Journal of the American College of Cardiology* 45(12):2034-2041.

Notomi, Y., M. G. Martin-Miklovic, S. J. Oryszak, T. Shiota, D. Deserranno, Z. B. Popovic, M. J. Garcia, N. L. Greenberg and J. D. Thomas. 2006. "Enhanced ventricular untwisting during exercise: a mechanistic manifestation of elastic recoil described by Doppler tissue imaging." *Circulation* 113(21):2524-2533.

Notomi, Y., Z. B. Popovic, H. Yamada, D. W. Wallick, M. G. Martin, S. J. Oryszak, T. Shiota, N. L. Greenberg and J. D. Thomas. 2008. "Ventricular untwisting: a temporal link between left ventricular relaxation and suction." *American Journal of Physiology.Heart and Circulatory Physiology* 294(1):H505-13.

Notomi, Y., R. M. Setser, T. Shiota, M. G. Martin-Miklovic, J. A. Weaver, Z. B. Popovic, H. Yamada, N. L. Greenberg, R. D. White and J. D. Thomas. 2005. "Assessment of left ventricular torsional deformation by Doppler tissue imaging: validation study with tagged magnetic resonance imaging." *Circulation* 111(9):1141-1147.

Notomi, Y., G. Srinath, T. Shiota, M. G. Martin-Miklovic, L. Beachler, K. Howell, S. J. Oryszak, D. G. Deserranno, A. D. Freed, N. L. Greenberg, A. Younoszai and J. D. Thomas. 2006. "Maturational and adaptive modulation of left ventricular torsional biomechanics: Doppler tissue imaging observation from infancy to adulthood." *Circulation* 113(21):2534-2541.

O'Keefe, J. H.,Jr, H. Abuissa, P. G. Jones, R. C. Thompson, T. M. Bateman, A. I. McGhie, B. M. Ramza and D. M. Steinhaus. 2005. "Effect of chronic right ventricular apical pacing on left ventricular function." *The American Journal of Cardiology* 95(6):771-773.

Park, S. J., C. Miyazaki, C. J. Bruce, S. Ommen, F. A. Miller and J. K. Oh. 2008. "Left ventricular torsion by two-dimensional speckle tracking echocardiography in patients with diastolic dysfunction and normal ejection fraction." *Journal of the American Society of Echocardiography : Official Publication of the American Society of Echocardiography* 21(10):1129-1137.

Prinzen, F. W., C. H. Augustijn, T. Arts, M. A. Allessie and R. S. Reneman. 1990. "Redistribution of myocardial fiber strain and blood flow by asynchronous activation." *The American Journal of Physiology* 259(2 Pt 2):H300-8.

Prinzen, F. W., W. C. Hunter, B. T. Wyman and E. R. McVeigh. 1999. "Mapping of regional myocardial strain and work during ventricular pacing: experimental study using magnetic resonance imaging tagging." *Journal of the American College of Cardiology* 33(6):1735-1742.

Russel, I. K., M. J. Gotte, G. J. de Roest, J. T. Marcus, S. R. Tecelao, C. P. Allaart, C. C. de Cock, R. M. Heethaar and A. C. van Rossum. 2009. "Loss of opposite left ventricular basal and apical rotation predicts acute response to cardiac resynchronization therapy and is associated with long-term reversed remodeling." *Journal of Cardiac Failure* 15(8):717-725.

Saito, M., H. Okayama, K. Nishimura, A. Ogimoto, T. Ohtsuka, K. Inoue, G. Hiasa, T. Sumimoto, J. Funada, Y. Shigematsu and J. Higaki. 2009. "Determinants of left ventricular untwisting behaviour in patients with dilated cardiomyopathy: analysis by two-dimensional speckle tracking." *Heart (British Cardiac Society)* 95(4):290-296.

Schwaab, B., Frohlig, G., Alexander, C., Kindermann, M., Hellwig, N., Schwerdt, H., et al. (1999). Influence of right ventricular stimulation site on left ventricular function in atrial synchronous ventricular pacing. *Journal of the American College of Cardiology,* 33(2) 317-323.

Sengupta, P. P., B. K. Khandheria, J. Korinek, J. Wang and M. Belohlavek. 2005. "Biphasic tissue Doppler waveforms during isovolumic phases are associated with asynchronous deformation of subendocardial and subepicardial layers." *Journal of Applied Physiology (Bethesda, Md.: 1985)* 99(3):1104-1111.

Sharma, A. D., C. Rizo-Patron, A. P. Hallstrom, G. P. O'Neill, S. Rothbart, J. B. Martins, M. Roelke, J. S. Steinberg, H. L. Greene and DAVID Investigators. 2005. "Percent right ventricular pacing predicts outcomes in the DAVID trial." *Heart Rhythm : The Official Journal of the Heart Rhythm Society* 2(8):830-834.

Shaw, S. M., D. J. Fox and S. G. Williams. 2008. "The development of left ventricular torsion and its clinical relevance." *International Journal of Cardiology* 130(3):319-325.

Sogaard, P., H. Egeblad, W. Y. Kim, H. K. Jensen, A. K. Pedersen, B. O. Kristensen and P. T. Mortensen. 2002a. "Tissue Doppler imaging predicts improved systolic performance and reversed left ventricular remodeling during long-term cardiac resynchronization therapy." *Journal of the American College of Cardiology* 40(4):723-730.

Sogaard, P., H. Egeblad, A. K. Pedersen, W. Y. Kim, B. O. Kristensen, P. S. Hansen and P. T. Mortensen. 2002b. "Sequential versus simultaneous biventricular resynchronization for severe heart failure: evaluation by tissue Doppler imaging." *Circulation* 106(16):2078-2084.

Sorger, J. M., B. T. Wyman, O. P. Faris, W. C. Hunter and E. R. McVeigh. 2003. "Torsion of the left ventricle during pacing with MRI tagging." *Journal of Cardiovascular Magnetic Resonance : Official Journal of the Society for Cardiovascular Magnetic Resonance* 5(4):521-530.

Stambler, B. S., K. Ellenbogen, X. Zhang, T. R. Porter, F. Xie, R. Malik, R. Small, M. Burke, A. Kaplan, L. Nair, M. Belz, C. Fuenzalida, M. Gold, C. Love, A. Sharma, R. Silverman, F. Sogade, B. Van Natta, B. L. Wilkoff and ROVA Investigators. 2003. "Right ventricular outflow versus apical pacing in pacemaker patients with congestive heart failure and atrial fibrillation." *Journal of Cardiovascular Electrophysiology* 14(11):1180-1186.

Suffoletto, M. S., K. Dohi, M. Cannesson, S. Saba and J. Gorcsan 3rd. 2006. "Novel speckle-tracking radial strain from routine black-and-white echocardiographic images to quantify dyssynchrony and predict response to cardiac resynchronization therapy." *Circulation* 113(7):960-968.

Sweeney, M. O., A. J. Bank, E. Nsah, M. Koullick, Q. C. Zeng, D. Hettrick, T. Sheldon, G. A. Lamas and Search AV Extension and Managed Ventricular Pacing for Promoting Atrioventricular Conduction (SAVE PACe) Trial. 2007. "Minimizing ventricular pacing to reduce atrial fibrillation in sinus-node disease." *The New England Journal of Medicine* 357(10):1000-1008.

Sweeney, M. O., A. S. Hellkamp, K. A. Ellenbogen, A. J. Greenspon, R. A. Freedman, K. L. Lee, G. A. Lamas and MOde Selection Trial Investigators. 2003. "Adverse effect of ventricular pacing on heart failure and atrial fibrillation among patients with normal baseline QRS duration in a clinical trial of pacemaker therapy for sinus node dysfunction." *Circulation* 107(23):2932-2937.

Takeuchi, M., H. Nakai, M. Kokumai, T. Nishikage, S. Otani and R. M. Lang. 2006. "Age-related changes in left ventricular twist assessed by two-dimensional speckle-tracking imaging." *Journal of the American Society of Echocardiography : Official Publication of the American Society of Echocardiography* 19(9):1077-1084.

Thackray, S. D., K. K. Witte, N. P. Nikitin, A. L. Clark, G. C. Kaye and J. G. Cleland. 2003. "The prevalence of heart failure and asymptomatic left ventricular systolic dysfunction in a typical regional pacemaker population." *European Heart Journal* 24(12):1143-1152.

Tomioka, H., O. J. Liakopoulos, G. D. Buckberg, N. Hristov, Z. Tan and G. Trummer. 2006. "The effect of ventricular sequential contraction on helical heart during pacing: high septal pacing versus biventricular pacing." *European Journal of Cardio-Thoracic Surgery : Official Journal of the European Association for Cardio-Thoracic Surgery* 29 Suppl 1:S198-206.

Tops, L. F., M. J. Schalij, E. R. Holman, L. van Erven, E. E. van der Wall and J. J. Bax. 2006. "Right ventricular pacing can induce ventricular dyssynchrony in patients with atrial fibrillation after atrioventricular node ablation." *Journal of the American College of Cardiology* 48(8):1642-1648.

Tops, L. F., M. S. Suffoletto, G. B. Bleeker, E. Boersma, E. E. van der Wall, J. Gorcsan 3rd, M. J. Schalij and J. J. Bax. 2007. "Speckle-tracking radial strain reveals left ventricular dyssynchrony in patients with permanent right ventricular pacing." *Journal of the American College of Cardiology* 50(12):1180-1188.

Torrent-Guasp, F., M. J. Kocica, A. Corno, M. Komeda, J. Cox, A. Flotats, M. Ballester-Rodes and F. Carreras-Costa. 2004. "Systolic ventricular filling." *European Journal of Cardio-Thoracic Surgery : Official Journal of the European Association for Cardio-Thoracic Surgery* 25(3):376-386.

Tse, H. F. and C. P. Lau. 1997. "Long-term effect of right ventricular pacing on myocardial perfusion and function." *Journal of the American College of Cardiology* 29(4):744-749.

Tse, H. F., C. Yu, K. K. Wong, V. Tsang, Y. L. Leung, W. Y. Ho and C. P. Lau. 2002. "Functional abnormalities in patients with permanent right ventricular pacing: the effect of sites of electrical stimulation." *Journal of the American College of Cardiology* 40(8):1451-1458.

Vatankulu, M. A., O. Goktekin, M. G. Kaya, S. Ayhan, Z. Kucukdurmaz, R. Sutton and M. Henein. 2009. "Effect of long-term resynchronization therapy on left ventricular remodeling in pacemaker patients upgraded to biventricular devices." *The American Journal of Cardiology* 103(9):1280-1284.

Victor, F., Leclercq, C., Mabo, P., Pavin, D., Deviller, A., de Place, C., et al. (1999). Optimal right ventricular pacing site in chronically implanted patients: a prospective randomized crossover comparison of apical and outflow tract pacing. *Journal of the American College of Cardiology*, 33(2)311-316.

Wilkoff, B. L., J. R. Cook, A. E. Epstein, H. L. Greene, A. P. Hallstrom, H. Hsia, S. P. Kutalek, A. Sharma and Dual Chamber and VVI Implantable Defibrillator Trial Investigators. 2002. "Dual-chamber pacing or ventricular backup pacing in patients with an implantable defibrillator: the Dual Chamber and VVI Implantable Defibrillator (DAVID) Trial." *JAMA : The Journal of the American Medical Association* 288(24):3115-3123.

Wyman, B. T., W. C. Hunter, F. W. Prinzen and E. R. McVeigh. 1999. "Mapping propagation of mechanical activation in the paced heart with MRI tagging." *The American Journal of Physiology* 276(3 Pt 2):H881-91.

Yamano, T., T. Kubo, S. Takarada, K. Ishibashi, K. Komukai, T. Tanimoto, Y. Ino, H. Kitabata, K. Hirata, A. Tanaka, T. Imanishi and T. Akasaka. 2010. "Advantage of right ventricular outflow tract pacing on cardiac function and coronary circulation in comparison with right ventricular apex pacing." *Journal of the American Society of Echocardiography : Official Publication of the American Society of Echocardiography* 23(11):1177-1182.

Yu, C. M., G. B. Bleeker, J. W. Fung, M. J. Schalij, Q. Zhang, E. E. van der Wall, Y. S. Chan, S. L. Kong and J. J. Bax. 2005. "Left ventricular reverse remodeling but not clinical improvement predicts long-term survival after cardiac resynchronization therapy." *Circulation; Circulation* 112(11):1580-1586.

Yu, C. M., J. Y. Chan, Q. Zhang, R. Omar, G. W. Yip, A. Hussin, F. Fang, K. H. Lam, H. C. Chan and J. W. Fung. 2009. "Biventricular pacing in patients with bradycardia and normal ejection fraction." *The New England Journal of Medicine* 361(22):2123-2134.

Yu, C. M., J. W. Fung, Q. Zhang, C. K. Chan, Y. S. Chan, H. Lin, L. C. Kum, S. L. Kong, Y. Zhang and J. E. Sanderson. 2004. "Tissue Doppler imaging is superior to strain rate imaging and postsystolic shortening on the prediction of reverse remodeling in both ischemic and nonischemic heart failure after cardiac resynchronization therapy." *Circulation; Circulation* 110(1):66-73.

Yu, C. M., Q. Zhang, Y. S. Chan, C. K. Chan, G. W. Yip, L. C. Kum, E. B. Wu, P. W. Lee, Y. Y. Lam, S. Chan and J. W. Fung. 2006. "Tissue Doppler velocity is superior to displacement and strain mapping in predicting left ventricular reverse remodelling response after cardiac resynchronisation therapy." *Heart (British Cardiac Society); Heart (British Cardiac Society)* 92(10):1452-1456.

Zanon, F., E. Bacchiega, L. Rampin, S. Aggio, E. Baracca, G. Pastore, T. Marotta, G. Corbucci, L. Roncon, D. Rubello and F. W. Prinzen. 2008. "Direct His bundle pacing preserves coronary perfusion compared with right ventricular apical pacing: a prospective, cross-over mid-term study." *Europace : European Pacing, Arrhythmias, and Cardiac Electrophysiology : Journal of the Working Groups on Cardiac Pacing, Arrhythmias, and Cardiac Cellular Electrophysiology of the European Society of Cardiology* 10(5):580-587.

Zhang, Q., F. Fang, G. W. Yip, J. Y. Chan, Q. Shang, J. W. Fung, A. K. Chan, Y. J. Liang and C. M. Yu. 2008a. "Difference in prevalence and pattern of mechanical dyssynchrony in left bundle branch block occurring in right ventricular apical pacing versus systolic heart failure." *American Heart Journal* 156(5):989-995.

Zhang, X. H., H. Chen, C. W. Siu, K. H. Yiu, W. S. Chan, K. L. Lee, H. W. Chan, S. W. Lee, G. S. Fu, C. P. Lau and H. F. Tse. 2008b. "New-onset heart failure after permanent right ventricular apical pacing in patients with acquired high-grade atrioventricular block and normal left ventricular function." *Journal of Cardiovascular Electrophysiology* 19(2):136-141.

7

# Noninvasive Imaging of Cardiac Electrophysiology (NICE)

Michael Seger[1], Bernhard Pfeifer[1] and Thomas Berger[2]
[1]*Institute of Electrical, Electronic and Bioengineering, UMIT – The Health and Life Sciences University*
[2]*Division of Internal Medicine III/Cardiology, Medical University Innsbruck Austria*

## 1. Introduction

### 1.1 General description and aim of NICE

Many clinically relevant types of cardiac dysfunctions can be diagnosed by a proper knowledge of the spatio-temporal spread of cardiac electrical excitation, such as supraventricular and ventricular tachycardias. This knowledge supports the cardiologist to apply the optimal treatment strategy for the individual patient.

Computer modeling of bioelectric activity has been of interest in cardiac electrophysiology for several decades (Gulrajani R. M., 1988; Johnson J. R., 1997; Modre R. et al., 2001). Additionally, noninvasive imaging of the electrical excitation from recorded electrocardiograms (ECGs) has become a diagnosis tool in clinical electrophysiology (Modre R. et al., 2003; Ramanathan C. et al., 2004). Noninvasive imaging of the electrical function requires the combination of four dimensional anatomical (three dimensions: space) and ECG mapping (one dimension: time) data. This allows computation of the so-called electrocardiographic inverse problem. This means to calculate the unknown sources (e.g., cardiac electrophysiological parameters) by considering the measured – and thus known – anatomical and ECG data in an appropriate manner.

NICE – **N**oninvasive **I**maging of **C**ardiac **E**lectrophysiology – has been developed for investigating and assessing the electrophysiological cardiac status of humans in a noninvasive manner over the past 25 years at Graz Technical University (Graz, Austria), Medical University Innsbruck (Innsbruck, Austria) and UMIT (Hall in Tirol, Austria). Selected publications reflecting the related development and progress of this method are (Berger T. et al., 2006; 2005; 2011; Fischer G. et al., 2000; 1999; Messnarz B., Seger M., Modre R., Fischer G., Hanser F. & Tilg B., 2004; Modre R. et al., 2006; 2003; Pfeifer B. et al., 2008; 2006; Renhardt M. et al., 1992; Seger M. et al., 2004; Tilg B., Hanser F., Modre-Osprian R., Fischer G., Messnarz B., Berger T., Hintringer F., Pachinger O. & Roithinger F. X., 2002; Tilg B. et al., 1992; Wach P. et al., 2001; 1997).

In brief, NICE enables the computation of electrophysiologically and clinically meaningful parameters, such as cardiac activation times (ATs) or the spatio-temporal transmembrane potential distribution on both the atrial or ventricular surfaces. All the related steps necessary to obtain this information are accomplished exclusively in a noninvasive fashion. Thus

- interventional procedures for diagnostic purposes can be avoided and therefore the risk of complications can be reduced,
- a diagnosis based on the results of NICE can help the cardiologist to plan appropriate therapeutical treatment strategies,
- post-interventional analyses can be performed at higher and more detailed spatial resolutions as compared to the 12-lead standard ECG, and
- patient individual screening or monitoring of changes of electrophysiological behaviour (e.g., CRT) can be performed.

An individual patient-specific model of cardiac electrophysiology gives important information about clinically relevant parameters of atrial and ventricular electroanatomic activation. For this purpose a distinct knowledge of different mathematical, physical and medical disciplines, related methods and applications is essential. The most relevant disciplines involved in NICE are (examples of corresponding activities related to NICE are given in brackets)

- *biomedical signal processing* (filtering, baseline correction and extraction of the relevant portions of the recorded multi-channel ECG signals),
- *biomedical image processing* (segmentation of the patient individual volume conductor model based on medical imaging modalities (e.g., Magnetic Resonance Imaging (MRI)) including heart, chest, lungs, blood masses; registration of the electrodes' positions on the volume conductor model),
- *modelling and simulation of biophysical systems and compounds* (bidomain theory for the biophysical description of the electric sources generated by the myocytes),
- *electrical engineering* (Maxwell's equations applied to describe bioelectrical phenomena and thus to relate the electrical sources to the measured ECG signals),
- *solving techniques applied to inverse problems* (the problem formulation of NICE is ill-posed and requires therefore application of regularization techniques),
- *numerical mathematics* (discretization of the patient's geometry and of the related Maxwell's equations according to the chosen method, e.g., Boundary-Element-Method (BEM), Finite-Element-Method (FEM) or hybride cellular automata based approaches),
- *experimental and clinical electrophysiology* (data analysis, interpretation of the results and implications, future perspectives and possible clinical applications).

## 2. Methods

### 2.1 Mathematical/physical background

#### 2.1.1 Description of the problem

The most relevant measures which can be obtained noninvasively are the spatio-temporal distribution of

- epi-, endo- and/or myocardial electrical potentials $\varphi$ (performed by, e.g., (Ramanathan C. et al., 2004; 2003)),

- transmembrane voltages (difference of intra- and extracellular potentials $\varphi_m = \varphi_{intra} - \varphi_{extra}$; performed by, e.g., (Messnarz B., Tilg B., Modre R., Fischer G. & Hanser F., 2004)) or
- the cardiac activation times $\tau$ (time instant when the depolarization of the region of interest occurs; performed by, e.g., (Berger T. et al., 2006; 2011)).

These parameters can be calculated for the outer and inner surfaces of the heart (on the epi- and endocardia) and/or within the myocardium. In case of NICE, the cardiac activation times are determined both on the epi- and endocardia.

The cardiac activation times are related to the ECG on the body surface (also termed Body Surface Potential Mapping – BSPM). Therefore, an appropriate model formulation can be applied. In the following subsections the mathematical derivation for final determination of cardiac activation times $\tau(\mathbf{x})$ (with $\mathbf{x} \in \Omega$ or $\Gamma \subset \mathbb{R}^3$; $\Gamma$ representing the cardiac surfaces (epi-, endocardia), $\Omega$ represents the whole cardiac volume) is presented in a more detailed manner.

### 2.1.2 Bidomain theory

According to (Geselowitz D. B. & Miller 3rd W. T., 1983) a physical description for the behavior of electrically active tissue – thus also the heart – on a macroscopic scale can be represented by the so-called *bidomain theory*. In Fig. 1 the modeling assumptions for the continuum model

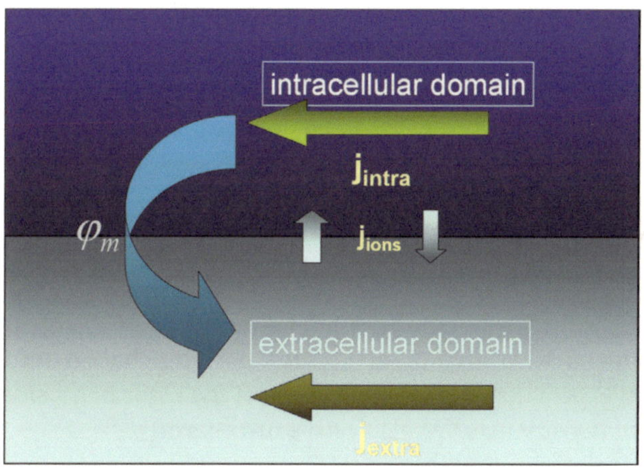


Fig. 1. A schematic snapshot of the intra- and extracellular domain for the *bidomain continuum model* is shown. The intracellular space is separated from the extracellular space by the cellular membrane. Ion currents are able to pass through the membrane via specific ion channels ($j_{ions}$). Current densities occur within the cell ($j_{intra}$) and outside the cell in the interstitial space ($j_{extra}$). The voltage measured as difference between the intracellular and the extracellular potentials is termed transmembrane potential $\varphi_m = \varphi_{intra} - \varphi_{extra}$.

derivating the bidomain theory are shown. As the cardiac fibers (myocytes) are connected to each other via highly conductive *gap-junctions* it is assumed, that intra- and extacellular spaces can be smeared over the whole heart. That means, there is no need to model each cardiac cell individually, but the values necessary to describe the electrical behavior are averaged over a small tissue volume. As an example, current density $j_x$ in direction of the x-axis can thus be calculated by the intracellular $I_{intra}$ and extracellular $I_{extra}$ current

$$j_x = \frac{I_{intra} + I_{extra}}{\Gamma} = -\frac{\Gamma_{intra}}{\Gamma} \cdot \sigma^*_{intra} \cdot \frac{\partial \varphi_{intra}}{\partial x} - \frac{\Gamma_{extra}}{\Gamma} \cdot \sigma^*_{extra} \cdot \frac{\partial \varphi_{extra}}{\partial x}. \quad (1)$$

The intracellular cross section is denoted by $\Gamma_{intra}$, the extracellular by $\Gamma_{extra}$ and the cross section of the whole cell by $\Gamma$. Scalars $\sigma^*_{intra}$ and $\sigma^*_{extra}$ represent the conductivities of the intra- and extracellular space, respectively, $\frac{\partial \varphi_{intra}}{\partial x}$ and $\frac{\partial \varphi_{extra}}{\partial x}$ denote the gradients of the corresponding potentials. Combining expressions $\frac{\Gamma_{intra}}{\Gamma} \cdot \boldsymbol{\sigma}^*_{intra}$ to $\boldsymbol{\sigma}_{intra}$, the effective intracellular conductivity, and $\frac{\Gamma_{extra}}{\Gamma} \cdot \boldsymbol{\sigma}^*_{extra}$ to $\boldsymbol{\sigma}_{extra}$, the effective extracellular conductivity, leads finally – for all three Cartesian coordinates – to

$$\boldsymbol{j} = -\boldsymbol{\sigma}_{extra}\mathrm{grad}(\varphi_{extra}) - \boldsymbol{\sigma}_{intra}\mathrm{grad}(\varphi_{intra}). \quad (2)$$

Introducing the transmembrane (or action) potential

$$\varphi_m = \varphi_{intra} - \varphi_{extra} \quad (3)$$

and the bulk conductivity, $\boldsymbol{\kappa}_B = \boldsymbol{\sigma}_{intra} + \boldsymbol{\sigma}_{extra}$, Equation (2) can be reorganized and rewritten to

$$\boldsymbol{j} = -\boldsymbol{\sigma}_{intra}\mathrm{grad}(\varphi_m) - \boldsymbol{\kappa}_B\mathrm{grad}(\varphi_{extra}). \quad (4)$$

Note that bold symbols represent in case of $\boldsymbol{j}$ a vector or in case of e.g., $\boldsymbol{\sigma}_{intra}$ tensors, which means that the electrical conductivities in general can be referred to as electrically anisotropic measures. Applying Equation (16) (the mathematical calculus why the divergence of $\boldsymbol{j}$ is set to zero will be explained in the next subsection 2.1.3), Equation (4) finally results in

$$\mathrm{div}[\boldsymbol{\kappa}_B\mathrm{grad}(\varphi_{extra})] = -\mathrm{div}[\boldsymbol{\sigma}_{intra}\mathrm{grad}(\varphi_m)]. \quad (5)$$

Equation (5) is an elliptical differential equation and also known as BIDOMAIN EQUATION. This equation represents the mathematical model description of electrical cardiac function on a continuum model level. Note, that (5) is – with according change of the values – the same equation as (17) with expression $-\boldsymbol{\sigma}_{intra}\mathrm{grad}(\varphi_m)$ on the right hand side of (5) representing the impressed current density (cardiac electrical source term) $\boldsymbol{j}^{(\mathrm{imp})}$.

The spatio-temporal distribution of $\varphi_m$ over and within the heart can be most commonly computed by, e.g., cellular automata approaches ((Barbosa C. R. H., 2003; He B. et al., 2002; Hintermüller C. et al., 2004; Saxberg B. E. & Cohen R. J., 1990)). This is of particular interest, when the effects of varying different parameters of the model description on the potentials measured on the torso is the focus of interest, i.e., when solving the forward problem of electrocardiography (see also chapter 2.1.6 describing the forward problem in more detail). When, however, the electrical activation time $\tau$ (i.e., the time instant, when the depolarization of the action potential takes place) is of interest, Equation (5) still can be used as the biophysical problem description with a mathematical additional function $\varphi_m(t) = \mathrm{f}(\tau)$ relating the transmembrane potential's shape to the activation time.

**2.1.3 Relation of the transmembrane potential $\varphi_m$ with the (extracellular) potential $\varphi$**

The general MAXWELL'S EQUATIONS in differential form are:

$$
\begin{aligned}
&\mathrm{div}(\boldsymbol{D}) = \varrho && \text{Coulomb's law} \\
&\mathrm{rot}(\boldsymbol{H}) = \boldsymbol{j} + \tfrac{\partial \boldsymbol{D}}{\partial t} && \text{Ampere's law} \\
&\mathrm{rot}(\boldsymbol{E}) = -\tfrac{\partial \boldsymbol{B}}{\partial t} && \text{Faraday's law} \\
&\mathrm{div}(\boldsymbol{B}) = 0 && \text{Absence of magnetic monopoles,}
\end{aligned}
\tag{6}
$$

with $\boldsymbol{D}$ describing the electrical displacement, $\boldsymbol{H}$ the magnetic field, $\boldsymbol{E}$ the electrical field, $\varrho$ the electrical charge volume density and $\boldsymbol{j}$ the current surface density. The relations between $\boldsymbol{E}$, $\boldsymbol{D}$ and $\boldsymbol{H}$, $\boldsymbol{B}$ are given by

$$\boldsymbol{D} = \varepsilon \boldsymbol{E} + \boldsymbol{P} \tag{7}$$

$$\boldsymbol{B} = \mu(\boldsymbol{H} + \boldsymbol{M}), \tag{8}$$

where $\boldsymbol{P}$ describes electrical polarization, $\boldsymbol{M}$ magnetization, $\varepsilon = \varepsilon_r \varepsilon_0$ is the electric permittivity, $\mu = \mu_r \mu_0$ is the magnetic permeability. Subscript "$r$" indicates the relative (matter depending), index "0" the value for the permeability and permittivity of the free space. Finally, with the sum

$$\boldsymbol{j} = \boldsymbol{j}^{(\mathrm{imp})} + \boldsymbol{j}^{(\mathrm{ind})} \tag{9}$$

($\boldsymbol{j}^{(\mathrm{imp})}$ is the vector holding impressed or active currents; $\boldsymbol{j}^{(\mathrm{ind})}$ describes the induced or passive current density) we gain the whole set of equations describing the behavior of electromagnetic fields in matter in the most general form. Equation

$$\boldsymbol{j}^{(\mathrm{ind})} = \boldsymbol{\kappa} \boldsymbol{E} \tag{10}$$

is also termed OHM'S LAW and allows computation of the induced current density applying the electric conductivity tensor $\boldsymbol{\kappa}$.

The following assumptions about modeling electrical function of biological tissue are made:

- Electrical field strengths are not too high $\Rightarrow$ biological tissue is assumed to behave linear with regard to its electrical properties.
- Capacitive as well as inductive effects can be neglected $\Rightarrow$ biological tissue can be described to be purely resistive.
- Due to low frequency components reflecting cardiac electrical activity ($\leqslant$ several kHz) temporal derivatives of Equation (6) can be neglected (quasi-static approximation of Maxwell's equations).

The discussion and justification for the assumptions can be found in, e.g, Geselowitz D. B. (1967); Gulrajani R. M. & Mailloux G. E. (1983); Malmivuo J. & Plonsey R. (1995); Roth B. J. (1991). Applying these assumptions, consequently MAXWELL'S EQUATIONS lead to

$$\operatorname{div}(\boldsymbol{D}) = \varrho \tag{11}$$
$$\operatorname{rot}(\boldsymbol{H}) = \boldsymbol{j} \Rightarrow \operatorname{div}(\boldsymbol{j}) = \operatorname{div}[\operatorname{rot}(\boldsymbol{H})] = 0 \tag{12}$$
$$\operatorname{rot}(\boldsymbol{E}) = 0 \Leftrightarrow \boldsymbol{E} = -\operatorname{grad}(\varphi) \tag{13}$$
$$\operatorname{div}(\boldsymbol{B}) = 0. \tag{14}$$

Consequently, employing (10), Equation (9) can be rewritten as

$$\boldsymbol{j} = \boldsymbol{j}^{(\mathrm{imp})} - \boldsymbol{\kappa}\operatorname{grad}(\varphi) \text{ and with} \tag{15}$$
$$\operatorname{div}(\boldsymbol{j}) = 0 \tag{16}$$

the fundamental equation for biological tissue (with the constraints mentioned above) can be derived:

$$\operatorname{div}[\boldsymbol{\kappa}\operatorname{grad}(\varphi)] = \operatorname{div}(\boldsymbol{j}^{(imp)}). \tag{17}$$

For the special case, that the conductivity $\boldsymbol{\kappa}$ is assumed to be isotropic only, Equation (17) reduces to POISSON'S EQUATION

$$\kappa\Delta(\varphi) = \operatorname{div}(\boldsymbol{j}^{(imp)}), \tag{18}$$

for source-holding domains (i.e., electrically active regions like the heart), whereas for regions having passive properties only (source-free domains), which is reflected by a homogeneous term on the right hand side of Equation (17) leading to LAPLACE'S EQUATION

$$\kappa\Delta(\varphi) = 0. \tag{19}$$

Comparing Equation (17) with (5)

$$\begin{aligned} \operatorname{div}[\boldsymbol{\kappa}\operatorname{grad}(\varphi)] &= \operatorname{div}(\boldsymbol{j}^{(imp)}) \quad \text{with} \\ \operatorname{div}[\boldsymbol{\kappa}_B\operatorname{grad}(\varphi_{extra})] &= -\operatorname{div}[\boldsymbol{\sigma}_{intra}\operatorname{grad}(\varphi_m)] \end{aligned} \tag{20}$$

the following relations of the values between the Maxwell's equations based and the bidomain based derivation can be identified: i) $\boldsymbol{\kappa}_B \leftrightarrow \boldsymbol{\kappa}$, ii) $\varphi_{extra} \leftrightarrow \varphi$, and iii) $-\boldsymbol{\sigma}_{intra}\operatorname{grad}(\varphi_m) \leftrightarrow \boldsymbol{j}^{(imp)}$.

Due to i) the bulk conductivity $\boldsymbol{\kappa}_B = \boldsymbol{\sigma}_{intra} + \boldsymbol{\sigma}_{extra}$ and due to ii) the extracellular potentials $\varphi_{extra}$ can be interpreted as the passive electrical part, relation iii) reflects the fact, that the impressed currents are due to the intracellular conductivity multiplied by the negative gradient of the transmembrane voltages $\boldsymbol{j}^{(imp)} = -\boldsymbol{\sigma}_{intra}\operatorname{grad}(\varphi_m)$ reflecting the active electrical properties (responsible for generating the action potential in this modelling approach) of the heart.

As a consequence, the extracellular potentials $\varphi_{extra}$ on the boundary surfaces of the heart are potentials $\varphi$, which could be measured, e.g., on the endo- or epicardia by intracardiac electrodes. In the following the cardiac extracellular potentials will be denoted by $\varphi$, the intracellular conductivity tensor by $\boldsymbol{\sigma}_{in}$.

### 2.1.4 The boundary value problem

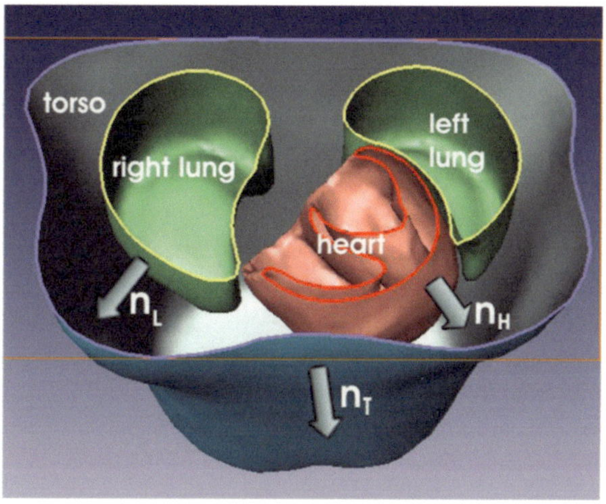


Fig. 2. Cutting plane through the volume conductor model of a patient in antero-oblique view displaying the corresponding boundary surfaces. Vectors $\boldsymbol{n}_{\mathrm{H}}$, $\boldsymbol{n}_{\mathrm{L}}$ and $\boldsymbol{n}_{\mathrm{T}}$ indicate the normal vectors of the related compartment perpendicular to the enclosed volume.

In order to be able to describe bioelectromagnetic phenomena within the human body, all relevant compartments of the volume conductor model (VCM) have to be taken into account. The volume conductor model is a representation of the patient individual geometry comprising the electrically most relevant compartments, which distinguish themselves by their different electrical properties, such as the electrical conductivity (Geselowitz D. B., 1967; Gulrajani R. M. & Mailloux G. E., 1983; Klepfer R. N. et al., 1997; Malmivuo J. & Plonsey R., 1995; Pullan A. J. et al., 2001): heart, bloodmasses within the heart's cavities, left and right lung, and torso. In Fig. 2 a schematic illustration of the boundaries of a volume conductor model is given. The equations

$$\mathrm{div}[\boldsymbol{\sigma}_{bm}\mathrm{grad}(\varphi_{bm})] = 0, \tag{21}$$
$$\mathrm{div}[\boldsymbol{\sigma}_{L}\mathrm{grad}(\varphi_{L})] = 0, \text{ and} \tag{22}$$
$$\mathrm{div}[\boldsymbol{\sigma}_{T}\mathrm{grad}(\varphi_{T})] = 0 \tag{23}$$

form together with Eqation (5) the set of differential equations describing the electrical behavior of each compartment of the volume conductor model, i.e., heart, bloodmasses (abbreviation: *bm*; conductivity $\boldsymbol{\sigma}_{bm}$; not shown in Fig. 2), lungs (*L*; conductivity $\boldsymbol{\sigma}_{L}$), and torso (*T*; conductivity $\boldsymbol{\sigma}_{T}$). Note, that the right hand side of each equation (Eqations (21)–(23)) is 0, as these compartments own electrical passive properties only, hence the impressed current density vanishes.

In order to describe electrical behavior of the whole volume conductor model, boundary conditions have to be taken into account linking the – so far – separate compartments mathematically together. The following boundary conditions hold on the adjoining compartments' interfaces (termed 1 and 2):

- continuity of the potentials (consequence of Eqation 13)

$$\varphi_1 = \varphi_2 \text{ on intersection of compartments,} \tag{24}$$

  and

- continuity of the current densities perpendicular to the adjoining compartments' interfaces (except torso–outside; consequence of charge conservation):

$$\begin{aligned} \boldsymbol{\sigma}_1 \text{grad}(\varphi_1) \cdot \boldsymbol{n}_1 &= -\boldsymbol{\sigma}_2 \text{grad}(\varphi_2) \cdot \boldsymbol{n}_2 \text{ with} \\ \boldsymbol{n}_1 \cdot \boldsymbol{n}_2 &= -1. \end{aligned} \tag{25}$$

Equation (24) is also referred to as DIRICHLET – the potential is defined – Eqation (25) as NEUMANN BOUNDARY CONDITION, where the gradient of the potential is defined. As the outer surface of the torso is surrounded by air (electrical conductivity $\boldsymbol{\sigma}_{outside} = 0$) the related NEUMANN BOUNDARY CONDITION leads to

$$\boldsymbol{\sigma}_T \text{grad}(\varphi_T) \cdot \boldsymbol{n}_T = 0. \tag{26}$$

For a definite solution of the sought potentials, also a DIRICHLET'S BOUNDARY CONDITION on the torso's surface has to be formulated, as (26) defines only the gradient of the potential. It is advantageous to consider the Wilson central terminal (WCT) for a DIRICHLET'S CONDITION, which in clinical practice defines the zero potential, i.e., the sum of potentials of the right arm (RA), left arm (LA) and left leg (LL) (Fischer G. et al., 2002):

$$\varphi_{RA} + \varphi_{LA} + \varphi_{LL} = 0. \tag{27}$$

### 2.1.5 Solving the boundary value problem

For solving the sets of Eqation (5)–(23) considering the boundary conditions (24)–(27) to an individual torso geometry, numerical approaches have to be employed. Several numerical methods can be applied, like, e.g., the finite difference, the finite volume, the boundary element (BEM) or the finite element method (FEM). It depends mainly on the intended application, the computational power available and on the basic modeling strategy, which type of numerical solving technique should be used.

In case, that the electrical conductivities of all compartments are modeled to be homogeneous and isotropic, the BEM is the first choice. This approach needs the boundary value problem stated above to be defined in integral from. It has, however, the advantage that only boundary surfaces enclosing a volume of homogeneous isotropic conductivity have to be approximated by, e.g., triangles, whereas using the FEM the whole volume has to be approximated by suitable elements (e.g., tetrahedral elements).

In general and independent from the applied numerical method the equations are transformed into a set of linear algebraic equations by discretization of all compartments of the volume conductor model (e.g., (Fischer G. et al., 2000; Seger M. et al., 2005)). Without loss of generality the related matrix equation is shown here employing the FEM for the case of tetrahedral elements used for discretization:

$$\boldsymbol{R}\boldsymbol{\Phi} = \boldsymbol{S}\boldsymbol{\Phi}_{\boldsymbol{m}}. \tag{28}$$

Matrix $\boldsymbol{R}$ is the $(m \times m)$ *left stiffness matrix* ($m$ is the number of tetrahedral nodes of the whole volume) reflecting the properties of the passive compartments, $\boldsymbol{S}$ is the $(m \times s)$ *right stiffness matrix* ($s$ is the number of source nodes), but only a $(s \times s)$ submatrix reflects the active properties of the cardiac tissue (electrically active region) as stated by (5). The passive compartments, (electrical behavior described by Equations (21) – (23)) are represented by zero-entries in $m - s$ rows of $\boldsymbol{S}$. The stiffness matrices are – in case FEM is applied – *symmetric, positive semi-definite* and *sparse*, which allows to store only the non-zero entries of the matrices and thus optimizing utilization of computer memory (Press W. H. et al., 2002). The $(m \times t)$ matrix $\boldsymbol{\Phi}$ holds the potentials in all nodes for $t$ time steps, $\boldsymbol{\Phi}_{\boldsymbol{m}}$ is a $(s \times t)$ matrix consisting of the transmembrane potentials in each (cardiac) source node.

The Wilson central terminal in (27) can be considered by assembling a *terminal-element-matrix* to the global stiffness matrix $\boldsymbol{R}$ employing the potential definition vector $\boldsymbol{w}$ (Fischer G. et al., 2002):

$$\boldsymbol{w}^T\boldsymbol{\Phi} = 0, \qquad \tilde{\boldsymbol{R}} = \boldsymbol{R} + \omega \boldsymbol{w}\boldsymbol{w}^T, \quad \omega > 0. \tag{29}$$

Vector $\boldsymbol{w}$ – the interpolation vector of the torso's surface nodes nearest located to the Wilson terminal electrodes – is *sparse*, as at most three entries (in case of tetrahedral elements) differ from zero. A suitable choice for the positive weighting factor $\omega$ is achieved by taking the corresponding pivot elements of $\boldsymbol{R}$ in order to guarantee that entries of $\tilde{\boldsymbol{R}}$ are in the same order of magnitude as $\boldsymbol{R}$. Thus the properties of $\tilde{\boldsymbol{R}}$, i.e., symmetry and sparseness, are conserved. After this manipulation the *positive definite* matrix $\tilde{\boldsymbol{R}}$, can be inverted, yielding for the node potentials of the volume conductor model:

$$\boldsymbol{\Phi} = \tilde{\boldsymbol{R}}^{-1}\boldsymbol{S}\boldsymbol{\Phi}_{\boldsymbol{m}}, \tag{30}$$

with $\tilde{\boldsymbol{R}}^{-1}\boldsymbol{S}$ representing the *node field matrix*. Introducing the *interpolation matrix* $\boldsymbol{N}$, which relates the $e$ electrode potentials $\boldsymbol{\Phi}_e$ $(e \times t)$ to all node potentials

$$\boldsymbol{\Phi}_e = \boldsymbol{N}\boldsymbol{\Phi} \implies \boldsymbol{\Phi}_e = \boldsymbol{N}\tilde{\boldsymbol{R}}^{-1}\boldsymbol{S}\boldsymbol{\Phi}_{\boldsymbol{m}}, \tag{31}$$

the *lead field matrix* (or also termed *transfer matrix*) $\boldsymbol{L}$ can be written as

$$\boldsymbol{L} = \boldsymbol{N}\tilde{\boldsymbol{R}}^{-1}\boldsymbol{S}. \tag{32}$$

In case the BEM is applied the discrete formulation, when applying, e.g., linear triangular elements for approximation of the boundary surfaces, the following matrix equation is gained:

$$\boldsymbol{H}\boldsymbol{\Phi} = \boldsymbol{\Phi}_m, \tag{33}$$

where $\boldsymbol{H}$ $(h \times n)$ represents the so-called *double layer matrix*, matrix $\boldsymbol{\Phi}$ $(n \times t)$ contains the potentials in all $n$ boundary surface nodes of the mesh for $t$ time steps and $\boldsymbol{\Phi}_m$ $(h \times t)$ holds the transmembrane potentials in all $h$ source nodes for $t$ time steps. In contrast to the left stiffness matrix $\boldsymbol{R}$, which occurs in the finite element method, matrix $\boldsymbol{H}$ is dense and rectangular. It is, however, also singular, which is due to the fact, that the potentials on the boundary surfaces of the torso are only determined by NEUMANN'S BOUNDARY CONDITION. Thus, similar to the FEM, a DIRICHLET'S BOUNDARY CONDITION has to be integrated in the double layer matrix $\boldsymbol{H}$. This is done by including a zero-potential definition vector (determined by, e.g., the electrodes comprising the *Wilson-central-terminal*), which is described in detail in (Fischer G. et al., 2002). After this manipulation, matrix $\tilde{\boldsymbol{H}}$ can be inverted employing standard matrix inversion techniques, like, e.g., the Gaussian elimination method, yielding for the potentials $\boldsymbol{\Phi}$ in all nodes of the conductivity interfaces, especially on the torso surface:

$$\boldsymbol{\Phi} = \tilde{\boldsymbol{H}}^{-1}\boldsymbol{\Phi}_m. \quad (34)$$

The computation of the potentials in $e$ electrodes $\boldsymbol{\Phi}_e$ is performed in a similar way as applying the FEM:

$$\boldsymbol{\Phi}_e = \boldsymbol{N}\tilde{\boldsymbol{H}}^{-1}\boldsymbol{\Phi}_m, \quad (35)$$

where the interpolation matrix $\boldsymbol{N}$ $(e \times n)$ relates each location of the electrodes to the corresponding nearest boundary surface nodes, and $\boldsymbol{N}\tilde{\boldsymbol{H}}^{-1} = \boldsymbol{L}$ represents the *lead field matrix* computed employing the BEM.

### 2.1.6 Forward and inverse problem of electrocardiography

The framework elaborated so far can now be employed for two fields:

- the forward (or direct) problem of electrocardiography and
- the inverse problem of electrocardiography.

The forward problem in this context means, that the effect is to be computed which is due to a known cause, in the inverse problem the effect is known and one is seeking for the cause responsible for this effect. In either case a mathematical model based description has to be developed to be able to link effect and cause.

#### 2.1.6.1 Forward problem

For the forward problem this description is the lead field matrix $\boldsymbol{L}$, which represents the mathematical relationship between the electrical cardiac sources $\boldsymbol{\Phi}_{\text{source}}$, e.g., the transmembrane potentials, and the effect $\boldsymbol{\Phi}_{\text{effect}}$, e.g., the potentials measured by the electrodes:

$$\boldsymbol{\Phi}_{\text{effect}} = \boldsymbol{L}\boldsymbol{\Phi}_{\text{source}}. \quad (36)$$

Thus – when the sources are assumed to be the transmembrane potentials – solving the forward problem of electrocardiography is possible for individual heart, lungs and torso geometries (computation of the lead field matrix by means of the above described methods) when also the spatio-temporal distribution of the transmembrane potentials is known. The transmembrane potential distribution can be computed by, e.g., a cellular automaton taking various properties depending on different cardiac tissue types into account (Barbosa C. R. H., 2003; He B. et al., 2002; Modre R. et al., 2006).

Apart from the transmembrane potential source formulation, other electrical cardiac source formulations are employed: the so-called epicardial potential (more precisely: pericardial) (Greensite F. & Huiskamp G., 1998; Ramanathan C. et al., 2004). In the epicardial potential formulation the potentials on the heart surface (i.e., on the epicardial surface only) are modeled to be electrical sources, which means, that – with respect to the bidomain theory – only extracellular potentials have to be taken into account for solving the forward problem. This formulation can be extended geometrically to the whole heart surface formulation, where not only the epicardial but also the endocardial extracellular potential distribution is modeled as electrical cardiac source. The major problem, however, employing these two latter methods in the forward modeling is the fact, that computing the potentials on the body surface requires knowledge of the potential distribution on the heart surfaces, which cannot directly be linked to the cardiac action potentials. Therefore, most commonly current dipoles are used in order to represent cardiac electrical activation.

2.1.6.2 Inverse problem

The computation of an underlying source leading to an observed and measured effect requires the knowledge of the relationship between source and effect and available data representing the effect. The mathematical relationship is established by the lead field matrix $\boldsymbol{L}$, the measured data reflecting the effect is represented by the matrix $\boldsymbol{\Phi}_{\text{effect}}$ in (36). It is, however, not straightforward to compute the sources by simply inverting the lead field matrix $\boldsymbol{L}$ in (36). This is due to the fact that the inverse problem of electrocardiography is ill posed, which means, that at least one of the following conditions (HADAMARD'S DEFINITION of well posedness) is broken:

- for all admissible (source) data a solution exists,
- for all admissible (source) data the solution is unique and
- the solution depends continuously on the (source) data.

In case of the inverse electrocardiographic problem at least the two last criteria are not fulfilled. Thus, in general, the inverse solution is neither unique nor continuously depending on the data. Therefore methods have to be applied which deliver a reasonable source distribution $\boldsymbol{\Phi}_{\text{source}}$, like, e.g., *regularization techniques*. Regularizing means in this context to impose constraints onto the electrical sources in question and thus to confine the solution space. The effect in terms of computing the cardiac activation sequence is, that only physiologically meaningful epi- and endocardial breakthroughs are allowed to occur (spatial regularization). The regularization is controlled by a regularization parameter, which has to be determined in order to achieve an optimal distribution of the cardiac sources.

An even stricter confinement of the solution space can be achieved by incorporating a-priori information about essential physiological properties of the transmembrane potential (temporal regularization). In the following, only one inverse approach is described in more detail as this method is the one used in NICE. It is not intended to reflect the entire spectrum of inverse algorithms employed in the field of electrophysiology, as this is far beyond the focus of this chapter. A detailed elaboration about inverse problems in general can be found, e.g., in (Engl H. W. et al., 1996).

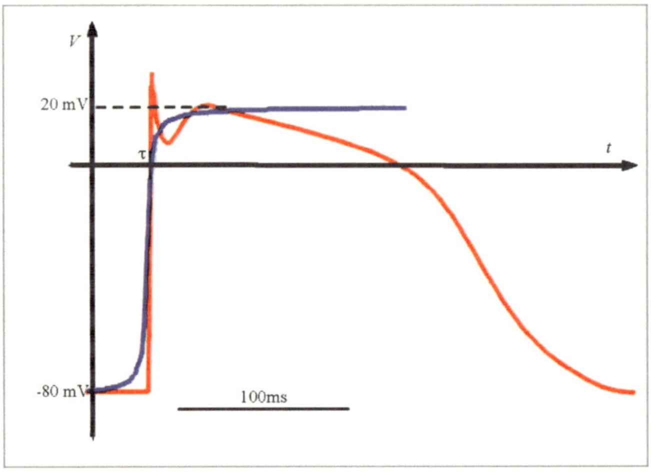


Fig. 3. Measured action potential (red) of a ventricular myocyte (mid-myocardial cell) and the corresponding time course of an approximated one (blue) employing Equation (37). Parameter $\tau$ represents the related activation time.

Activation time imaging – Noninvasive imaging of cardiac electrical function – NICE

The transmembrane potential's shape is described by an arctan-like-function (see Fig. 3). The transmembrane potential denoted by $\varphi_m$ can be approximated by

$$\varphi_m(\tau, t) = \frac{u}{2}\left\{1 + \frac{2}{\pi}\mathrm{atan}\left[\pi\frac{t-\tau}{w}\right]\right\} + a, \qquad (37)$$

where $\varphi_m(\tau, t)$ is computed at each source point on the cardiac surface with the parameters resting membrane potential $a$ (a value of $= 0.09$ V has been used in our computations), action potential amplitude $u$ ($= 0.1$ V), rise time $w$ ($= 2 \cdot 10^{-3}$ s) and activation time $\tau$. Equation (37) is an approximation of the time course of the action potential, but it has the advantage, that the number of parameters to be determined in the inverse computation is reduced to only one: the activation time.

The functional to be minimized with respect to $\tau$ is (Modre R. et al., 2001; 2002)

$$\|\boldsymbol{L}\Phi_m - \boldsymbol{D}\|_F^2 + \lambda^2\|\Delta\tau\|_2^2 \longrightarrow \text{min.} \qquad (38)$$

The *surface Laplacian* $\Delta$ (Huiskamp G. J., 1991) in (38) represents the regularization term and is introduced in order to avoid an unphysiological activation pattern by smoothing the solution of the activation time map. Parameter $\lambda$ determines the amount of regularization and is calculated employing the L-curve method (Hansen P. C., 2001), weighting the residual norm on the left hand side of (38) against the spatial regularization term leading to an L-shaped curve. The optimal solution is said to be found, when the curve exposes the corner of the L-shape. As the relationship between matrix $\boldsymbol{D}$ with the dimensions (number of electrodes $\times$ depolarization time instants) contains the measured ECG data in the electrodes and $\|\cdot\|_F$ represents the FROBENIUS' NORM. activation time and transmembrane potential is non-linear, the resulting problem to be solved is an ill-posed, non-linear, inverse problem and requires, e.g., a quasi-Newton-method to be properly solved. As a starting vector for the solution to be searched for the result of the *critical point theorem* is employed (Huiskamp G. & Greensite F., 1997).

The numerical solution was based on the Boundary Element Method with the chosen electrical (isotropic) conductivity values for each compartment:

- heart:
  - effective intracellular conductivity: 0.1 $Sm^{-1}$
  - bulk conductivity: 0.2 $Sm^{-1}$ (i.e. the sum of effective intra- and extracellular conductivity according to the bidomain model)
- lungs: 0.08 $Sm^{-1}$
- cavitary blood masses: 0.6 $Sm^{-1}$
- chest: 0.2 $Sm^{-1}$

The non-linear problem can be solved by a sequence of linearised ill-posed problems(Modre R. et al., 2001).

A computationally optimized and slightly different approach for solving the inverse problem in terms of computing the cardiac activation times can be found in (Fischer G., Pfeifer B., Seger M., Hintermüller C., Hanser F., Modre R., Tilg B., Trieb T., Kremser C., Roithinger F. X. & Hintringer F., 2005). The major differences are, that a sigmoidal function as template function for the transmembrane potential is applied and the regularization strategy for finding the optimal inverse solution is not based on the L-curve method but on starting with a high value for the regularization parameter $\lambda$, and successively using the resulting activation time map for the next iterative computation with a reduced value of $\lambda$. This procedure is repeated until $\lambda$ is set to zero in the last step and the final computed activation time map is regarded as the solution to the ill-posed inverse problem.

### 2.2 Clinical background

In clinical routine the diagnosis of cardiac arrhythmias, infarction or related disorders is based on the standard 12-lead ECG. The interpretation of the standard ECG by the cardiologist allows in general to obtain a clinical diagnosis using a rough measure of the heart's electrophysiological properties. The surface ECG lacks precise geometrical information of the underlying spatiotemporal electroanatomical substrate. If a more accurate or detailed information about the electroanatomical activation of the heart can be obtained (e.g., the localization of an accessory pathway situated on the ventricles' basis) a more detailed or appropriate procedure can be applied. Up to date, this information can be obtained by an invasive procedure with a catheter and – in most of the cases – an electro-anatomic mapping system (e.g., CARTO™ (Biosense Webster, Inc.)) in an electrophysiology laboratory, which is, however, linked to some risks for the patient due to the intervention. Therefore, it would be favourable to determine relevant cardiac electrophysiological parameters in a fully noninvasive fashion.

A relevant parameter for diagnosis of cardiac arrhythmias is the cardiac activation time. A cardiac activation time map on the epi-, endo- and myocardium enables to, e.g.,

- determine of the origin of cardiac focal events (e.g., atrial and ventricular ectopies, accessory pathways),
- localize scar tissue (e.g, ischemic heart disease)
- determine macroreentry based tachycardias (e.g., atrial flutter)
- discover the starting point and/or rotor evolution of atrial fibrillation,
- plan interventional procedures (electrophysiology study (EPS), pacemaker or implantable cardioverter defibrillator (ICD) implantatations, cardiac resynchronization therapy (CRT)).

An additional benefit of NICE is the fact that it does not rely on stable arrhythmias. NICE allows single-beat calculation of electroanatomical activation of the heart. This is, for several reasons, of special clinical interest as many arrhythmias do not show stable activation patterns.

The activation time map represents the spatio-temporal spread of electrical excitation (i.e., the progression of the action potential's depolarization phase) for epi/endocardial as well as for midmyocardial tissue and has the property to offer detailed information with sufficient geometrical accuracy for further diagnostic and therapeutical interventions.

### 2.3 NICE – Workflow definition – technical background

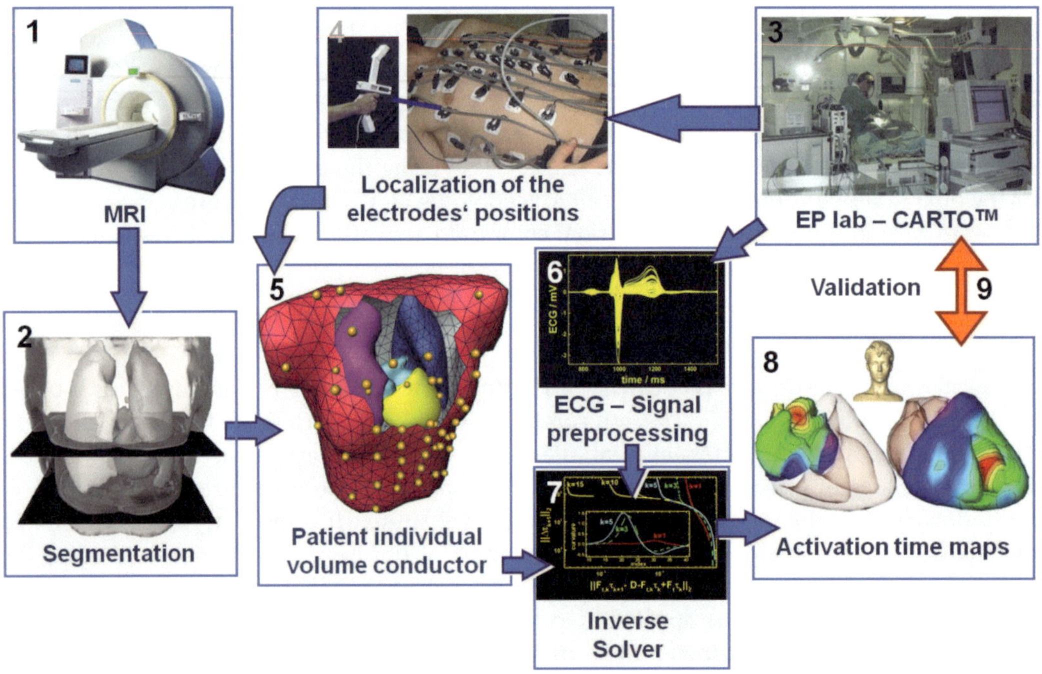


Fig. 4. The workflow scetch as applied for NICE during the validation studies performed in the electrophysiology lab. The sequences are indicated by numbers 1 – 9. For a detailed description of the workflow please refer to the text.

The workflow which was applied for the clinical validation studies (see also section 3.1) is depicted in Fig. 4. The workflow for the results given in section 3.2 and 3.3 (cardiac resynchronization therapy) is shown in Fig. 4. For all studies presented in this chapter written informed consent of the patients was acquired. All studies were approved by the local ethics committee.

### 2.3.1 Magnetic resonance imaging, segmentation and the patient individual volume conductor model (steps 1, 2 and 5 in Fig. 4)

For generation of the patient individual volume conductor model the anatomy of the patient has to be acquired.

To create a volume conductor model in order to estimate the electrical spread in the human heart, those compartments need to be considered, which show to have a major influence on the bioelectrical properties (Bradley C. et al., 2000). With respect to NICE these compartments are:

- chest (medium electrical conductivity, surface electrodes),
- lungs (low electrical conductivity, filled with air),
- atrial and ventricular blood masses (high electrical conductivity),
- atrial and ventricular myocardium (medium electrical conductivity, electrical sources).

The image acquisition was performed by MRI using a Magnetom-Vision-Plus 1.5 T (Siemens Medical Solutions) scanner. The atrial and ventricular geometry was recorded in CINE-mode during breath-hold (expiration, short-axis scans, 4 – 6 mm spacing). The shapes of the lungs and the torso were recorded in T1-Flash-mode during breath-hold (expiration, long-axis scans, 10 mm spacing).

For localization and coupling of the mapping electrodes vitamin E capsules were used. These markers are clearly visible within the MRI images and can therefore be easily identified. Seven markers (anatomical landmarks on the anterior and lateral chest wall) were used to couple the locations of the electrodes to the MRI frame. Eleven capsules were attached on the back, in order to tag the positions of the posterior electrodes, which were not accessible during the electrophysiology study. A volume conductor model with electrode positions visualized by spheres is depicted in Fig. 5. The next step was the volume conductor modeling task using two volume data sets. The short-axis data was used for modeling intracardiac blood masses, the ventricles' myocardium and the atria. The axial data set was used for modeling the lungs and chest surface.

Due to the variety of the different compartments the volume conductor model requires different compartment-specific approaches as there is no uniform segmentation approach capable of extracting different compartments (Pfeifer B. et al., 2005; 2008; 2006; 2007). Furthermore, there are two pre-processed data sets (short-axis scan and axial scan) to handle this modeling task.

To meet these requirements, the Medical Segmentation Toolkit (MST) was developed (Pfeifer B. et al., 2005; 2008; 2006). The Medical Segmentation Toolkit enables an easy integration of a variety of state-of-the-art frameworks and segmentation methods. The framework facilitates the development of segmentation pipelines to extract different compartments semiautomatically after initial parameter settings. After extraction the compartments were coupled together to the volume conductor model. This modeling part

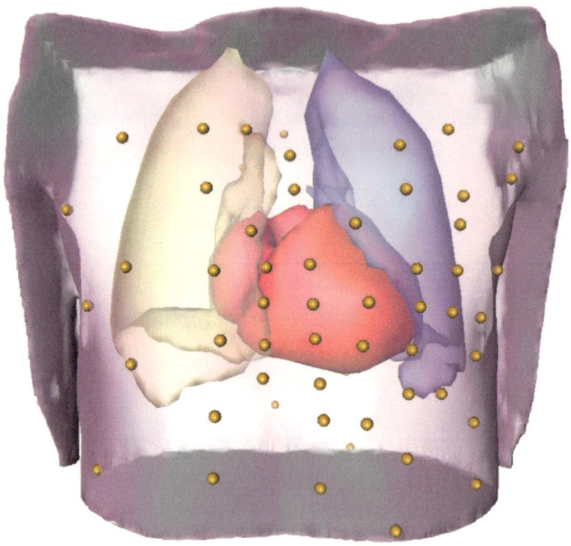

Fig. 5. Volume conductor model generated from 3-D cine MRI data with two axial MR scans with overlaid electrode positions (yellow spheres) in an anterior-posterior view. The thorax and the left (blue) and right (yellow) lungs are displayed in transparent style. Parts of the atria (velvet) are hidden by the ventricles (red).

needed to be done in a short time period because the time between the MRI procedure and the catheter intervention was normally limited by two hours. In clinical routine this time interval should be as short as possible to allow "online" data acquisition (i.e., computation of the cardiac electrical activation times directly at the catheter laboratory) (Seger M. et al., 2004).

### 2.3.2 Electrophysiology lab, localization of electrode position (steps 3, 4 and 6 in Fig. 4)

The Mark-8 body surface potential mapping system (Biosemi V. O. F.) is an online portable computer acquisition system with data transmission by optical fibre (SippensGroenewegen A. et al., 1998; Tilg B., Hanser F., Modre-Osprian R., Fischer G., Messnarz B., Berger T., Hintringer F., Pachinger O. & Roithinger F. X., 2002). Electrode signals are amplified and AD converted with a 16-bit converter at a sample rate of 2,048 Hz per channel. A radiotransparent carbon electrode array (University of Amsterdam, The Netherlands) was used to record unipolar ECG data from 62 torso sites (anterior chest: 41; posterior chest: 21). The Wilson central terminal defined the reference potential. The positions of the anterior and lateral electrodes and of the seven anterior reference (sternum, left and right rib cage) landmarks were digitized employing the FASTRAK® digitizing system (Polhemus, Inc.). The same seven markers were also digitized with the CARTO™ system, providing coordinate transformation of the invasively obtained data to the MRI frame. The derived ECG signals were then pre-filtered , baseline corrected and the necessary portions of the ECGs (i. e., P-wave for reconstruction of atrial, QRS-complex for reconstruction of ventricular activation times) were extracted employing a self developed software framework implemented in MATLAB® (The MathWorks, Inc.) based on the investigation of the root mean square (RMS) of all non-corrupted channels of the recorded ECG signals (Berger T. et al., 2006; 2011). Channels were excluded if their signal to noise ratio was low or when electrodes could not be attached to the patient's chest due to medical reasons (e.g., electrode's position at the implant site of the pacemaker).

#### 2.3.3 Computation of the activation time imaging map and validation (steps 7, 8 and 9 in Fig. 4)

Cardiac activation time maps were computed employing inverse solvers (Fischer G., Hanser F., Pfeifer B., Seger M., Hintermüller C., Modre R., Tilg B., Trieb T., Berger T., Roithinger F. X. & Hintringer F., 2005; Modre R. et al., 2001). Electrically isotropic conductivities were assumed for all compartments of the volume conductor model (therefore the boundary element method was applied for computing the lead field matrix). According to previous data (Modre R. et al., 2006) this is a justified assumption also for the cardiac intra- and extracellular conductivities having neglectable influence on the solution of the inverse problem for determining cardiac activation times.

For example, NICE allows the cardiologist to localize the insertion site of an accessory pathway prior to invasive intervention (e.g., Wolff-Parkinson-White (WPW) Syndrome) (Berger T. et al., 2006; Modre R. et al., 2001; 2002; Tilg B., Fischer G., Modre R., Hanser F., Messnarz B., Schocke M., Kremser C., Berger T., Hintringer F. & Roithinger F. X., 2002). Using radiofrequency ablation the insertion site of the accessory pathway was disconnected (Morady F., 1999). After this, the successful ablation site within the CARTO™ map was used for validation of the NICE derived insertion site of the accessory pathway (Berger T. et al., 2006).

## 3. Results

NICE enables the visualization of atrial and ventricular electroanatomical activation (Berger T. et al., 2006; Modre R. et al., 2003). NICE was validated by comparing the electroanatomic activation sequences with data obtained by invasive electroanatomical mapping (CARTO™ ). Thus, a quantitative estimation of the mean localization error of NICE was performed. The corresponding findings are shown in the first part of the results' section. Assessment of cardiac resynchronization therapy has been the second major focus of future applications of NICE in clinical electrophysiology and will be described in the second part of the results' section. In the third part first preleminary results of the activation time map of a newly developed pacemaker device are presented.

### 3.1 Electrophysiology laboratory – validation of NICE

Modre et al. (Modre R. et al., 2003) tested the hypothesis that human atrial activation time imaging is feasible with sufficient spatial and temporal resolution. For the first time, noninvasive atrial activation time imaging was performed in a clinical environment and validated with electroanatomic mapping, invasively localized pacing sites, and pacing at anatomic markers (e.g., pulmonary veins). One example of the results of this study is given in Fig. 6 for activation time imaging of sinus rhythm and in Fig. 7 showing the activation time map for pacing within the right atrial appendage. The activation time map on the

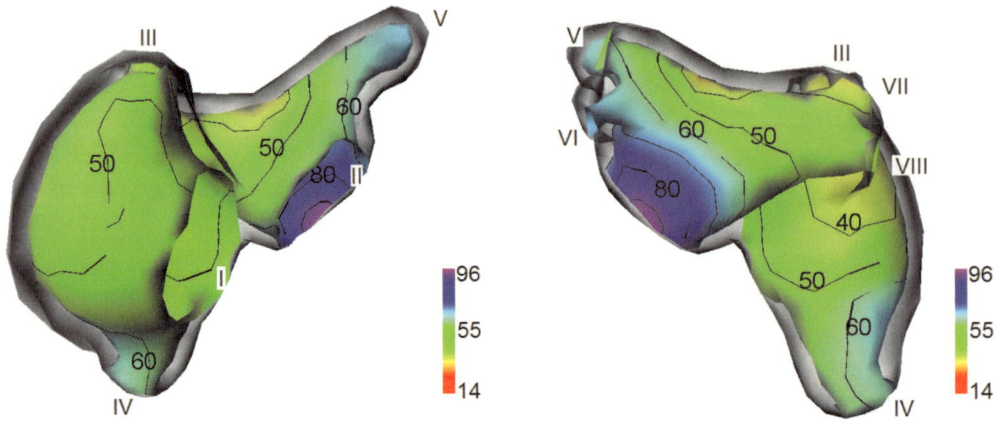


Fig. 6. Atrial endocardial activation time map for sinus rhythm. The isochrones (given in ms) are displayed in intervals of 10 ms, the numbers at the color maps represent ms. Left panel displays the atria in a anterior-posterior, right panel in a posterior-anterior view. The epicardia are displayed in transparent style. Roman numbers indicating anatomical locations of: I. . . tricuspid annulus; II. . . mitral annulus; III. . . vena cava superior; IV. . . vena cava inferior; V. . . left upper pulmonary vein; VI. . . left lower pulmonary vein; VII. . . right upper pulmonary vein; VIII. . . right lower pulmonary vein.

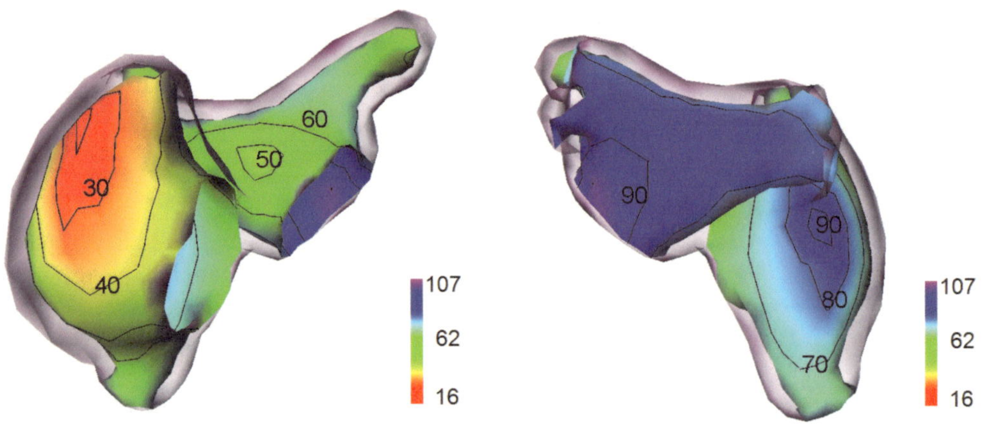


Fig. 7. Atrial endocardial activation time map for pacing in the right atrial appendage. The isochrones (given in ms) are displayed in intervals of 10 ms, the numbers at the color maps represent ms. Left panel displays the atria in a anterior-posterior, right panel in a posterior-anterior view. The epicardia are displayed in transparent style.

endocardium for pacing within the right atrial appendage of the right atrium shows one breakthrough point at the high right atrium close to the breakthrough point on the epicardium at 20 msec. In the right atrium, activation propagated from the high right atrium to the inferior vena cava and the superior vena cava. Finally, the posterior wall of the right atrium was activated 90 msec after pacing. Depolarization ofthe left atrium started 50 msec after the pacing spike. The latest activation of the atria was found at the posterior wall of the left atrium near the mitral annulus 100 msec after pacing. The individual complex anatomic model of the atria of each patient in combination with high-quality mesh optimization and precise data coupling enabled accurate activation time imaging, resulting in a localization error for the estimated pacing sites of 10 mm in the worst case. (Modre R. et al., 2003)

The aim of the study by Berger et al. (Berger T. et al., 2006) was to test the hypothesis that noninvasive ventricular activation mapping was feasible in the clinical setting of a catheter laboratory with sufficient spatial and temporal resolution. For the first time, noninvasive mapping of human ventricular pre-excitation was performed and the results were validated by invasive 3-D electroanatomic mapping (CARTO™ ).

Seven patients (3 female; mean age 29 $\pm$ 9 years) with overt ventricular pre-excitation underwent electrophysiologic examination and subsequent radiofrequency catheter ablation of the accessory pathway. All patients had structurally normal hearts which was confirmed by prior transthoracic echocardiography.

The reconstructed activation time maps of ventricular pre-excitation were validated with the catheter-based electroanatomic data (CARTO™) and anatomical markers. For quantitative analysis, the ablation site positions were digitized and coupled with the computer model as described in (Modre R. et al., 2003; Tilg B., Fischer G., Modre R., Hanser F., Messnarz B., Schocke M., Kremser C., Berger T., Hintringer F. & Roithinger F. X., 2002). The last (successful) ablation site was used to calculate the spatial and temporal accuracy of NICE. The position error of the NICE-based activation mapping was defined as the distance between the site of earliest activation on the reconstructed NICE map and the successful ablation site on the CARTO™ map. The color coded activation time maps of three patients of this study is shown in Fig. 8.
The root mean square (RMS) distances between the computed location of the accessory pathway insertion site and the successful ablation sites for all seven patients were 18.7 $\pm$ 5.8 mm for normal AV conduction and 18.7 $\pm$ 6.4 mm during adenosine-induced block. These results have to be interpreted carefully with special attention to the fact of the dispersion of ablation sites during clinical routine. For quantification of this measure the RMS distance between the unsuccessful ablation sites and the localization of successful radiofrequency application was computed, which was found to be 14 $\pm$ 5 mm for all seven patients. Moreover, conventional radiofrequency ablation catheters create lesions with an estimated size of 5 to 8 mm (Simmons W. N. et al., 1996). Taking these circumstances into account, the localization of the accessory pathways' insertion sites computed by NICE showed a strong concordance with the invasively determined successful ablation sites. (Berger T. et al., 2006)

### 3.2 Cardiac resynchronization therapy

Cardiac resynchronization therapy (CRT) has developed as an established treatment of patients with severe heart failure refractory to optimal medical therapy. Large clinical trials showed a significant benefit on mortality and on morbidity in patients with wide QRS complex in NYHA class III and severely impaired left ventricular ejection fraction (LVEF) (Cleland J. G. et al., 2005).

In CRT a pacemaker or an ICD device is implanted and resynchronization of the ventricles is achieved by a synchronization of the timing of both left and right ventricular pacing (biventricular pacing). The right ventricular pacing electrode is in general placed in the right ventricular apical region. The left ventricular pacing electrode is positioned in the left lateral ventricular free wall. This electrode position can be achieved by placement of the electrode via the coronary sinus and coronary veins.

In a previous study we were able to visualize biventricular endocardial and epicardial activation in heart failure patients who underwent CRT. These activation sequences were compared to the activation sequences of a healthy control group by using NICE (Berger T. et al., 2011).

Ten patients (1 female, mean age 63 ± 6 years, NYHA class III and class IV, LVEF < 35 %) with congestive heart failure (ischemic n = 2) and left bundle branch block (LBBB) undergoing CRT and ten patients (4 females; mean age 31 ± 16 years, LVEF > 50 %) without structural heart disease and normal atrioventricular conduction undergoing an electrophysiology study (control) were included in the study. An ECG butterfly plot of 65 channels of one patient of this study is depicted in Fig. 9 for native (blue) rhythm and for biventricular paced rhythm (red). The dotted vertical lines indicate the extracted QRS-intervals for native rhythm and for biventricular pacing.

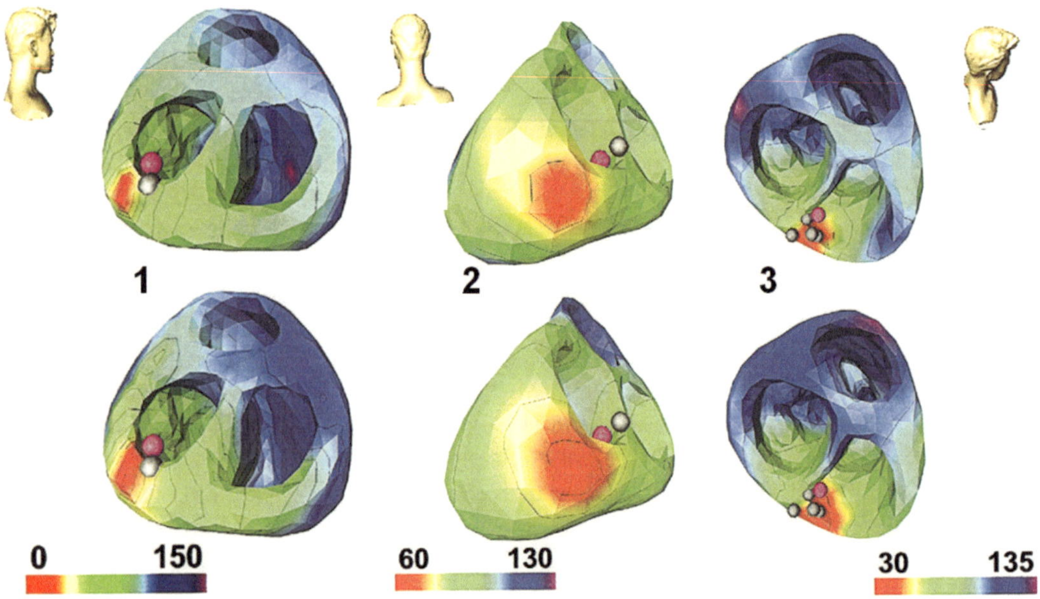


Fig. 8. The location of earliest ventricular activation as computed by NICE is indicated in red. The ablation points are denoted by grey markers, and the location of successful ablation is given by a purple marker, indicating the ventricular insertion site of the accessory pathway. Upper panels show activation sequences during normal atrioventricular (AV) conduction, lower panels show activation sequences during adenosine-induced AV block. Head icons indicate point of view. Red color indicates early, blue–velvet color late electrical activation (see also the colormaps at the bottom with the related activation times in ms).
From (Berger T. et al., 2006) with modification.

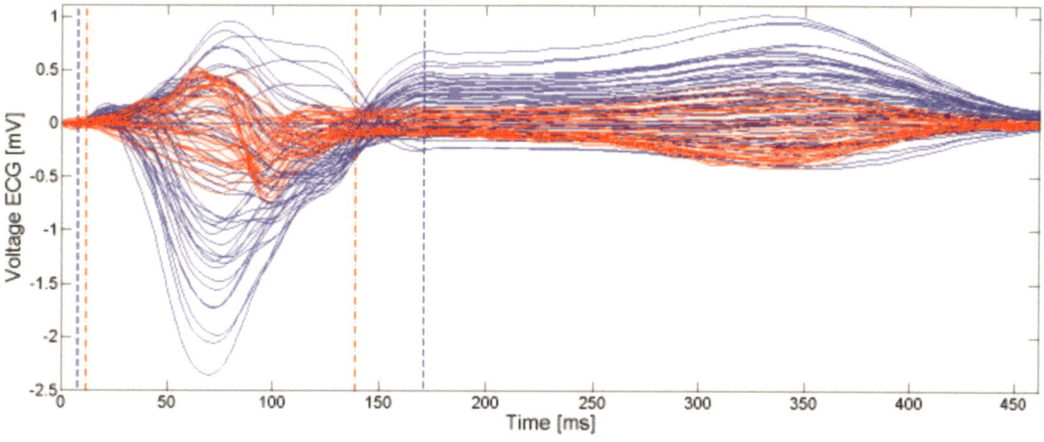


Fig. 9. Butterfly plot of the ECG of the 65-body surface ECG leads during native sinus rhythm (blue) and biventricular pacing (red) of one patient who participated in a CRT-study. The dotted vertical lines indicate begin and end of the QRS complex. From (Berger T. et al., 2011).

The activation time maps for a patient with left bundle branch block (LBBB) is shown in Fig. 10 for native rhythm (left upper panel), right ventricular pacing (RV pacing; right upper panel), left ventricular pacing (LV pacing; left lower panel) and biventricular pacing (right lower panel). The QRS durations clearly indicate an improvement by biventricular pacing as compared to the native rhythm, which could also be confirmed by the activation time maps. There is obviously a high correlation between the intrinsic activation map of a LBBB patient and the activation time map of a control patient during RV pacing. This finding can be related to the fact that in a patient with LBBB the electrical activation starts within the right ventricle and the left ventricle is activated with a temporal delay. This typical activation pattern is similar to the activation pattern during RV pacing. (Berger T. et al., 2011)

The endo-, epicardial and septal breakthrough times in the left and right ventricles could also be determined using NICE. The corresponding times for the LBBB patients and the control group are depicted in Table 1. NICE revealed significant differences between the control and the LBBB patient cohort which is in concordance with previous results (Rodriguez L. M. et al., 2003).

### 3.3 NICE applied to a CRT patient with novel quadripolar LV pacing lead

New developments in electrode design allows more sophisticated options in stimulation of the left ventricle. One of these new devices uses a left-ventricular pacing lead with four distinct electrodes (VectSelect Quartet™, St. Jude Medical). The activation time maps for both the left and the right ventricle using different LV pacing vectors were investigated noninvasively by NICE. This new technique allows selecting between 10 different pacing vectors by combination of the LV electrodes and the RV coil. The implanted leads are displayed in Fig. 11 acquired by fluoroscopy after succesful CRT implantation.

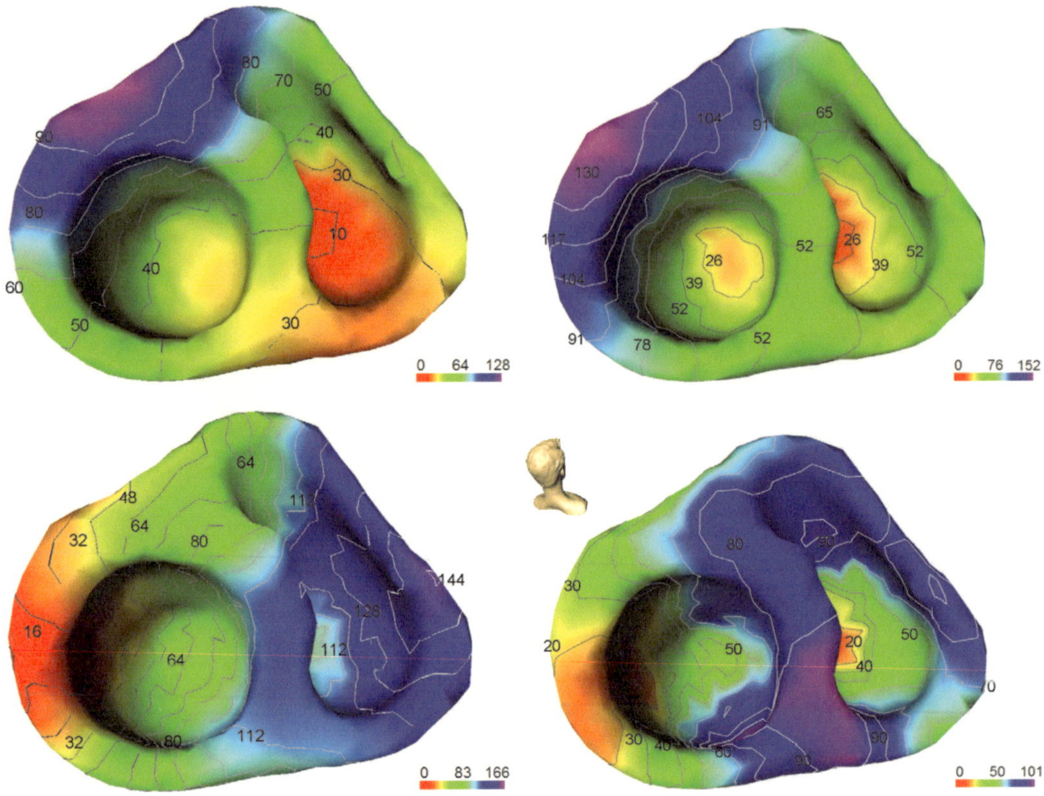


Fig. 10. Activation time maps (isochrones given in ms after first onset of depolarization) showing the left and the right ventricles of a patient with left bundle branch block who underwent CRT in a cranial view (note the head icon indicating the spatial orientation). Left upper panel depicts the activation time map due to native rhythm, right upper panel shows the activation time map during RV pacing, lower left panel shows the activation time map during LV pacing, lower right panel during biventricular pacing. Red color indicates early electrical activation, velvet color indicates areas of late electrial activation. The corresponding QRS durations were: native rhythm: 128 ms; RV pacing: 152 ms; LV pacing: 166 ms; bivent pacing: 101 ms. Note the different scaling of the colormaps for each of the four activation time maps.

The activation time maps determined by NICE are depicted in Fig. 12 for two selected left ventricular pacing sites:

- lead 1 (Distal 1) to lead 2 (Mid 2) defined as pacing vector 1, and
- lead 4 (Proximal 4) to RV coil defined as pacing vector 10

(see Fig. 11 for the locations of the related pacing leads in the 2-D fluoroscopic picture).

| | right ventricle | | | left ventricle | | |
|---|---|---|---|---|---|---|
| | endo [ms] | epi [ms] | septal [ms] | endo [ms] | epi [ms] | septal [ms] |
| control intrinsic | 12 ± 13* | 19 ± 13* | 20 ± 10* | 17 ± 10*† | 24 ± 16*† | 16 ± 10*† |
| control RV pacing | 0 ± 1* | 14 ± 6* | 12 ± 11* | 41 ± 13* | 36 ± 16* | 34 ± 11* |
| LBBB intrinsic | 7 ± 10† | 10 ± 8† | 17 ± 12† | 46 ± 19†‡ | 49 ± 16†‡ | 36 ± 13† |
| LBBB RV pacing | 0 ± 0†‡ | 15 ± 6‡ | 16 ± 6‡ | 50 ± 18§ | 51 ± 17§ | 37 ± 10 |
| LBBB biventricular pacing | 16 ± 13‡ | 28 ± 12†‡ | 30 ± 11†‡ | 17 ± 7‡§ | 1 ± 2‡§ | 40 ± 11 |

Table 1. Endocardial and epicardial left- and right ventricular breakthrough times in milliseconds after QRS-onset (0 ms) during intrinsic rhythm and different pacing modes of control group versus LBBB patients. Symbols '*', '†', '‡', and '§' represent a significant column-wise difference (p-value $< 0.05$) between the corresponding different pacing procedures and rhyhtms. From (Berger T. et al., 2011).

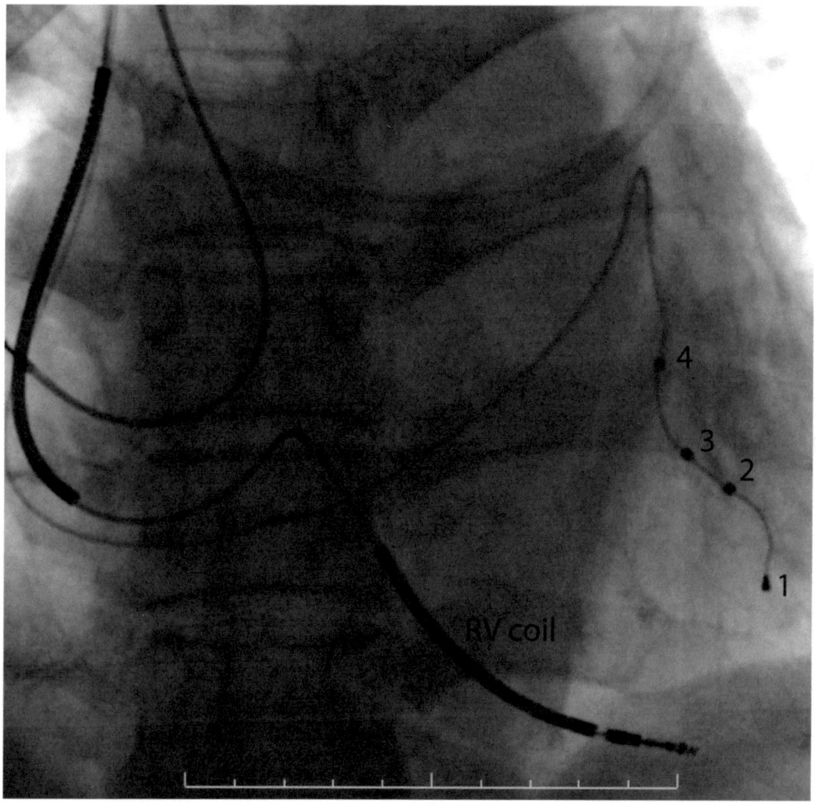


Fig. 11. 2-D picture showing the leads of the Promote Quadra™ device (St. Jude Medical) acquired by fluoroscopy in an anterior-posterior view. The four electrodes on the left ventricular lead (inserted via the coronary sinus) are clearly visible in this picture. The numbers indicate the postion of the distinct electrodes of the left lead. The RV coil is located in the right ventricle and is also part of some of the possible stimulation vectors.

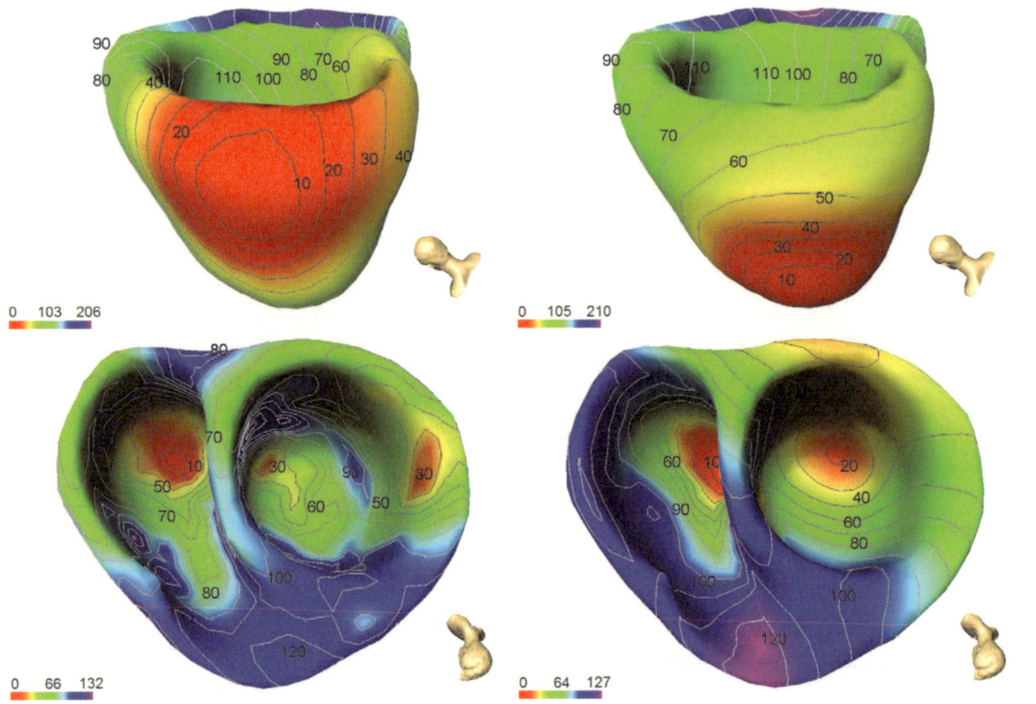


Fig. 12. Activation time maps for left ventricular pacing only (upper panels) and pacing in the right ventricular apex and at the left ventricular lateral wall (lower panels). Note the head icon for spatial orientation. For both figures on the left hand side left ventricular pacing was performed with pacing vector 10 (Proximal 4 to RV coil; see Fig. 11 for the related leads' positions), the figures on the right hand side show the results for left ventricular pacing employing vector 1 (Distal 1 to Mid 2).

## 4. Discussion and conclusion

NICE allows to determine the electrical activation times in a fully noninvasive fashion by combining 3-D geometrical data (acquired by MRI, CT, ultrasound etc.) with a high-resolution multi-channel ECG recording system. As the problem is ill-posed regularization has to be applied. In case of NICE for regularization in the time domain an arcus-tangens-function is introduced in order to mimick the depolarization sequence of a myocyte. Geometrial regularization is achieved by a 2$^{nd}$ order Tikhonov regularization applying the surface Laplacian.

Studies confirmed that NICE can be applied in a clinical environment for solving electrophysiologically relevant problems (Berger T. et al., 2006; 2005; 2011; Modre R. et al., 2004; 2003; Seger M. et al., 2004; Tilg B., Hanser F., Modre-Osprian R., Fischer G., Messnarz B., Berger T., Hintringer F., Pachinger O. & Roithinger F. X., 2002).

NICE enables an accurate estimation of atrial activation times. This was shown in a recent study (Modre R. et al., 2003) which showed a high correlation between the reconstructed activation time maps (NICE) and a catheter-based electroanatomic maps (CARTO™ ) in the right atrium during coronary sinus pacing. This finding and the high localization accuracy

during pacing from different clearly defined pacing sites implicate that atrial activation time imaging of focal events is feasible with sufficient spatial and temporal resolution. (Modre R. et al., 2003)
In the work of Berger et al. (Berger T. et al., 2006) noninvasive electrocardiographic imaging of ventricular pre-excitation was performed in the clinical setting of a catheter laboratory. The results obtained by NICE were validated using invasive 3-D electroanatomic mapping of patients with WPW syndrome. The results showed a strong concordance between the reconstructed activation sequences and the anatomical localization of the accessory bundle insertion site as assessed by invasive electroanatomic mapping. The ventricular activation maps reconstructed by NICE were obtained within a computation time of a few minutes. Clinically important steps such as signal processing, classification of QRS morphology, target beat selection and baseline correction were performed with a high level of automation. These findings and the sufficient localization accuracy of the ventricular insertion sites of the accessory pathways (as indicated by the similarity of ventricular activation sequences obtained with NICE and CARTO™) during sinus rhythm as well as during adenosine-induced AV nodal block demonstrated that also mapping of focal ventricular events was feasible. (Berger T. et al., 2006)
Radiofrequency catheter ablation has become the standard treatment for patients with symptomatic WPW syndrome and has success rates of well over 90 % (Schilling R. J., 2002). Noninvasive imaging of the ventricular activation sequence is of special interest for catheter ablation treatment of patients with AV accessory pathways. It supports the identification of the location of the insertion site of the accessory pathway, which is the target substrate for ablation, within a few minutes. Therefore, NICE-based electroanatomic mapping helps to decrease procedure duration, to improve ablation outcome, and to prevent potential complications. In contrast to other electroanatomic imaging techniques, NICE enables single-beat electroanatomic mapping, which is crucial for mapping unstable focal arrhythmias.

In a recent study performed in CRT patients (Berger T. et al., 2011) NICE was used for simultaneous imaging of endocardial and epicardial ventricular activation during native sinus rhythm as well as during different ventricular pacing modes for the first time. Due to limitations of current mapping techniques, there are only limited data available about the effects of different pacing modes on biventricular endocardial and epicardial activation in humans (Auricchio A. et al., 2004; Lambiase P. D. et al., 2004). In this study (Berger T. et al., 2011) control patients showed a deterioration of the ventricular activation sequence during RV pacing comparable to the activation sequence of congestive heart failure (CHF) patients with complete LBBB during native sinus rhythm. During RV pacing the septal, as well as the endocardial and epicardial activation times of the left ventricle were markedly delayed as compared to native sinus rhythm. The septal activation sequence changed from left-to-right during native conduction to a right-to-left septal activation pattern which is in accordance to previous data (Rodriguez L. M. et al., 2003). The earliest LV activation was observed close to the septum mimicking the activation pattern of LBBB patients. Moreover, RV pacing resulted in an increase of total RV and LV activation duration. This increase in ventricular activation duration during RV pacing may be due to cell-to-cell coupled propagation of the activation wavefront until connecting to the intrinsic conduction system and spreading via the Purkinje system. In CHF patients the delay between right and left ventricular endocardial and epicardial activation was significantly prolonged due to complete LBBB as compared to control patients. In CHF patients biventricular pacing did not affect the direction of transseptal activation respectively the timing of the LV septal breakthrough although the RV septal breakthrough was delayed as compared to native sinus rhythm. This indicates that the major effect of CRT is achieved by preceding the left ventricle by stimulation close to the site of latest left ventricular activation rather than affecting propagation via the intrinsic conduction system. Therefore, optimal placement of the left ventricular lead is crucial and stimulation as close as possible to the site of latest left ventricular activation (during native rhythm) should be aimed at. Epicardial pacing at the left lateral wall and simultaneous endocardial pacing at the right ventricular apex during CRT resulted in a significant decrease of LV total activation duration. Interestingely, total activation duration of the right ventricle was not changed during CRT. This study revealed also differences in propagation velocities of the ventricular activation between the CHF and control group. Left ventricular propagation velocities were significantly decreased in CHF patients as compared to control patients. This is in accordance with the results by Rodriguez et al. (Rodriguez L. M. et al., 2003) who found reduced conduction velocities in patients with congestive heart failure. Both CHF and control patients did not show a significant difference in propagation velocities of the right ventricles. This finding may indicate that the underlying substrate of ventricular dyssynchrony was located mainly within the left ventricle in the CHF patients included into our study. This may be different in patients with arrhythmogenic heart disease or hypertrophic cardiomyopathy. (Berger T. et al., 2011)

In conclusion all these findings show that NICE is a promising tool for noninvasive imaging of electroanatomic activation of the heart. The results indicate that NICE can be a valuable tool in clinical routine. Atrial as well as ventricular cardiac electrical activation can be determined with high accuracies.

The major future challenges will be the extension of activation time reconstruction also for midmyocardial structures. Therefore anisotropic cardiac electrical conductivities have to be considered in the forward problem formulation. Additionally, the inverse problem formulation (regularization term) has to be properly adapted. Implementation of scar tissue into the cardiac model is also a topic for future developments to improve this model-based noninvasive imaging technique.

## 5. References

Auricchio A., Fantoni C., Regoli F., Carbucicchio C., Goette A., Geller C., Kloss M. & Klein H. (2004). Characterization of left ventricular activation in patients with heart failure and left bundle-branch block, *Circulation* 109(9): 1133–1139.

Barbosa C. R. H. (2003). Simulation of a plane wavefront propagating in cardiac tissue using a cellular automata model, *Physics in Medicine and Biology* 48(24): 4151–4164.

Berger T., Fischer G., Pfeifer B., Modre R., Hanser F., Trieb T., Roithinger F. X., Stuehlinger M., Pachinger O., Tilg B. & Hintringer F. (2006). Single-beat noninvasive imaging of cardiac electrophysiology of ventricular pre-excitation, *Journal of the American College of Cardiology* 48(10): 2045–2055.

Berger T., Hanser F., Hintringer F., Poelzl G., Fischer G., Modre R., Tilg B., Pachinger O. & Roithinger F. X. (2005). Effects of cardiac resynchronization therapy on ventricular repolarization in patients with congestive heart failure, *Journal of Cardiovascular Electrophysiology* 16(6): 611–617.

Berger T., Pfeifer B., Hanser F. F., Hintringer F., Fischer G., Netzer M., Trieb T., Stühlinger M., Dichtl W., Baumgartner C., Pachinger O. & Seger M. (2011). Single-beat noninvasive imaging of ventricular endocardial and epicardial activation in patients undergoing CRT, *PLoS ONE* 6(1).

Bradley C., Pullan A. & Hunter P. (2000). Effects of material properties and geometry on electrocardiographic forward simulations, *Annals of Biomedical Engineering* 28(7): 721–741.

Cleland J. G., Daubert J. C., Erdmann E., Freemantle N., Gras D., Kappenberger L. & Tavazzi L. (2005). The effect of cardiac resynchronization on morbidity and mortality in heart failure, *New England Journal of Medicine* 352(15): 1539–1549.

Engl H. W., Hanke M. & Neubauer A. (1996). *Regularization of Inverse Problems*, Kluwer, Dordrecht.

Fischer G., Hanser F., Pfeifer B., Seger M., Hintermüller C., Modre R., Tilg B., Trieb T., Berger T., Roithinger F. X. & Hintringer F. (2005). A signal processing pipeline for noninvasive imaging of ventricular preexcitation, *Methods of Information in Medicine* 44(4): 508–515.

Fischer G., Pfeifer B., Seger M., Hintermüller C., Hanser F., Modre R., Tilg B., Trieb T., Kremser C., Roithinger F. X. & Hintringer F. (2005). Computationally efficient noninvasive cardiac activation time imaging, *Methods of Information in Medicine* 44(5): 674–686.

Fischer G., Tilg B., Modre R., Hanser F., Messnarz B. & Wach P. (2002). On modeling the wilson terminal in the boundary and finite element method, *IEEE Transactions on Biomedical Engineering* 49(3): 217–224.

Fischer G., Tilg B., Modre R., Huiskamp G. J. M, ., Fetzer J., Rucker W. & Wach P. (2000). A bidomain model based bem-fem coupling formulation for anisotropic cardiac tissue, *Annals of Biomedical Engineering* 28(10): 1229–1243.

Fischer G., Tilg B., Wach P., Modre R., Leder U. & Nowak K. (1999). Application of high-order boundary elements to the electrocardiographic inverse problem, *Computer Methods and Programs in Biomedicine* 58(2): 119–131.

Geselowitz D. B. (1967). *On bioelectric potentials in inhomogeneous volume conductor*, The Art of Computer Programming, Biophysics Journal.

Geselowitz D. B. & Miller 3rd W. T. (1983). A bidomain model for anisotropic cardiac muscle, *Annals of Biomedical Engineering* 11(3–4): 191–206.

Greensite F. & Huiskamp G. (1998). An improved method for estimating epicardial potentials from the body surface, *IEEE Transactions on Biomedical Engineering* 45(1): 98–104.

Gulrajani R. M. (1988). Models of the electrical activity of the heart and computer simulation of the electrocardiogram, *Critical Reviews in Biomedical Engineering* 16(1): 1–66.

Gulrajani R. M. & Mailloux G. E. (1983). A simulation study of the effects of torso inhomogeneities on electrocardiographic potentials, using realistic heart and torso models, *Circulation Research* 52(1): 45–56.

Hansen P. C. (2001). *Computational Inverse Problems in Electrocardiography*, WIT Press, Southampton, chapter The L-curve and its use in the numerical treatment of inverse problems, pp. 119–142.

He B., Li G. & Zhang X. (2002). Noninvasive three-dimensional activation time imaging of ventricular excitation by means of a heart-excitation model, *Physics in Medicine and Biology* 47(22): 4063–4078.

Hintermüller C., Fischer G., Seger M., Pfeifer B., Hanser F., Modre R. & B., T. (2004). Multi-lead ECG electrode array for clinical application of electrocardiographic inverse problem, *Annual International Conference of the IEEE Engineering in Medicine and Biology Society. IEEE Engineering in Medicine and Biology Society*, Vol. 3, San Francisco, USA, pp. 1941–1944.

Huiskamp G. & Greensite F. (1997). A new method for myocardial activation imaging, *IEEE Transactions on Biomedical Engineering* 44(6): 433–446.

Huiskamp G. J. (1991). Difference formulas for the surface laplacian on a triangulated surface, *Journal of Computational Physics* 95(2): 477–496.

Johnson J. R. (1997). Computational and numerical methods for bioelectric field problems, *Critical Reviews in Biomedical Engineering* 25(1): 1–81.

Klepfer R. N., Johnson C. R. & Macleod R. S. (1997). The effects of inhomogeneities and anisotropies on electrocardiographic fields: a 3-D finite-element study, *IEEE Transactions on Biomedical Engineering* 44(8): 706–719.

Lambiase P. D., Rinaldi A., Hauck J., Mobb M., Elliott D., Mohammad S., Gill J. S. & Bucknall C. A. (2004). Non-contact left ventricular endocardial mapping in cardiac resynchronisation therapy, *Heart* 90(1): 44–51.

Malmivuo J. & Plonsey R. (1995). *Bioelectromagnetism*, Oxford University Press, Oxford.

Messnarz B., Seger M., Modre R., Fischer G., Hanser F. & Tilg B. (2004). A comparison of noninvasive reconstruction of epicardial versus transmembrane potentials in consideration of the null space, *IEEE Transactions on Biomedical Engineering* 51(9): 1609–1618.

Messnarz B., Tilg B., Modre R., Fischer G. & Hanser F. (2004). A new spatiotemporal regularization approach for reconstruction of cardiac transmembrane potential patterns, *IEEE Transactions on Biomedical Engineering* 51(2): 273–281.

Modre R., Seger M., Fischer G., Hintermüller C., P., Hanser F. & Tilg B. (2006). Cardiac anisotropy: Is it negligible regarding noninvasive activation time imaging?, *IEEE Transactions on Biomedical Engineering* 53(4): 569–580.

Modre R., Tilg B., Fischer G., Hanser F., Messnarz B., Seger M., Hintringer F. & Roithinger F. X. (2004). Ventricular surface activation time imaging from electrocardiogram mapping data, *Medical and Biological Engineering and Computing* 42(2): 146–150.

Modre R., Tilg B., Fischer G., Hanser F., Messnarz B., Seger M., Schocke M., Berger T., Hintringer F. & Roithinger F. X. (2003). Atrial noninvasive activation time imaging of paced rhythm data, *Journal of Cardiovascular Electrophysiology* 14(7): 712–719.

Modre R., Tilg B., Fischer G. & Wach P. (2001). An iterative algorithm for myocardial activation time imaging, *Computer Methods and Programs in Biomedicine* 64(1): 1–7.

Modre R., Tilg B., Fischer G. & Wach P. (2002). Noninvasive myocardial activation time imaging: A novel inverse algorithm applied to clinical ECG mapping data, *IEEE Transactions on Biomedical Engineering* 49(10): 1153–1161.

Morady F. (1999). Radio-frequency ablation as treatment for cardiac arrhythmias, *New England Journal of Medicine* 340(7): 534–544.

Pfeifer B., Hanser F., Hintermüller C., Modre - Osprian R., Fischer G., Seger M., Mühlthaler H., Trieb T. & Tilg B. (2005). C++ framework for creating tissue specific segmentation pipelines, *Medical Imaging: Visualization, Image-Guided Procedures, and Display. Proceedings SPIE*, Vol. 5744, San Diego, USA, pp. 317–328.

Pfeifer B., Hanser F., Seger M., Fischer G., Modre-Osprian R. & Tilg B. (2008). Patient-specific volume conductor modeling for Non-Invasive Imaging of Cardiac Electrophysiology, *Open Medical Informatics Journal* 2: 32–41.

Pfeifer B., Seger M., Hintermüller C., Fischer G., Hanser F., Modre R., Mühlthaler H. & Tilg B. (2006). Semiautomatic volume conductor modeling pipeline for imaging the cardiac electrophysiology noninvasively, *Medical image computing and computer-assisted intervention: MICCAI ... International Conference on Medical Image Computing and Computer-Assisted Intervention*, Vol. 9 (Pt 1), Copenhagen, Denmark, pp. 588–595.

Pfeifer B., Seger M., Hintermüller C., Fischer G., Mühlthaler H., Modre - Osprian R. & Tilg B. (2007). Aam-based segmentation for imaging cardiac electrophysiology, *Methods of Information in Medicine* 46:III(1): 36–42.

Press W. H., Teukolsky S. A., Vetterling W. T. & Flannery B. P. (2002). *Numerical recipies in C++ the art of scientific computing*, 2nd edn, Cambridge University Press.

Pullan A. J., Cheng L. K., Nash M. A., Bradley C. P. & Paterson D. J. (2001). Noninvasive electrical imaging of the heart: Theory and model development, *Annals of Biomedical Engineering* 29(10): 817–836.

Ramanathan C., Ghanem R. N., Jia P., Ryu K. & Rudy Y. (2004). Noninvasive electrocardiographic imaging for cardiac electrophysiology and arrhythmia, *Nature in Medicine* 10(4): 422–428.

Ramanathan C., Jia P., Ghanem R., Calvetti D. & Rudy Y. (2003). Noninvasive electrocardiographic imaging (ECGI): application of the generalized minimal residual (GMRes) method, *Annals of Biomedical Engineering* 31(8): 981–994.

Renhardt M., Wach P., Dienstl F., Fleischmann P., Killmann R. & Tilg B. (1992). Computersimulation des Elektro- und Magnetokardiogramms bei Ischämie und infarkt, *Biomedizinische Technik/Biomedical Engineering* 37(s1): 36–38.

Rodriguez L. M., Timmermans C., Nabar A., Beatty G. & Wellens H. J. (2003). Variable patterns of septal activation in patients with left bundle branch block and heart failure, *Journal of Cardiovascular Electrophysiology* 14(2): 135–141.

Roth B. J. (1991). Electrical conductivity values used with the bidomain model of cardiac tissue, *IEEE Transactions on Biomedical Engineering* 44(4): 326–328.

Saxberg B. E. & Cohen R. J. (1990). Cellular automata models for reentrant arrhythmias, *Journal of Electrocardiology* 23(Suppl.): 95.

Schilling R. J. (2002). Which patient should be referred to an electrophysiologist: supraventricular tachycardia, *Heart* 87(3): 299–304.

Seger M., Fischer G., Modre R., Messnarz B., Hanser F. & Tilg B. (2005). Lead field computation for the electrocardiographic inverse problem – finite elements versus boundary elements, *Computer Methods and Programs in Biomedicine* 77(3): 241–252.

Seger M., Fischer G., Modre R., Pfeifer B., Hanser F., Hintermüller C., Roithinger F. X., Hintringer F., Trieb T., Schocke M. & Tilg B. (2004). On-line noninvasive localization of accessory pathways in the EP lab, *Medical image computing and computer-assisted intervention: MICCAI ... International Conference on Medical Image Computing and Computer-Assisted Intervention*, Vol. 2, St. Malo, France, pp. 502–509.

Simmons W. N., Mackey S., He D. S. & Marcus F. I. (1996). Comparison of gold versus platinum electrodes on myocardial lesion size using radiofrequency energy, *Pacing and Clinical Electrophysiology* 19(4): 398–402.

SippensGroenewegen A., Roithinger F. X., Peeters H. A., Linnenbank A. C., van Hemel N. M., Steiner P. R. & Lesh M. D. (1998). Body surface mapping of atrial arrhythmias: atlas of paced p wave integral maps to localize the focal origin of the right atrial tachycardia, *Journal of Electrocardiology* 31(Suppl.): 85–91.

Tilg B., Fischer G., Modre R., Hanser F., Messnarz B., Schocke M., Kremser C., Berger T., Hintringer F. & Roithinger F. X. (2002). Model-based imaging of cardiac electrical excitation in humans, *IEEE Transactions on Medical Imaging* 21(9): 1031–1039.

Tilg B., Hanser F., Modre-Osprian R., Fischer G., Messnarz B., Berger T., Hintringer F., Pachinger O. & Roithinger F. X. (2002). Clinical ECG mapping and imaging of cardiac electrical excitation, *Journal of Electrocardiology* 35(4, part B): 81–87.

Tilg B., Renhardt M., Fleischmann P. & Wach P. (1992). Modellierung der Leitfähigkeitsanisotropie im Herzen zur EKG- und MKG-berechnung, *Biomedizinische Technik/Biomedical Engineering* 37(s1): 33–35.

Wach P., Modre R., Tilg B. & Fischer G. (2001). An iterative linearized optimization technique for non-linear ill-posed problems applied to cardiac activation time imaging, *COMPEL: The International Journal for Computation and Mathematics in Electrical and Electronic Engineering* 20(3): 676–688.

Wach P., Tilg B., Lafer G. & Rucker W. (1997). Magnetic source imaging in the human heart: estimating cardiac electrical sources from simulated and measured magnetocardiogram data, *Medical and Biological Engineering and Computing* 35(3): 157–166.

8

# Past, Present and Future Catheter Technologies and Energy Sources for Atrial Fibrillation Ablation

Inderpal Singh, Adam Price, Zachary Leshen and Boaz Avitall
*University of Illinois at Chicago, IL*
*USA*

## 1.Introduction

Atrial fibrillation (AF) is one of the most common tachyarrhythmias, with an incidence that continues, especially among the elderly where it affects upto 7% of the population. Due to the associated morbidities, including the risk of stroke, heart failure and impaired quality of life, numerous modalities have emerged for the treatment of atrial fibrillation. In recent years, an increasing number of patients are being treated with catheter ablation in an effort to restore sinus rhythm and decrease the associated co-morbidities. Compared to other treatment modalities, primarily that of pharmacotherapy, ablation of AF offers the unique opportunity to restore sinus rhythm and its associated benefits without the associated risks of anti-arrhythmic medications. These benefits, however, must be weighed against the known risks of ablation, which include perforation, cardiac tamponade, pulmonary vein stenosis and esophageal injury. It has been well described previously that premature atrial contractions (PACs) originating from the pulmonary veins are an important trigger for the initiation of AF. The sources of these PAC s are believed to be related to the presence of left atrial myocardial tissue that extends into the pulmonary vein. Consequently, most ablation strategies attempt to achieve electrical isolation of the pulmonary veins for the treatment of paroxysmal AF. Different energy sources combined with innovative catheter technologies are likely to improve the success rates of AF ablation.

## 2. Radiofrequency lesions

Radiofrequency (RF) energy is currently the most widely used energy source for performing catheter ablation procedures. RF generators deliver alternating current at frequencies too high to depolarize the myocardium between 500 and 1000 KHz (Haines 1993 and Skanes et al 2003). When using a 4mm catheter ablation tip, the radiofrequency energy used (20 to 50 W) is often generated from a 550 KHz electrosurgical unit and is delivered for 30-120 seconds (Manolis et al 1994). Most commonly the RF power is delivered between a 8F 4-8mm catheter ablation tip and a dispersive reference patch applied to the skin. The application of RF energy between the small ablation tip and the dispersive electrode results in the greatest resistance to the current flow at the catheter tip to tissue interface. This results in resistive heating, and consequently leads into lesion formation at the catheter to tissue interface. Deep tissue heating is consequence of conductive heating which is responsible for deep lesion formation. Conductive heating diminishes as a function of $1/r^4$ where 'r' equals the distance from the point of maximal resistive heating (Hoffmann et al 1992 and Avitall et al 2004). Tissue temperatures above 45 °C result in increase in cytosolic calcium concentration due to increased permeability, while sarcoplasmic ATPase is inhibited at temperatures above 50°C. Above 50°C, irreversible tissue damage has been documented (Haines DE 1993 and Inesi et al 1973). At 60°C, collagen denaturation occurs, with loss of elasticity and compliance of the ablated tissues.

### 2.1 RF ablation non irrigated tip catheter

The depth of lesion size increases as the temperature increase at the interface up to 100°C. Above this temperature, the plasma starts boiling resulting in coagulum formation at the tip. This can lead to clot embolization, a sudden increase in impedance, loss of thermal conductivity, and ineffective tissue heating. Non-irrigated catheters are available with 4-5mm and 8mm length tip ablation electrodes with an integrated thermocouple to monitor the tip temperature. With the 8mm catheter, a large portion of the electrode is exposed to flowing blood which cools the tip allowing for the application of higher RF power and the creation of larger lesions.

A thermocouple is integrated at the tip for monitoring the temperature during ablation. The new generation RF generators can help to titrate the power up and down until the desired tip temperature is reached. This is called temperature guided RF ablation (Skanes et al, 2003). Nowadays the generators are capable of opting between temperature guided or power guided RF ablation. The risk of a thromboembolism after LARFA (Left atrial radiofrequency ablation) is 1.1%, with most events occurring within 2 weeks after the procedure using 8mm tip catheter. (Oral et al 2006)

### 2.2 Irrigated tip electrode catheter

The irrigated tip electrode catheter (Figure 1) has 4-5mm ablation electrode. The presence of irrigation helps to keep the temperature at the tissue-electrode interface lower, thereby permitting improved delivery of RF energy to deeper tissues. Ultimately, this can facilitate the creation of more complete, and transmural, radiofrequency lesions. Additionally, irrigation at the site of ablation has also helped to minimize thrombus formation at the ablation site as well. The saline used for irrigation can be circulated within the electrode (closed loop system), or open irrigation system that flushes saline through openings in the ablation electrode (Budde et al 1987, Grumbrecht et al 1998, Kongsgaard et al 1997, matsudairi et al 2003, Nakagawa et al 1998, Wittkampf et al 1989 and Yokoyama et al 2006). A major limitation of this catheter is the poor correlation of the tip temperature with the tissue temperature, often resulting in RF being curtailed and therefore incomplete lesions are made. The incidence of silent thromboembolic event in post ablation atrial fibrillation patients is 8.3% in irrigated tip catheter, 38.9% in duty cycled multielectrode catheter and 5.6% in cryoballoon (Gaita et al 2011). The duty cycled and cryoballoon ablation catheters have further been explained in the chapter.

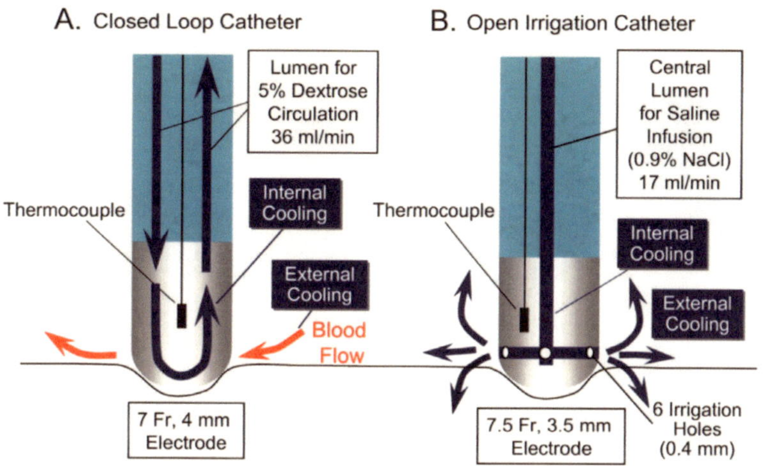


Fig. 1. Irrigated closed loop and open irrigation electrode catheter (Yokoyama et al 2006).

## 3. Irrigated tip catheter with contact sensor

RF ablation is dependent on good tissue contact where the ablation electrode is firmly embedded in the targeted tissue. The contact angle and the force between the tip of the catheter and the tissue surface play a major role in the characteristics of the lesion. Irrigated tip catheters with contact sensors can be used to estimate the contact force and angle (Figure 2). The catheter tip in this case is equipped with a deformable body that makes contact with the myocardial tissue. When subject to contact forces exerted by the tissue, the deformable body translates these forces into changes in wavelengths by optical fibers present within the catheter. Ultimately, these changes in wavelength are transformed via a computer algorithm to display both catheter vectors as well as contact force. The benefit of this catheter is that the combination of appropriate angle and force can be used to generate maximum transmurality with minimum incidence of steam pop and thrombus formation. (Schmidt et al 2009)

## 4. Spiral catheter

Another example of a catheter that is designed to specifically isolate the pulmonary vein (PV) Ostia resembles a corkscrew shape (Figure 3). This catheter is equipped with four 12 mm coil electrodes, with two thermistors placed at the edges of each coil to regulate the RF power, adjusting to the maximal sensed temperature from each thermistor (Avitall et al 2005). Standard radiofrequency generator with specialized interface was used.

The ablation catheter is introduced into the PVs via a 9F sheath. Once the tip of the catheter is in the PV, the sheath is withdrawn while maintaining the catheter position in the PV. As shown below, the spiral catheter expands within the vein and the coil electrodes are embedded within and under the orifice of the PV [figure 4]. Prior studies using this catheter demonstrated no visible PV narrowing during final PV angiography. PV circumferential lesions were documented in PVs and no PV stenosis was documented. One drawback however was the requirement to rotate the catheter position to create a circumferential lesion.

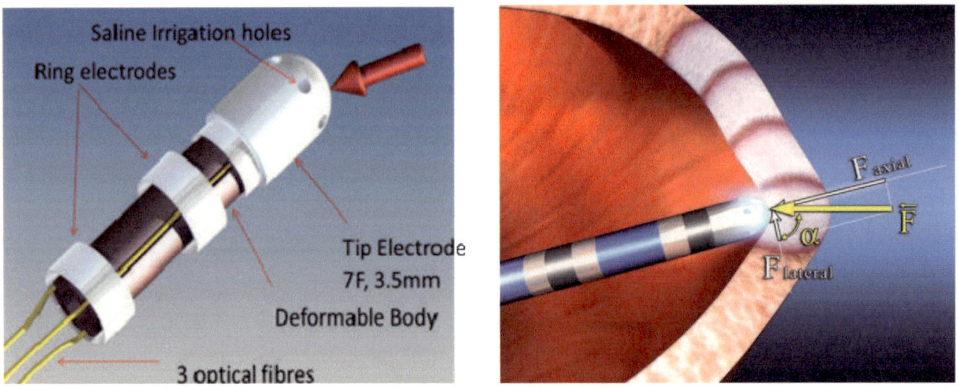


Fig. 2. Irrigated tip catheter with Contact sensor (Yokoyama et al 2008).

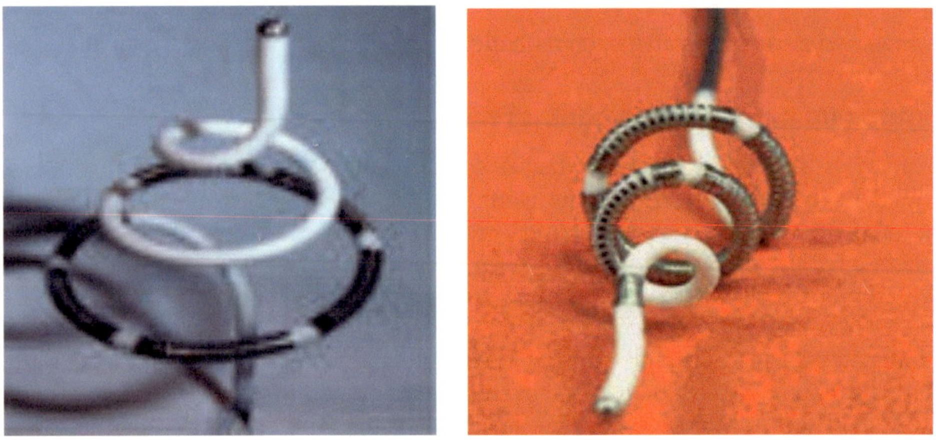

Fig. 3. PV ostia spiral catheter (Avitall et al 2005).

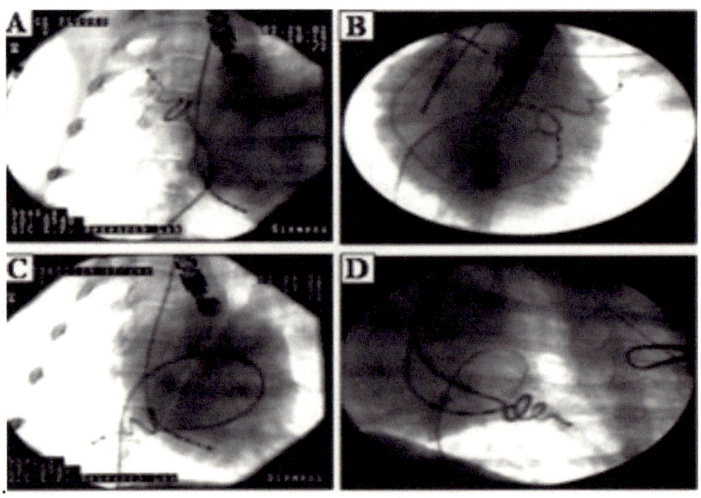


Fig. 4. Spiral catheter in Pulmonary veins, the spiral catheter expands within the vein and the coil electrodes are embedded within and under the orifice of the PV.

## 5. The duty cycled multi electrode catheter

The pulmonary vein ablation catheter (PVAC) or duty cycled multi electrode catheter (Ablation Frontiers, Inc., Carlsbad, CA, USA) is a 9F, over-the-wire, circumlinear (diameter 25mm), decapolar mapping and ablation catheter (Figure 5). The 3mm long platinum electrodes have an outer diameter of approximately 1.5mm and are spaced 3mm apart. Each electrode contains a thermocouple positioned on the surface contact side of the electrode. The catheter has 2 control handles. One allows bidirectional deflection of the shaft and the other is used to move the distal tip forward along the 0.032 mm guidewire, allowing a change of the catheter from its circular shape to a spiral configuration and finally to a longitudinal shape. The catheter is advanced through the sheath in its longitudinal shape and then deployed in the atria with the guidewire positioned in the vein (Boersma et al 2008). The GENius RF generator (Ablation Frontiers, Inc., Carlsbad, CA, USA) is a multichannel, dutycycled RF generator capable of independently delivering energy simultaneously to a maximum of 12 electrodes. RF energy can be delivered in unipolar (between ablation electrode and reference patch) and bipolar (between 2 adjacent ablation electrodes) configurations. Pairs of electrodes can be selected independently. During RF application, energy delivery is controlled by a software algorithm that modulates power to reach the user-defined target temperature (60°C), but always limits power to a maximum of 10W per electrode. In this way, the ablation is "temperature controlled". Although this ablation technology limits the peak power to 10W, lower than with a non-irrigated 4 mm tip catheter, the current density applied at the tissue surface is approximately the same due to the smaller surface area of the electrodes. One limitation however is that achieving PV isolation requires rotation of the catheter to create overlapping circumferential lesions (Boersma et al 2008). Boersma et al studied 98 patients with paroxysmal or persistent AF to evaluate the feasibility and safety of this multielectrode catheter. All targeted PVs were isolated using this catheter, and follow-up after 6 months without antiarrhythmic drugs showed freedom from AF in 83% of patients. This study also demonstrated that fluoroscopy and procedural time appear to be shorter than those associated with current AF ablation techniques, without the need for sophisticated mapping and/or steering modalities (Wijffels et al 2009).

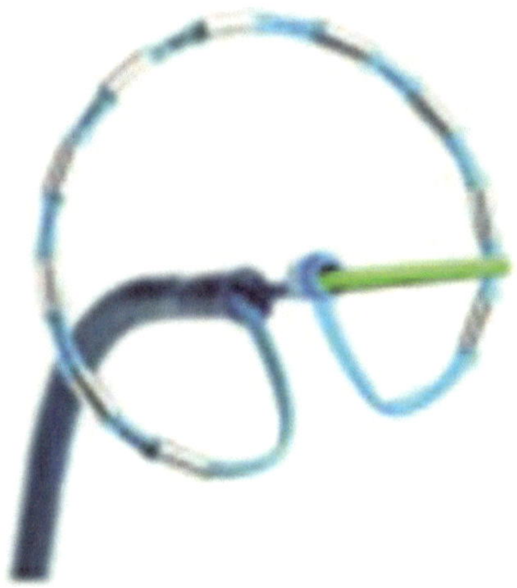

Fig. 5. PVAC (Decapolar Mapping and Ablation Catheter) (Wijffels et al.).

## 6. Loop catheter

The loop catheter design for the creation of linear lesions in an effort to ablate AF was introduced in 1997. There are two main loop catheter systems, mostly used for experimental studies (Boston Scientific, EP Technologies, Sunnyvale, CA, USA) (Avitall et al 1999). Both catheter designs are shown in Figure 6. The first catheter system has twenty four 4mm ring electrodes that can create loops in the atria. In an effort to increase the efficiency of the ablation system, the second loop catheter was designed with fourteen 12-mm long coil electrodes 2 mm apart, equipped with two thermistors that were positioned at the two edges of each coil. The power is regulated to the maximal temperature measured between the two thermistors. Depending on the magnitude of the pullwire retraction and the size of the catheter portion extending from the sheath, the electrode portion of the catheter can form loops of various sizes. The body of the catheter applies pressure on the thin atrial walls and forces them to stretch around the catheter, maintaining consistent electrode-tissue contact along the entire length of the ablation portion of the catheter. Since the forces that are applied to the atrial walls are distributed along the catheter shaft around the loop, it is presumed that no single point is exposed to excessive forces. A locking mechanism holds the catheter and pullwire firmly in position. (Avitall et al 2002).

The most important determinant in the effective creation of a RF lesion is the electrode-tissue contact. Using the variable loop concept, the globular shaped atrial chambers will adapt around the catheter providing continuous contact. When using temperature control with this technology, over 90% of the lesions created in both atria were both contiguous and transmural while minimizing the incidence of significant rises in impedance. The catheter can be used to create linear lesions 6 mm wide and up to 16 cm long with minimal manipulation. Linear lesions were made by ablating at individual electrodes. Having multiple ablation electrodes on a single shaft allows for minimal catheter manipulation in creating long linear lesions and, therefore, may reduce both thromboembolic risk and radiation exposure. Once the catheter is in place, it remains in position for the duration of the power application to all of the electrodes (Avitall et al 2002).

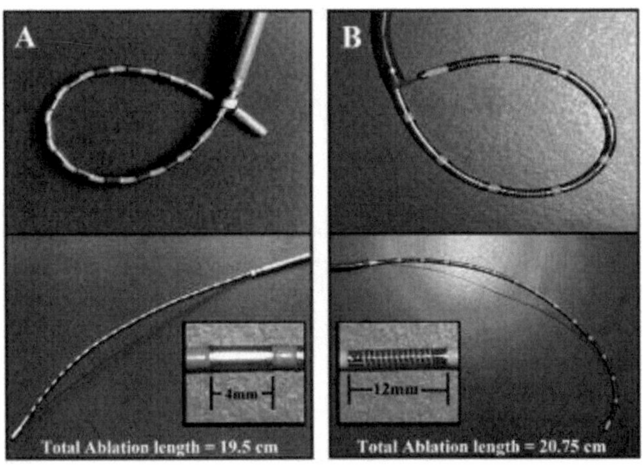


Fig. 6. The loop catheter system. (A) 8F with 24 4-mm-long ring electrodes spaced 4 mm apart. (B) 8F with 14 12-mm-long coil electrodes spaced 2-mm apart. A soft, braided pull wire attached to the distal tip of the catheter can be retracted into the long guiding sheath to deflect the catheter tip to create a loop of various sizes. (Avitall et al 1999).

## 7. Laser AF ablation

A laser is a device that emits light (electromagnetic radiation) through a process of optical amplification based on the stimulated emission of photons. Emitted laser light is notable for its high degree of spatial and temporal coherence, unattainable using other technologies. Since duration and intensity of a laser can be controlled, it penetrates the tissue and scatters after getting absorbed in the tissue. Photon energy causes the vibrational excited state of surrounding molecules. This leads to generation of heat resulting in lesion creation. Laser energy can create deeper lesions with less reliance on thermal diffusion and can reduce tissue vaporization and coagulum formation. Because of its focused nature, it minimizes the collateral atrial tissue damage (Littman et al 1993). Two types of laser namely, Nd- YAG and Diode laser have been used in clinical application. Between them Diode laser with a wavelength of 980 nm, can minimize endocardial disruption. (Littman et al 1993)

### 7.1 Visually guided Laser balloon catheter

Identification of the left atrial-pulmonary vein junction remains challenging, and additionally, creating contiguous lesions in a point by point manner to isolate the pulmonary veins (PV) is quite difficult. Balloon catheters provide an advantage in overcoming the challenge of charring and clot formation allowing for more precise lesion creation (Reddy et al 2004). The visually guided balloon catheter (Figure 7a) has an optic fiber head at the proximal end of the balloon and is equipped with an endoscope, permitting a visual angle of 110 degrees. When adequate tissue contact is made, tissue blanching will occur. If there is poor contact, however, then only free flowing blood is seen through the endoscope. Once the PV ostium is visualized, the next step is to use the optical fiber to target the laser arc at the appropriate tissue site. Correct identification of the ostium is critical to prevent formation of thrombus, which occurs when laser energy is focused on red blood cells. Keeping this in mind, the difference in the color of the light reflected is observed (seen as an arc) by the tissue and blood allows for assessment of contact. A red arc reflects contact with both tissue and blood, while green arc (Figure 7b) reflects balloon contact with tissue representing the target of ablation using this balloon technology. Once the arc is appropriately positioned to target the tissue of interest, a continuous 980-nm arc of laser energy is delivered. To avoid the overheating of myocardial tissue, sterile cooling fluid is circulated inside the balloon. Multiple arcs of ablation are applied to "stitch" individual lesions together to achieve a continuous circumferential lesion set.

Studies utilizing visually guided balloon catheter ablation demonstrated long-term freedom from recurrence of atrial fibrillation at 67%, a rate comparable to that achieved with radiofrequency ablation (Reddy et al 2004**).** The delivery of deeper ablation energies in the pulmonary vein results in an increased risk of PV stenosis. The interface of the laser balloon catheter remains well outside the PV with the arc is projected on the ostium resulting in a decreased risk creating PV stenosis.

To prevent esophageal injury intraoperative temperature monitoring of the esophagus is done. If the temperature rises then the arc is either advanced or retracted.In addition there is less incidence of pericardial tamponade because of the controlled energy delivery. (Reddy et al 2004).

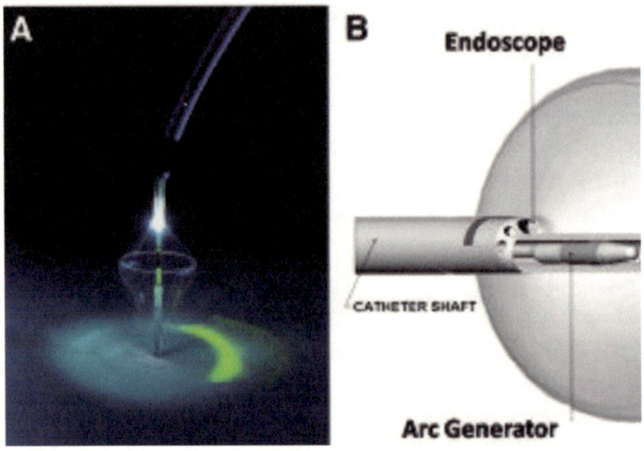


Fig. 7a. Panel A visually guided balloon catheter displaying the green laser arc. In panel B Distal end of the catheter is shown. Catheter shaft endoscope and arc generator can be seen. (Reddy et al 2008).

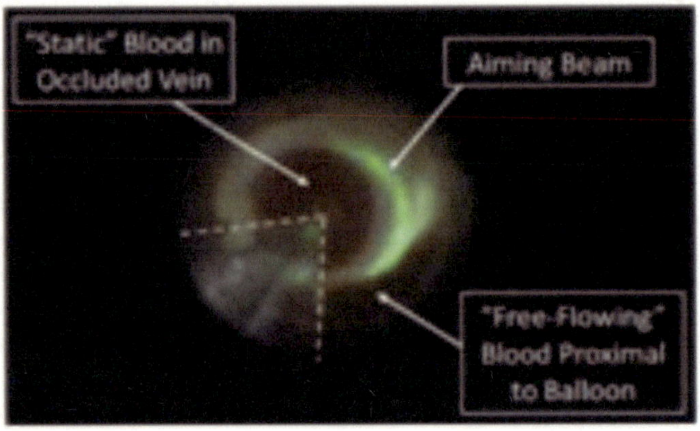


Fig. 7b. In this figure, the arc of laser can be seen. The green light signifies the tissue and red light signifies the blood in the vein.

## 8. High intensity focused ultrasound balloon system

The High intensity focused ultrasound balloon system (HIFU) is a dual balloon in balloon design (Figure 8). The steerable HIFU catheter, a 10F catheter equipped with a 24mm diameter balloon, is advanced over the guidewire to the PV orifice, assisted by fluoroscopy and phased array intracardiac ultrasound (ICE) guidance. The anterior balloon is filled with fluid and the posterior with carbon dioxide. The interface created by the fluid and gas becomes the reflective interface of the ultrasound waves. The radially directed ultrasound energy is reflected forward to create a circumferential zone of concentrated ablative energy just beyond the face of the balloon. The mechanism of lesion formation is based on the conversion of the high intensity focused acoustic energy which causes molecular vibration that releases thermal energy in cardiac tissue. The steep tissue temperature gradient (2-5 °C per second) reaches 65-100°C with little heating of the adjacent tissue. (Okumura et al 2008 and Kennedy et al 2003)

The balloon technology allows complete, 360° delivery of circumferential energy around the PV orifice, which may simplify the procedure. The balloon catheter has a predictable focused zone with very rapid achievement of lethal tissue temperatures. Power titration may control energy delivery and limit its impact on collateral tissue. This also highlights the need for careful monitoring of device positioning within the context of the geometry of the vein and adjacent structures. Use of balloons larger than the PV orifice may prevent injury of phrenic nerve or distal pulmonary veins.

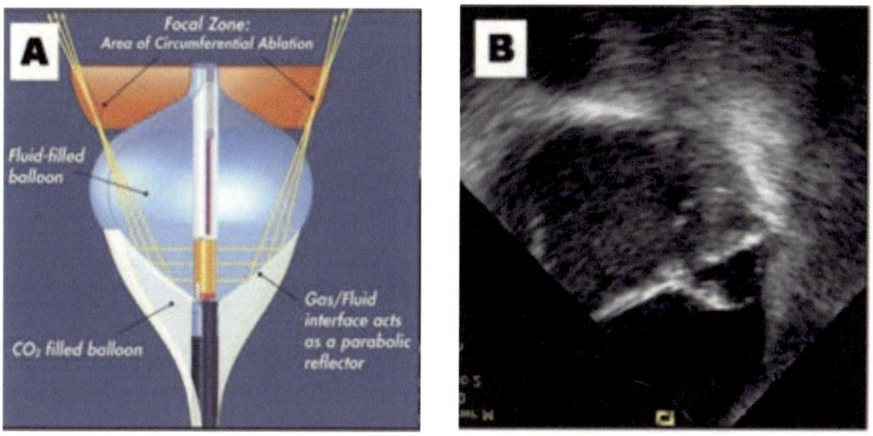


Fig. 8 A. High-intensity focused ultrasound balloon ablation system. B: An ICE catheter is placed within the coronary to visualize the HIFU catheter positioned at the ostium of the left inferior PV. (Reddy et al 2004).

## 9. Cryothermal energy

Cryotechnology has been used for cardiac ablation for three decades, but catheter based ablation has been a more recent development. Cryothermal energy produces lesions through hypothermic exposure, which is a very different mechanism of tissue injury as compared to heat ablation. Cryolesions are generated by application of a cryoprobe cooled with liquid nitrous oxide for 2 - 5 minutes (Stobie et al 2003).

Progressive cooling of cardiac tissue slows down conduction and eventually blocks electrical activity when temperatures are reduced to 0 to -20°C. Permanent lesions are created when temperatures are reduced to -60 to -80 °C (Becker et al 2004).

Applying the cryoprobe to the tissue surface causes the formation of a hemisphere of frozen tissue, or iceball. Ice crystals formed are seen both intracellularly and extracellularly. The primary mechanism of cell death is fatal structural change in subcellular organelles and the mitochondrial membrane. The electron transport system, which normally utilizes the mitochondrial membrane, stops working, this leads to irreversible mitochondrial damage, and ultimately cell death characterized by coagulative necrosis. Extracellular ice causes additional compression and distortion of adjacent cytoplasmic components and nuclei.

Histpathologically RF lesions cause complete disruption of elastic fibers in comparison to normal appearing elastic fibers in cryolesions. Esophageal injury can occur in both RF and cryo, however cryo tissue injury is often benign and reversible. RF is compared with

Cryoablation in the table 2 below. Moreover, tensile strength of the tissue remains intact in cryolesions. The potential advantages of cryoablation over RF for ablation include a low risk of endocardial disruption, reduced incidence of thrombus formation, and stable adhesion of the catheter tip to the endocardium during freezing (Arora et al 2009).

### 9.1 Cryoballoon

New cryoballoon technology can safely and effectively electrically isolate the PVs (Avitall et al 2004). Avitall et al studied the original cryo balloon technology and found that after multiple consecutive cryolesions no PV stenosis was noted 3 months after ablation. After cryo ablation, PV electrograms were eliminated and tissue recovery exhibits no cartilage formation. Acute tissue hemorrhage and hemoptysis are short term complications of cryoablation. Arctic front cardiac cryoablation catheter developed by CryoCath is shown in the figure 9. It creates cryo lesions by delivering liquid N2O into the semi compliant balloon (23mm - 28mm diameter) and it is currently FDA approved for human PV isolation.

| | Advantages | Disadvantages |
|---|---|---|
| Cryoablation | 1. Marked differences in lesion morphology (minimal collagen formation).<br>2. Preserved atrial contraction and size.<br>3. Marked reduction in the risk of stroke (no char).<br>4. Assessment of arrhythmogenic source prior to ablation (cool mapping). | 1. Pressurized gas system.<br>2. Complexity of control and delivery<br>3. Potential gas toxicity to the operator and patient.<br>4. Cooling of the patient.<br>5. Intramural hemorrhage and risk of hemoptysis.<br>6. Requires tissue contact |
| Radiofrequency Ablation | 1. Simple, well-proven technology.<br>2. Ability to assess contact.<br>3. Assessment of temperature.<br>4. Limited tissue damage. | 1. Difficulty of uniform assessment of tissue contact.<br>2. Significant amount of collagen and cartilage/calcification.<br>3. Moderate risk of stroke, PV stenosis.<br>4. Atrial shrinkage.<br>5. Moderate reduction in atrial mechanical function. |

Table 1. Comparison of cryoablation vs radiofrequency ablation (Yiu et al 2006).

## 10. Virtual electrode and visualization catheter

In the Virtual and visual electrode catheter a unipolar tip electrode is present with an endoscope circumferential to the tip it has a hood made up of a flexible elastopolymer membrane at the proximal end. This hood carries the circumferential light source bands for illumination. Consequently, this catheter provides the means of directly visualizing the target tissue that needs to be ablated. It is helpful in maintaining the contiguity of the lesions and also decreases the total procedure time.

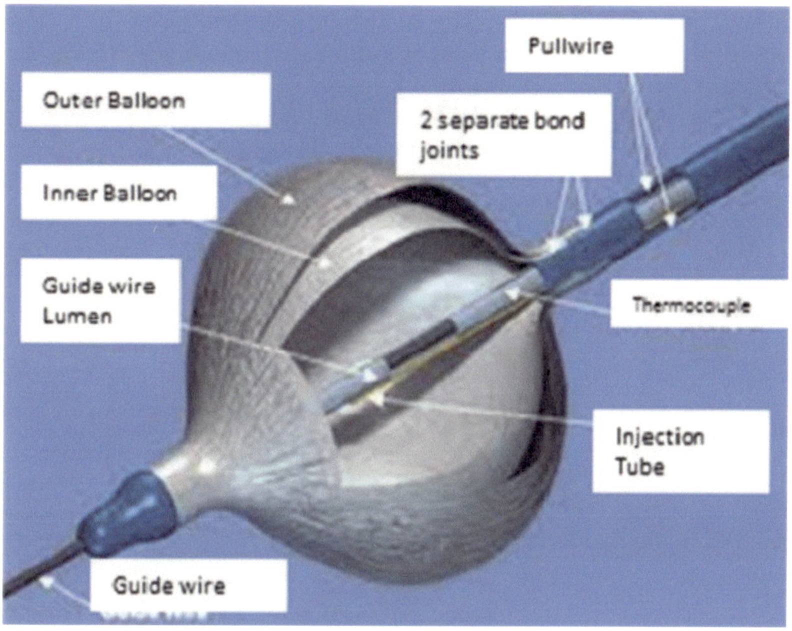


Fig. 9. Cryoballoon.

Additionally, ablation time can be controlled by visualizing blanching at the site where ablation is taking place, which is indicative of lesion formation (Figure 10 and 11). This catheter is constantly irrigated to evacuate the blood collection in the hood to increase the visibility of the tissue and also to cool the tip. Increased power leads to bubble formation in the hood and darkening of the tissue. Such lesions often result in steam pop. As a result, bubble formation and darkening of the tissue could be an indicator for lowering the power (Ahmed et al 2010).

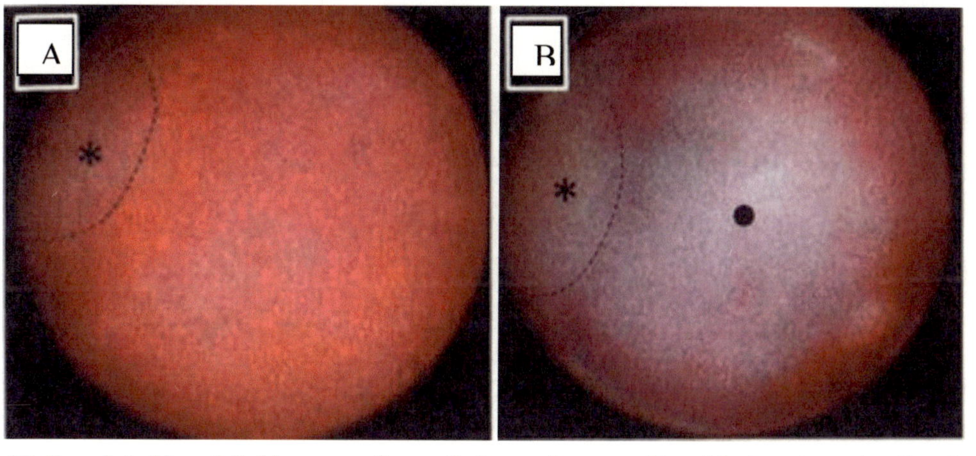


Fig. 10. Panel A: Visual field as seen through the endoscope. Pre ablation tissue is all red. Panel B: Post ablation tissue is pale as seen by the endoscopic visual field. * shows the previous ablation lesion with panel B demonstrating visualization of lesion contiguity (Ahmed et al 2011).

Identified limitations of this catheter relate to technical difficulties of fixing the hood at the tissue interface, especially at rough surface of atrial tissue and edges around the pulmonary veins. The nature of the elastopolymer coating results in slippage of the catheter. It has also been seen to collapse, likely related to the force generated during lesion formation, requiring catheter replacement in certain cases (Ahmed et al 2011).

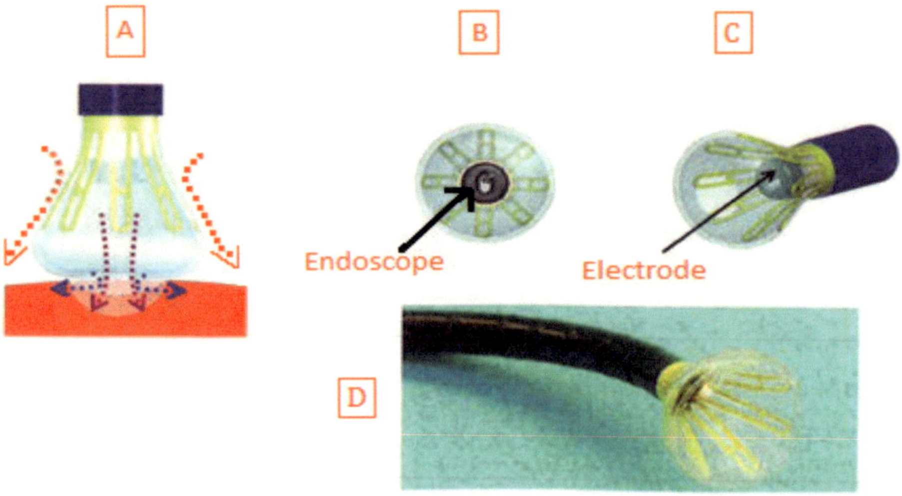


Fig. 11 A. Blue lines indicate the saline irrigation, purple lines indicate radiofrequency; Red lines indicate the flowing blood .B, C, D Virtual and visual electrode catheter from different angles. Hood with source of illumination can be seen clearly in panel C, endoscope and electrodes in the center are clearly visible in panel B. (Ahmed et al 2011).

Besides the technical limitations, current studies using this technology are limited by their small sample size, lack of application to atrial fibrillation and concerns over the volume of irrigation fluid delivered during the course of an ablation using this technology (Ahmed et al 2011).

## 11. Microwave

Microwave energy is an electromagnetic spectrum occupying the frequency range between 500 MHz - 100 MHz. When this electromagnetic radiation comes in contact with the biological tissues, it causes bipolar molecules (particularly water molecules) to oscillate and rotate under the influence of alternating electromagnetic radiation. This oscillation results in the conversion into kinetic energy, and finally collision of molecules cause heat energy formation (Johnson et al 1972). This (microwave induced) heat forms in deeper tissues as compared to RF where heat flows down the tissue interface to the deeper tissues via conductive heating, decreasing as a function of distance ($1/r^4$). Microwave energy excites deeper tissues resulting in deep high temperature and larger lesions.

In fact, microwave induced scar seems to be the endpoint of two distinct pathways. The first pathway is the direct effect of microwave radiation, while the second is a result of ischemic damage.

| Features | Radiofrequency | Microwave |
|---|---|---|
| Clinical experience | +++ | + |
| Potential for endocardial Disruption | High | Low/ Medium |
| Thrombogenicity | High | Medium |
| Mapping capability | Limited | NO |
| Ability to create transmural lesion | Require optimal Contact | Optimal contact/ antenna orientation required |
| Lesion size | ++ | +++ |
| Linear lesion | ++ | ++++ |
| Perforation rate | Low | Low |
| Procedure time | Shorter | Longer |
| Injury to adjacent structures: | | |
| Phrenic nerve | +++ | Unknown |
| Esophagus | +++ | ++ |
| Coronary artery | +++ | + |
| PV stenosis | +++ | No |

Table 2.Comparison of Radiofrequency ablation and microwave ablations (Yiu et al 2006).

## 12. Conclusion

To date, many patients with refractory supraventricular tachyarrythmias have been successfully ablated without complications, however successful ablation of atrial fibrillation continues to pose unique problems to the cardiac electrophysiologist. While progress has been made on identification of the triggers and underlying substrate of atrial fibrillation, the tools necessary to isolate and ablate AF lags behind our knowledge of the mechanisms underlying this arrhythmia. The ideal catheter should possess the best mapping resolution to target the tissues of interest, create reliable transmural and contiguous lesions, and clearly discriminate between successful and unsuccessful lesion formation and maturation. Furthermore, the ideal catheter technology should be easily steered and adapt to the atrial anatomy reducing the procedure time. Further benefits of such an approach would be decreasing excessive exposure of radiation to the physician and the patient in the EP lab. So far, balloon devices seem to offer a unique promise, however lesion transmurality is still a question.

## 13. References

Avitall B., Lafontaine D., Rozmus G., Adoni N., Le K., Dehnee A., Urbonas A.; The safety and efficacy of multiple consecutive cryo lesions in canine pulmonary veins-left atrial junction. Heart Rhythm, (2004) Volume 1, Issue 2, Pages 203 - 209.

Avitall B., Urboniene D., Rozmus G., Lafontaine D., Helms R., and Urbonas A.; New Cryotechnology for Electrical Isolation of the Pulmonary Veins. J Cardiovasc Electrophysiol (March 2003) Volume 14 Issue 3, Pages 281 - 286.

Avitall B, Helms R, Koblish J, Seiben W, Kotov AV, Gupta GN. The creation of linear contiguous lesions in the atria with an expandable loop catheter. JACC 1999; 33(4):972-984.

Avitall B, Urbonas A, Urboniene D, Rozmus G, Helms R. Linear lesions provide protection from atrial fibrillation induction with rapid atrial pacing. J of Cardiovasc Electrophysiol 2002; 13:455-62.

Avitall B, Aleksonis D, Koblish J, Chicos A, Mykytsey A, Taimisto M. New RF J shaped catheter design for creation of circumferential linear lesions and PVs isolation. Heart Rhythm, 2005 2 (5): S154.

Ahmed Humera, BA, Neuzil Petr, MD, Skoda Jan, MD, Sediva Luce, MD Kralovec Stepan, Reddy Y Vivek MD Initial clinical experience with a novel visualization and virtual electrode radiofrequency ablation catheter to treat atrial flutter 2011 heart rhythm Page 361-367

Arora Pawan K. MBBS, Hansen James C MD, Price Adam D. MD, Koblish Josef , Avitall Boaz MD PhD,FHRS An Update on the Energy Sources and Catheter Technology for the Ablation of Atrial Fibillation 2010 JAFib

Arora PK, Hansen JC, Latchamsetty R, Avitall B. Is Cryo a better energy source than radiofrequency for AF ablation in preventing esophageal injury?J Atrial Fibrillation 2009; 1(6): 321-327

Becker, R., & Schoels, W., Ablation of atrial f rhythmibrillation: Energy sources and navigation tools: A review. Journal of Electro cardiology, (2004), 37, 55–62.

Boersma LVA, Wijffels MCEF, Oral H, Wever EFD, Morady F: Pulmonary vein isolation by duty-cycled bipolar and unipolar radiofrequency with a multielectrode ablation catheter. Heart Rhythm 2008; 5:1635-1642.

Budde T, Borggrefe M, Podczeck A, Jacob B, Langwasser J, Frenzel H, Breithard G. Radiofrequency ablation: an improvement of ablation techniques in comparison to direct-current delivery. In: Breithardt G, Borggrefe M, Zipes DP, eds. *Nonpharmacological Therapy of Tachyarrhythmias.* Mount Kisco, NY: Futura Publishing Company Inc; 1987:221–241

Haines David, Watson Denny Tissue Heating During Radiofrequency Catheter Ablation: A Thermodynamic Model and Observations in Isolated Perfused and Superfused Canine Right Ventricular Free Wall 1989

Demolin JM, Eick OJ, Munch K, Koukkick E, Nakagawa H, Wittkampf FHM. Soft thrombus formation in radiofrequency catheter ablation. *Pacing Clin Electrophysiol.* 2003; 25:1219 -1222

Gaita Fiorenzo , M.D Franc Jean ¸ Leclercq Ois , M.D, Schumacher Burghard, M.D, Scaglione Marco , M.D, Toso Elisabetta , M.D, Halimi Franck, M.D, Schade Anja, M.D Froehner Steffen, M.D, Ziegler Volker, M.D, Sergi Domenico, M.D, Cesarani Federico, M.D and Blandino Alessandro, M.D Incidence of Silent Cerebral Thromboembolic Lesions After Atrial Fibrillation Ablation May Change According To Technology Used: Comparison of Irrigated Radiofrequency, Multipolar Nonirrigated Catheter and Cryoballoon (2011 J Cardiovasc Electrophysiol, Vol. pp. 1-8)

Gauri AJ,Knight BP. Catheter Ablation for Atrial Fibrillation; indian pacing electrophysiol j 2003 oct-dec;3(4):210-223

Grumbrecht S, Neuzner J, Pitschner HF. Interrelation of tissue temperature versus flow velocity in two different kinds of temperature controlled Catheter radiofrequency energy application. *J Interv Card Electrophysiol.* 1998; 2:211–219

Haines DE The biophysics of radiofrequency catheter ablationin the heart: The importance of temperature monitoring. Pacing Clin Electrophysiology 1993;16 ( 3 pt 2): 586-591

Hoffmann E, Haberl R, Pulter R, Gokel M, Steinbeck G. Biophysical parameters of radiofrequency catheter ablation, international J Cardiol (1992); 13:213-233.

Inesi G, Millman M, Eletr S. Temperature-induced transitions of function and structure in sarcoplasmic reticulum membranes. J Mol Biol. (Dec 25, 1973);81(4):483-504

Johnson CC, Guy AW. Nonionizing electromagnetic wave effects in biological materials and systems. Proc IEEE. 1972; 60:692-709.

Kongsgaard E, Steen T, Jensen O, Aass H, Amlie JP. Temperature guided Radiofrequency catheter ablation of myocardium: comparison of catheter Tip and tissue temperatures in vitro. *Pacing Clin Electrophysiol.* 1997; 20:1252–1260

Kennedy JE, MBBS, MRCS1, Haar G R ter , MSc, PhD, DSc2 and Cranston D , DPhil, FRCS3 High intensity focused ultrasound: surgery of the future? 2003 British Journal of Radiology (2003) 76, 590-599

Littmann L, Svenson RH, Chuang CH, Splinter R, Kempler P, Norton HJ, Tuntelder JR, Thompson M, Tatsis GP: Neodymium:YAG contact laser photocoagulation of the in vivo canine epicardium: Dosimetry, effects of various lasing modes, and histology. Lasers Surg Med 1993; 13:158-167.

Manolis, A, Wang, P, & Estes, M. Radiofrequency catheter ablation for cardiac tachyarrhythmias. Annals of Internal Medicine, (1994), 121, 452–461

Matsudaira K, Nakagawa H, Yamanashi SW, Wittkampf FHM, Pitha JV, Imai S, Lazzara R, Jackman WM. High incidence of thrombus formation Without impedance rise during radiofrequency ablation using electrode Temperature control. *Pacing Clin Electrophysiol.* 2003; 26:1227–1237

Nakagawa H, Wittkampf FHM, Yamanashi WS, Pitha JV, Imai S, Campbell B, Arruda M, Lazzara R, Jackman WM. Inverse relationship between electrode size and lesion size during radiofrequency ablation with active electrode cooling. *Circulation* 1998; 98:458–465

Nakagawa H, Yamanashi WS, Pitha JV, Arruda M, Wang X, Ohtomo K, Beckman KJ, McClelland JH, Lazzara R, Jackman WM. Comparison of in vivo tissue temperature profile and lesion geometry for radiofrequency ablation with a saline-irrigated electrode versus temperature control in a canine thigh muscle preparation. *Circulation.* 1995; 91:2264 –2273

Okumura Yasuo ,MD, PhD,Kolasa Mark MD Johnson Susan BS,Bunch t Jared M.D,Benheird Henz M.D.,Brien Christine J. O ,Dylan Miller MD and Douglas Packer MDMechanism of Tissue Heating During High Intensity Focused Ultrasound Pulmonary Vein Isolation: Implications for Atrial Fibrillation Ablation Efficacy and Phrenic Nerve Protection September 2008 J Cardiovasc Electrophysiol, Vol. 19, pp. 945-951

Oral Hakan Chugh Aman , Özayd1n Mehmet, Good Eric, Fortino Jackie , Sankaran Sundar, Reich Scott, Igic Petar , Elmouchi Darryl , Tschopp David , Wimmer Alan , Dey Sujoya , Crawford Thomas , Pelosi Frank , Jr, Jongnarangsin Krit, Bogun Frank and Morady Fred Risk of Thromboembolic Events After Percutaneous Left Atrial Radiofrequency Ablation of Atrial Fibrillation Circulation 2006, 114:759-765

Perzanowski C, Teplitsky L, Hranitzky PM, and Bahnson TD; Real-Time Monitoring of Luminal Esophageal Temperature During Left Atrial Radiofrequency Catheter

Ablation for Atrial Fibrillation: Observations About Esophageal Heating During Ablation at the Pulmonary Vein Ostia and Posterior Left Atrium. J Cardiovasc Electrophysiol, (February 2006) Vol. 17,pp. 166-170

Reddy Vivek Y., MD; Neuzil Petr , MD, PhD; Themistoclakis Sakis, MD; B. Danik Stephan , MD; Bonso Aldo , MD; Rossillo Antonio , MD; Raviele Antonio, MD; Schweikert Robert, MD; Ernst Sabine, MD; Kuck Karl-Heinz, MD; Natale Andrea, MDVisually-Guided Balloon Catheter Ablation of Atrial Fibrillation Experimental Feasibility and First-in-Human Multicenter Clinical Outcome circulation 2009, pp 12-20

Reddy VY, Houghtaling C, Fallon J, Fischer G, Farr N, Clarke J, McIntyre J, Sinofsky E, Ruskin JN, Keane D: Use of a diode laser balloon ablation catheter to generate circumferential pulmonary venous lesions in an open-thoracotomy caprine model. Pacing Clin Electrophysiol 2004; 27:52-57.

Reddy Vivek Y. MD Neuzil Petr MD†, d'Avila Andre MD, Laragy Margaret BS, Malchano Zachary J MS, Kralovec Stepan †, J. Kim Steven MS‡ and. Ruskin Jeremy N MD Balloon catheter ablation to treat paroxysmal atrial fibrillation: What is the level of pulmonary venous isolation? Heart Rhythm 2008;5:353–360

Schmidt B , Kuck KH, Shah D, Reddy V, Saoudi N, Herrara C, Hindricks G, Natale A, Jais P, Lambert H Toccato multi center clinical study using irrigated ablation catheter with integrated contact force sensor: first resultsHeart rhythm. 2009;6:S536

Stobie P. & Green M. Cryoablation for septal accessory pathways: Has the next ice age arrived? Journal of Cardiovascular Electrophysiology, (2003) 14, 830–831.

Skanes AC, Klein GJ, Krahn AD, Yee R. Advances in energy delivery. Coron Artery Dis. 2003 ;14 (1) : 15-23

Taylor Gregg W., G. Neal Kay, g Zheng Xiangshen , Bishop Sanford , Ideker Raymond E , Pathological Effects of Extensive Radiofrequency Energy Applications in the Pulmonary Veins in Dogs. Circulation. (2000);101:1736-1742

Wijffels MCEF, Oosterhout MV, Boersma LVA, Werneth R, Kunis C,Hu B, Beekman JDM, Vos MA. Characterization of In Vitro and In Vivo Lesions Made by a Novel Multichannel Ablation Generator and a Circumlinear Decapolar Ablation Catheter. October 2009 J Cardiovasc Electrophysiol, Vol. 20, pp. 1142-1148

Wittkampf FHM, Hauer RNW, Robles de Medina EO. Control of radiofrequency lesion size by power regulation. *Circulation*. 1989;80:962–968

Yokoyama Katsuaki , Nakagawa Hiroshi, Shah Dipen C, Lambert Giovanni Hendrik Leo Nicolas Aeby, Ikeda Atsushi, Pitha Jan V, Tushar Sharma, Lazzara Ralph and. Jackman Warren M Novel contact force sensor incorporated in irrigated radiofrequency ablation catheter Predicts Lesion Size and Incidence of Steam Pop and Thrombus ;Circulation: Arrhythmia and Electrophysiology Issue: Volume 1(5), December 2008, pp 354-362

Yiu KH, Lau CP, Lee K, Tse HF. Emerging energy sources for catheter ablation of atrial fibrillation. J Cardiovasc Electrophysiol 2006; 17:S56–61.

Yokoyama Katsuaki, MD, PhD; Nakagawa Hiroshi , MD, PhD;. Wittkampf Fred H.M, PhD;. Pitha Jan V , MD, PhD; Lazzara Ralph, MD; Jackman Warren M. , MD Comparison of Electrode Cooling Between Internal and Open Irrigation in Radiofrequency Ablation Lesion Depth and Incidence of Thrombus and Steam Pop Circulation Issue: January 2006, Volume 113(1), pp 11-19